The Innate Immune System: Strategies for Disease Control

The Innate Immune System: Strategies for Disease Control

Proceedings of the Uehara Memorial Foundation Symposium on the Innate Immune System: Strategies for Disease Control, held in Tokyo, Japan between 11 and 13 July 2005

Editors:

Masaru Taniguchi
RIKEN Research Center for Allergy and Immunology
Kanagawa
Japan

Shizuo Akira
Department of Host Defence
Research Institute for Microbial Diseases
Osaka University
Osaka
Japan

Toshinori Nakayama
Department of Immunology
Graduate School of Medicine
Chiba University
Chiba
Japan

ELSEVIER

2005

ELSEVIER B.V.
Radarweg 29
P.O. Box 211, 1000 AE Amsterdam
The Netherlands

ELSEVIER Inc.
525 B Street, Suite 1900
San Diego, CA 92101-4495
USA

ELSEVIER Ltd
The Boulevard, Langford Lane
Kidlington, Oxford OX5 1GB
UK

ELSEVIER Ltd
84 Theobalds Road
London WC1X 8RR
UK

First edition 2005

Library of Congress Cataloging in Publication Data
A catalog record from the Library of Congress has been applied for.

British Library Cataloguing in Publication Data
A catalogue record from the British Library has been applied for.

International Congress Series No. 1285
ISBN: 0-444-51981-5
ISSN: 0531-5131

∞ The paper used in this publication meets the requirements of ANSI/NISO Z39.48-1992 (Permanence of Paper).
Printed in The Netherlands.

International Congress Series 1285 (2005) v–vi

ELSEVIER

www.ics-elsevier.com

Preface

With the recent completion of the complete sequence of the entire human genome, we, in the Life Sciences, find ourselves confronted with increasing expectations fueled by remarkable progress in many areas of biological and biomedical research. In the field of immunology, progress in recent years has been most visible in innate immunity. Over the past few years, many members of the Toll-like receptor (TLR) family in mammals have been identified, characterized, and found to play crucial roles in the innate immune system. Especially, the elucidation of TLR-mediated signaling has helped to shed light upon the molecular events that take place during the initial phase of the immune response, an area that little had been known about until most recently. The second area that has seen considerable progress recently is the dendritic cell biology. Numerous subpopulations of dendritic cells in the mouse and human immune systems have now been identified. In particular, the identification of a dendritic cell population that exhibits immunoregulatory functions is an intriguing finding, with implications for both basic immunology and the clinical milieu. Various clinical trials using specifically manipulated dendritic cells as anti-tumor vaccines have been performed, and some promising results are now starting to emerge. Thirdly, rapid progress has considerably enlarged our knowledge and understanding of newly identified regulatory cell populations, such as NKT cells and $CD4^+$ $CD25^+$ regulatory T (Tr) cells. While NKT cells do not constitute a cell population within the innate immune system, their unique bridging function between the innate and acquired immune systems is now widely acknowledged. The immunoregulatory function of NKT cells, as well as Tr cells, has been described in various experimental systems, including those for allergic reactions, autoimmune diseases, anti-tumor responses, and tolerance induction for transplantation. An increasing body of data suggests the potential of using such cells in new treatment strategies for various immune-related diseases.

The Uehara Memorial Foundation Symposium 2005, entitled “The Innate Immune System: Strategies for Disease Control”, was convened in Tokyo from July 11th to July 13th, 2005. During the symposium, numerous new findings related to the three issues described above were reported. The following are the main topics that were addressed by the various distinguished speakers at the symposium:

1. Receptor signaling and function in innate immune responses
2. Interfaces between innate and acquired immunity
3. Manipulation of the innate immune system and new strategies for disease control.

0531-5131/ © 2005 Published by Elsevier B.V.
doi:10.1016/j.ics.2005.09.007

The aim of the symposium was to bring together leading scientists in the field from all over the world, and to discuss the latest research findings on molecular events in the innate immune system, the interface between innate and acquired immunity, and potential applications of recent findings. It was an explicit aim of this symposium to increase our understanding in this filed and further the development of novel strategies for disease control in the 21st century.

Finally, as the organizers of the symposium, we feel very pleased to be able to publish the proceedings of this exiting symposium and would like to thank Elsevier Co. Ltd. for this opportunity.

Masaru Taniguchi

Contents

Receptor signalling and function in innate immune responses

ELSEVIER

International Congress Series 1285 (2005) 3–9

www.ics-elsevier.com

Role of toll-like receptor–commensal interactions in intestinal inflammation

Seth Rakoff-Nahoum *, Ruslan Medzhitov

Yale University School of Medicine and Howard Hughes Medical Institute, Immunobiology, 300 Cedar St., TAC S-669 New Haven, CT 06510, USA

Abstract. Toll-like receptors (TLRs) play a critical role in host defense of infection. Recent studies demonstrate that in addition to their function in the immune system, TLRs have an important physiological role in the maintenance of the intestinal homeostasis. © 2005 Published by Elsevier B.V.

Keywords: TLR; Inflammation

TLRs are a family of receptors involved in the recognition of conserved molecular constituents on microorganism [1]. These structures, while termed pathogen associated molecular patterns (PAMPs), are in actuality ubiquitous to microorganisms, both those considered pathogenic and those that are not. At least 10 different TLRs have been identified in mammals. A number of TLR ligands have been identified so far, including TLR2 ligands lipotechoic acid (LTA) and bacterial lipoprotein (BLP), TLR4 ligand LPS, TLR3 ligand double-stranded RNA, and TLR5 ligand Flagellin [2,3].

Signaling through TLRs is crucial for the induction of the host response to infection by orchestrating both the innate and adaptive arms of the immune response. While many intracellular signaling adaptors for TLRs have been identified, signaling through the adaptor myeloid differentiation factor 88 (MyD88) has been shown to be of central importance to the initiation of innate and adaptive immunity. MyD88 coordinates signaling pathways that lead to the activation of NF-κB and MAP kinases and induction of inflammatory mediators, most notably IL-1β, TNF, IL-6, and IL-8 (in humans; KC-1 in

* Corresponding author. Tel.: +1 2037857541; fax: +1 2037371765.
E-mail address: ruslan.medzhitov@yale.edu (R. Medzhitov).

doi:10.1016/j.ics.2005.07.098

mice). The induction of these cytokines is crucial to the influx of inflammatory cells including neutrophils and monocytes to areas exposed to microorganisms [2,3].

TLR signaling on professional antigen-presenting cells (APCs) such as dendritic cells (DC) leads to the initiation of adaptive immune responses [4]. This occurs through various mechanisms. The first to be described was the up-regulation of the co-stimulatory molecules, CD80/CD86, crucial to the activation of naïve CD4 T cells [5]. Recently, we have shown that the production of IL-6 by DC in response to TLR engagement is responsible for providing signals to effector T cells that make them refractory to the suppression by regulatory T cells [6]. Together, these two mechanisms allow for the activation and clonal expansion of antigen-specific cells upon the detection of PAMPs by TLRs. T cell-mediated immune responses and effector functions can be classified into various categories, two of these being type 1 and type 2 responses. Type I responses are characterized by the production of IFN-γ by T helper type 1 (Th1) cells. This type of immune response is involved in immunity and host defense to intracellular pathogens. The induction of Th1 cells is thought to be dependent on the production of various cytokines by DC, most importantly IL-12, but also of factors known to play accessory and complementary roles in Th1 development such as IL-23, -27, -18 and type I interferons [7,8]. We have previously shown that TLR signaling plays a critical role in the induction of Th1 responses [9].

As PAMPs are present on all microbes, independent of their pathogenicity, the question arises as to how TLRs can distinguish between pathogenic versus non-pathogenic microorganisms and what are the outcomes of this discernment with regard to host responses.

Mammals are colonized with a myriad of unicellular organisms that comprise an indigenous microflora. While present at many of the interfaces with the external world, such as the oropharynx and skin, the overwhelming majority and diversity of the endogenous bacterial flora is at the distal alimentary tract, most notably at the colon. It is here that the over 10^{14} resident bacteria confer many benefits to intestinal biology comprising a truly mutualistic relationship [10]. The metabolism of nutrients and organic substrates, the development of intestinal epithelium, vasculature and lymphoid tissue, and the contribution to the phenomena of colonization resistance to pathogens are only a few of the ways in which the host benefits from the resident microflora present in the gut [11,12].

However, the presence of commensal bacteria within the gut appears to be of crucial importance in the pathoetiology of human inflammatory bowel diseases (IBD), which include Crohn's disease and ulcerative colitis. It is thought that these diseases are characterized by a chronic inflammation of the intestine due to defects in the homeostasis of immune responses to commensals [13]. Current knowledge suggests that this dysregulation is the result of environmental and host genetic factors involved in mucosal immune tolerance to commensals [14].

Evidence for the pathoetiology and pathogenesis of this class of diseases comes from studies of patients with IBD and animal models of mucosal inflammation. While the anatomical extent and nature of inflammation in UC and CD differ, both are characterized by the presence of infiltrating leukocytes, including neutrophils, macrophages, T and B cells, and destruction of the intestine.

Studies in humans with IBD show both signs of augmented activation of intestinal antigen-presenting cells and increased levels of both inflammatory and Th1 associated cytokines. Using isolation methods and immunohistochemistry, DC present in inflamed regions of the colons of people with Crohn's disease or ulcerative colitis have revealed increased expression of CD40 [15], CD80 [16] and CD86 [17] compared with non-diseased tissue. In both UC and CD there is increased synthesis of IL-1β, IL-6, IL-8 and TNF in the mucosa [18]. Colonic regions of active disease in CD are characterized by granulomas, consisting of T cells and macrophages. Analysis of inflamed intestinal mucosa of patients with Crohn's disease has revealed increased amounts of IFN-γ mRNA and increased spontaneous release of this cytokine compared with T cells from healthy colons [18]. Similar studies of tissue from active Crohn's lesions showed increased expression of IL-12 from lamina propria monocuclear cells (LPMCs) and of the IL-12Rβ2 chain on LP T cells [18]. In addition, higher levels of active STAT4, a transcription factor that is crucial to IL-12R signaling, is found in the colons of patients with CD [18].

Animal models of colitis reveal many aspects of the factors involved in mucosal inflammation and the homeostatic mechanisms that are involved in regulating immune tolerance to commensals. One important mechanism that prevents chronic stimulation of the leukocytes resident in the gut mucosa is the presence of an intact epithelial barrier that keeps antigens present in the lumen sequestered from the lamina propria. Animal models such as administration of dextran sulfate sodium (DSS) and trinitrobenzene–sulfonic acid with ethanol (TNBS+E) cause direct injury to colonic epithelium. Current theories on the pathogenesis of these types of colitis are that they result in disruption of the epithelial barrier and exposure of commensal constituents to host cells, resulting in the induction of inflammation and intestinal injury [19].

Evidence for recognition of commensal organisms by the intestinal immune system under normal conditions has been implicit from many findings. These include the formation of germinal center reactions in murine Peyer's patches upon weaning or after either bacterial monoassociation or conventionalization of germ-free animals [20] and the induction of natural [20] and specific IgA [21] by commensals. Two recent findings reveal a steady-state interaction between intestinal dendritic cells and commensals in that IL-23 was shown to be constitutively expressed by lamina propria DC of the mouse ileum, production of which was absent in germ-free mice [22] and Peyer's patch CD11b+ DC were shown to carry live commensal bacteria to mesenteric lymph nodes [23].

The spontaneous development of colitis in certain animal models, in which colitis does not develop when raised in the absence of an indigenous microflora, also suggests that there is steady-state recognition of commensal bacteria and that the consequences of this recognition are actively regulated resulting in tolerance and immune homeostasis. Such animal models include the transfer of CD45RB^{hi} T cells to lymphopenic (Rag2−/−) hosts, and animals with deletions of IL-2 or IL-10. While the mechanisms of the breach of commensal-dependent immune tolerance are distinct in each of the models, there is much evidence to suggest that the initiation of colitis involves a common etiology and pathogenesis. In particular, studies of these models have revealed a chronic inflammation localized to the large intestine characterized by unregulated production of inflammatory cytokines and Th1 responses.

Transfer of CD45Rb^{hi} T cells into lymphopenic hosts, such as Rag2−/− or SCID mice, results in a T cell-mediated colonic inflammation [24,25] which is dependent on the presence of commensals, as transfer into germ-free SCID or Rag−/− does not result in colitis [26]. In conventionally raised mice, the colitis induced by the transfer of CD45RB^{hi} T cells can be prevented by cotransfering CD25+ T cells as it has been shown that this population of T cells plays a regulatory function in the control of inflammation and effector T cell responses through a number of mechanisms including a contact-dependent inhibition, as well as the production of IL-10 and TGF-β [27,28]. Thus, it appears that CD25+ T regulatory (Tregs) cells play a critical role in the suppression of T cell responses stimulated by the presence of the commensal microflora in the steady state. The role of innate immune recognition of commensals in mediating this form of colitis has yet to be investigated. However, there is much evidence that suggests that unregulated regulation of Th1 responses initiated by a commensal–TLR axis is operative.

Firstly, as noted above, lymphopenic animals transferred with naïve T cells will not develop colitis in germ-free environments. Local dendritic cells from these colitic animals have the hallmarks of activation. Lamina propria DC have up-regulated surface expression of CD40, CD80 and CD86 in addition to expressing higher levels of IL-12 p40 and IL-23 p19 upon CD40 ligation [29]. Upon CD45rbhi transfer, OX40L (CD134L) DC have been shown to accumulate in mesenteric lymph nodes, a prerequisite for pathogenic T cell entry and/or proliferation in the colon [30]. Intestines of colitic animals have been shown to express increased amounts of IFNγ and TNF [31,32]. The pathogenic role of these cytokines has been demonstrated by amelioration of disease upon the use of anti-IFNγ antibodies [31] or when T cells were transferred to animals deficient in TNF [33]. This latter result demonstrated the role of factors produced by recipient cells in the pathogenesis of disease. In addition to TNF, other factors, particularly those known to be produced upon activation of antigen-presenting cells, such as macrophage migration inhibitory factor (MIF) [34] and IL-12, through studies in STAT4/Rag2 double deficient recipients [35], have been shown to be crucial in the development of colitis in this model.

Both animals deficient in IL-10 and IL-2 develop a spontaneous colitis when raised in conventional environments, and are colitis-free when reared under germ-free conditions [36,37]. Thus both IL-2 and IL-10 are involved in some aspect of immunoregulation in the gut.

IL-2 deficient animals suffer from a multi-organ autoimmune condition. However, investigations into the pathoetiology of these autoimmune manifestations, including hemolytic anemia, lymphoid hyperplasia and colitis, have revealed both overlapping and non-overlapping mechanisms of disease. All pathologies have been shown to be T cell dependent, however, colitis as opposed to anemia still develops in the absence of B cells [38]. Importantly, studies have shown that the development of colitis is dependent on the presence of an intestinal microflora, while anemia and lymphoid hyperplasia in organs such as the lung, liver, spleen and pancreas are not [37,39,40]. Two theories have received the most attention concerning the nature of the loss of immune regulation in IL-2−/− mice. These focus on two manners of T cell regulation, an "autonomous" mechanism of IL-2 dependent induction of Fas expression on activated T cells leading to activation induced cell death [41] and one based on an "assisted" mechanism in which T cell dysregulation in IL-2 mice is the result of the absence of thymic derived CD4+ CD25+ regulatory T cells in these mice [42].

Characterization of the colitis of IL-2 mice points to dysregulation of both inflammatory mediator and Th1 responses. Even before the onset of colitis which typically is of delayed onset (beginning at 8 weeks of age), colons of 1.5-week-old IL-2−/− mice show increased expression of IL-1α, IL-1β, IL-6, TNF and IFNγ compared with WT controls [43]. Colons and lamina propria T cells from IL-2−/− colons produced higher levels of IL-12 and IFNγ, respectively, than WT [44].

IL-10 null mice develop a chronic T cell-mediated intestinal inflammation that is dependent on the presence of commensal flora [36,45]. IL-10 has been shown to play a crucial role in the modulation of immune responses through the regulation of both arms of the immune response, the innate and adaptive. IL-10 acts on many cells including macrophages, DC, mast cells, epithelial cells, and T and B cells, in addition to many others. In particular, IL-10 has been shown to regulate the activation and maturation of macrophages and DC in response to microbes, by inhibiting the surface expression of MHC Class II, CD40, CD80 and CD86 and limiting the production of inflammatory cytokines and factors crucial to the development of Th1 responses, such as IL-12 [46]. In addition, IL-10 may act directly on Th1 cells to limit IFNγ production [46]. Accordingly, the spontaneous colitis seen in IL-10−/− mice seems to be due to the inability of IL-10 to regulate the activation of antigen-presenting cells and Th1 responses triggered by the presence of the microflora of the colon. Colons of IL-10−/− mice show aberrant expression of MHC Class II [47] and production of IL-1α, TNF, IL-6, NO and IFNγ compared with WT [47]. Isolated CD4+ T cells are of increased number and activation state [45,47] and produce increased amounts of IFNγ compared with WT LP T cells [47]. The pathologic role of this dysregulation immune activation has come from studies showing amelioration of disease using neutralizing antibodies to IL-12 and IFNγ [47,48]. Further evidence for the role of the commensal–TLR–Th1 axis in disease pathogenesis has come from studies performed using animals with a conditional deletion of STAT3 in cells of the myeloid lineage [49], a mediator of many of the immunoregulatory actions of IL-10 signaling, which develop a colitis similar to that of IL-10−/−, as disease was ameliorated by crossing these mice to mice deficient in IL-12p40 and TLR4 [50].

Our recent studies demonstrate that TLR–commensal interactions play a crucial role in normal intestinal physiology, but can also lead to intestinal inflammation and pathology when dysregulated. Thus a complex balance of TLR–commensal interactions is maintained under normal conditions.

References

[1] G.M. Barton, R. Medzhitov, Toll-like receptor signaling pathways, Science 300 (2003) 1524–1525.

[2] S. Akira, Mammalian toll-like receptors, Curr. Opin. Immunol. 15 (2003) 5–11.

[3] R. Medzhitov, Toll-like receptors and innate immunity, Nat. Rev., Immunol. 1 (2001) 135–145.

[4] G.M. Barton, R. Medzhitov, Control of adaptive immune responses by toll-like receptors, Curr. Opin. Immunol. 14 (2002) 380–383.

[5] R. Medzhitov, P. Preston-Hurlburt, C.A. Janeway Jr., A human homologue of the *Drosophila* Toll protein signals activation of adaptive immunity, Nature 388 (1997) 394–397.

[6] C. Pasare, R. Medzhitov, Toll pathway-dependent blockade of CD4+ CD25+ T cell-mediated suppression by dendritic cells, Science 299 (2003) 1033–1036.
[7] K.M. Murphy, S.L. Reiner, The lineage decisions of helper T cells, Nat. Rev., Immunol. 2 (2002) 933–944.
[8] G. Trinchieri, Interleukin-12 and the regulation of innate resistance and adaptive immunity, Nat. Rev., Immunol. 3 (2003) 133–146.
[9] M. Schnare, et al., Toll-like receptors control activation of adaptive immune responses, Nat. Immunol. 2 (2001) 947–950.
[10] D.J. Hentges, Human Intestinal Microflora in Health and Disease, Academic Press, New York, 1983 (xvii, 568 pp.).
[11] L.V. Hooper, J.I. Gordon, Commensal host–bacterial relationships in the gut, Science 292 (2001) 1115–1118.
[12] R.D. Berg, The indigenous gastrointestinal microflora, Trends Microbiol. 4 (1996) 430–435.
[13] R.J. Farrell, J.T. LaMont, Microbial factors in inflammatory bowel disease, Gastroenterol. Clin. North Am. 31 (2002) 41–62.
[14] D.K. Podolsky, Inflammatory bowel disease, N. Engl. J. Med. 347 (2002) 417–429.
[15] S.J. Bell, et al., Migration and maturation of human colonic dendritic cells, J. Immunol. 166 (2001) 4958–4967.
[16] A.J. Stagg, et al., The dendritic cell: its role in intestinal inflammation and relationship with gut bacteria, Gut 52 (2003) 1522–1529.
[17] S. Vuckovic, et al., CD40 and CD86 upregulation with divergent CMRF44 expression on blood dendritic cells in inflammatory bowel diseases, Am. J. Gastroenterol. 96 (2001) 2946–2956.
[18] I. Monteleone, et al., Immunoregulation in the gut: success and failures in human disease, Gut. 50 (Suppl 3) (2002) III60–III64.
[19] W. Strober, I.J. Fuss, R.S. Blumberg, The immunology of mucosal models of inflammation, Annu. Rev. Immunol. 20 (2002) 495–549.
[20] K.E. Shroff, K. Meslin, J.J. Cebra, Commensal enteric bacteria engender a self-limiting humoral mucosal immune response while permanently colonizing the gut, Infect. Immun. 63 (1995) 3904–3913.
[21] A.J. Macpherson, et al., A primitive T cell-independent mechanism of intestinal mucosal IgA responses to commensal bacteria, Science 288 (2000) 2222–2226.
[22] C. Becker, et al., Constitutive p40 promoter activation and IL-23 production in the terminal ileum mediated by dendritic cells, J. Clin. Invest. 112 (2003) 693–706.
[23] A.J. Macpherson, T. Uhr, Induction of protective IgA by intestinal dendritic cells carrying commensal bacteria, Science 303 (2004) 1662–1665.
[24] F. Powrie, et al., Phenotypically distinct subsets of CD4+ T cells induce or protect from chronic intestinal inflammation in C. B-17 scid mice, Int. Immunol. 5 (1993) 1461–1471.
[25] P.J. Morrissey, K. Charrier, Induction of wasting disease in SCID mice by the transfer of normal CD4+/CD45RBhi T cells and the regulation of this autoreactivity by CD4+/CD45RBlo T cells, Res. Immunol. 145 (1994) 357–362.
[26] R. Aranda, et al., Analysis of intestinal lymphocytes in mouse colitis mediated by transfer of CD4+, CD45RBhigh T cells to SCID recipients, J. Immunol. 158 (1997) 3464–3473.
[27] E.M. Shevach, CD4+ CD25+ suppressor T cells: more questions than answers, Nat. Rev., Immunol. 2 (2002) 389–400.
[28] S. Sakaguchi, Regulatory T cells: key controllers of immunologic self-tolerance, Cell 101 (2000) 455–458.
[29] T. Krajina, et al., Colonic lamina propria dendritic cells in mice with CD4+ T cell-induced colitis, Eur. J. Immunol. 33 (2003) 1073–1083.
[30] V. Malmstrom, et al., CD134L expression on dendritic cells in the mesenteric lymph nodes drives colitis in T cell-restored SCID mice, J. Immunol. 166 (2001) 6972–6981.
[31] F. Powrie, et al., Inhibition of Th1 responses prevents inflammatory bowel disease in scid mice reconstituted with CD45RBhi CD4+ T cells, Immunity 1 (1994) 553–562.
[32] F. Powrie, et al., A critical role for transforming growth factor-beta but not interleukin 4 in the suppression of T helper type 1-mediated colitis by CD45RB(low) CD4+ T cells, J. Exp. Med. 183 (1996) 2669–2674.

[33] N. Corazza, et al., Nonlymphocyte-derived tumor necrosis factor is required for induction of colitis in recombination activating gene (RAG)2(−/−) mice upon transfer of CD4(+)CD45RB(hi) T cells, J. Exp. Med. 190 (1999) 1479–1492.
[34] Y.P. de Jong, et al., Development of chronic colitis is dependent on the cytokine MIF, Nat. Immunol. 2 (2001) 1061–1066.
[35] S.J. Simpson, et al., T cell-mediated pathology in two models of experimental colitis depends predominantly on the interleukin 12/Signal transducer and activator of transcription (Stat)-4 pathway, but is not conditional on interferon gamma expression by T cells, J. Exp. Med. 187 (1998) 1225–1234.
[36] R. Kuhn, et al., Interleukin-10-deficient mice develop chronic enterocolitis, Cell 75 (1993) 263–274.
[37] B. Sadlack, et al., Ulcerative colitis-like disease in mice with a disrupted interleukin-2 gene, Cell 75 (1993) 253–261.
[38] A. Ma, et al., T cells, but not B cells, are required for bowel inflammation in interleukin 2-deficient mice, J. Exp. Med. 182 (1995) 1567–1572.
[39] N.V. Contractor, et al., Lymphoid hyperplasia, autoimmunity, and compromised intestinal intraepithelial lymphocyte development in colitis-free gnotobiotic IL-2-deficient mice, J. Immunol. 160 (1998) 385–394.
[40] M. Schultz, et al., IL-2-deficient mice raised under germfree conditions develop delayed mild focal intestinal inflammation, Am. J. Physiol. 276 (1999) G1461–G1472.
[41] L. Van Parijs, D.A. Peterson, A.K. Abbas, The Fas/Fas ligand pathway and Bcl-2 regulate T cell responses to model self and foreign antigens, Immunity 8 (1998) 265–274.
[42] T.R. Malek, et al., CD4 regulatory T cells prevent lethal autoimmunity in IL-2Rbeta-deficient mice. Implications for the nonredundant function of IL-2, Immunity 17 (2002) 167–178.
[43] I.B. Autenrieth, et al., Cytokine mRNA expression in intestinal tissue of interleukin-2 deficient mice with bowel inflammation, Gut 41 (1997) 793–800.
[44] R.O. Ehrhardt, et al., Induction and prevention of colonic inflammation in IL-2-deficient mice, J. Immunol. 158 (1997) 566–573.
[45] R.K. Sellon, et al., Resident enteric bacteria are necessary for development of spontaneous colitis and immune system activation in interleukin-10-deficient mice, Infect. Immun. 66 (1998) 5224–5231.
[46] K.W. Moore, et al., Interleukin-10 and the interleukin-10 receptor, Annu. Rev. Immunol. 19 (2001) 683–765.
[47] D.J. Berg, et al., Enterocolitis and colon cancer in interleukin-10-deficient mice are associated with aberrant cytokine production and CD4(+) TH1-like responses, J. Clin. Invest. 98 (1996) 1010–1020.
[48] N.J. Davidson, et al., IL-12, but not IFN-gamma, plays a major role in sustaining the chronic phase of colitis in IL-10-deficient mice, J. Immunol. 161 (1998) 3143–3149.
[49] K. Takeda, et al., Enhanced Th1 activity and development of chronic enterocolitis in mice devoid of Stat3 in macrophages and neutrophils, Immunity 10 (1999) 39–49.
[50] M. Kobayashi, et al., Toll-like receptor-dependent production of IL-12p40 causes chronic enterocolitis in myeloid cell-specific Stat3-deficient mice, J. Clin. Invest. 111 (2003) 1297–1308.

ELSEVIER

International Congress Series 1285 (2005) 10–14

www.ics-elsevier.com

Viral recognition and type I interferon production by Toll-like receptor and an RNA helicase, RIG-I

H. Kato [a], T. Kawai [b], S. Uematsu [a], O Takeuchi [a], S. Akira [a,*]

[a] *Department of Host Defense, Research Institute for Microbial Diseases, Osaka University, Japan*
[b] *Akira Innate Immunity, ERATO, JST, 3-1 Yamadaoka, Suita, Osaka 565-0871, Japan*

Abstract. Individual Toll-like receptor (TLR) recognizes distinct components derived from pathogens, and triggers inflammatory and immune responses including production of cytokines and chemokines as well as activation of dendritic cells. TLR recruits IL-1 receptor associated kinase (IRAK) via adaptor MyD88, and finally induces activation of NF-κB and MAP kinases. Although MyD88 is essential for the responses to all TLR ligands except for TLR3 ligand, the TLR3- and TLR4-mediated signaling possesses a MyD88-independent pathway, which is activated by another adaptor molecule, TRIF. The TRIF-dependent pathway activates IRF3 phosphorylation via TBK1/IKKi complex, which causes translocation of IRF3 from the cytoplasm to the nucleus, and finally induction of interferon-beta (IFN-β). TLR3 recognizes double-stranded RNA (dsRNA), however, TLR3-deficient cells still responded to dsRNA, indicating the presence of TLR3-independent recognition of dsRNA. Recently retinoic acid-inducible gene-I (RIG-I), a DExD/H box RNA helicase has been suggested to be involved in antiviral responses by recognizing dsRNA in the cytoplasm. We have generated RIG-I knock-out (KO) mice, and found that RIG-I is essential for induction of type I interferons (IFNs) after infection with RNA viruses in fibroblasts and myeloid dendritic cells (DCs). RIG-I induces type I IFNs by activating IRF3 via IkB kinase related kinases. In contrast, plasmacytoid DCs, which produce a vast amount of IFN-α after viral infection, use the TLR system rather than RIG-I for viral detection. Taken together, RIG-I and the TLR system exert antiviral responses in a cell type specific manner. © 2005 Published by Elsevier B.V.

Keywords: Toll-like receptor; RNA virus; Retinoic acid-inducible gene-I; Type I interferon

* Corresponding author.
E-mail address: sakira@biken.osaka-u.ac.jp (S. Akira).

0531-5131/ © 2005 Published by Elsevier B.V.
doi:10.1016/j.ics.2005.07.102

1. TLR signaling and TIR domain-containing adaptor molecules

Toll-like receptors (TLRs) play essential roles in innate immune responses [1,2]. TLR signaling is initiated by the recruitment of cytoplasmic adaptor molecules to the receptor. These adaptors possess a TIR domain, and associate with the TIR domain of TLR/IL-1R via a homophilic interaction. To date, 5 TIR domain-containing adaptor molecules have been identified in mammals, including myeloid differentiation factor 88 (MyD88), TIR domain-containing adaptor inducing IFNβ (TRIF), TIR domain-containing adaptor protein (TIRAP)/MyD88 adaptor-like (MAL), TRIF-related adaptor molecule (TRAM) and sterile α and HEAT-Armadillo motifs (SARM). Four of these adaptors (MyD88, TRIF, TIRAP/Mal and TRAM) are known to be involved in TLR signaling in mammals. Among the adaptor molecules, MyD88 and TRIF regulate the activation of the two main signaling pathways leading to the production of proinflammatory cytokines and type I interferons (IFNs), respectively. In addition, cell type-specific recruitment of signaling machinery to each receptor is also important for the adaptive response to TLR ligands.

2. Type I IFNs production by TLRs

Toll-like receptors (TLRs) are critical for sensing invading pathogens and evoking immune responses. Antipathogenic host defense is mediated by the rapid induction of type I IFNs and proinflammatory cytokines, leading to subsequent activation of adaptive immune responses [3,4].

DCs are subcategorized into two subsets, conventional and plasmacytoid DCs by their expressions of different surface molecules. Conventional DCs (cDCs) express various TLRs, including TLR3, and stimulation with TLR ligands results in the production of IFNs and proinflammatory cytokines. Ligand stimulation of TLR3 or TLR4, poly I:C or LPS, induces the expression of IFNβ and IFN-inducible genes from cDCs, indicating that TRIF-dependent pathway mainly functions to induce type I IFNs in response to TLR stimulation.

A recently identified subset of DCs, plasmacytoid DCs (pDCs), is characterized for their potent ability to secrete IFN-α [5,6]. pDCs express high levels of TLR7 and TLR9, but not TLR3. Ligand stimulation of TLR7 and TLR9 results in the production of IFNα. Among the TLR9 ligands, A/D-type CpG-DNAs, but not conventional B/K-type CpG-DNAs, are potent inducers of IFNα, although the production of proinflammatory cytokines is vigorously induced by both types of CpG-DNAs [7]. Interestingly, the type I IFN induction in pDCs is independent of TBK1. In pDCs, MyD88 was found to directly associate with IRF-7, which then undergoes modifications such as phosphorylation and ubiquitination [8,9]. IRAK4, IRAK1 and TRAF6 are also recruited to the complex. $MyD88^{-/-}$ and $IRAK4^{-/-}$ pDCs failed to activate both NF-κB and IRF-7 in response to TLR9 ligands. In contrast, IRAK-1 plays a key role in the expression of type I IFNs, but not proinflammatory cytokines [10]. In $IRAK1^{-/-}$ pDCs, TLR9-mediated nuclear translocation of IRF-7 was specifically abrogated. In addition, IRAK1 can phosphorylate IRF-7 in vitro, suggesting that IRAK1 possibly functions as an IRF-7 kinase. The activated IRF-7 induces the expression of IFNα genes.

3. Viral recognition by TLRs and RIG-I

Among 12 reported TLRs, TLR3, TLR4, TLR7, TLR8 and TLR9 are involved in the recognition of viral components. In mice viral ds RNA, fusion protein of respiratory syncytial virus, ss RNA and genomic DNA from Herpes species and murine cytomegalovirus are recognized by TLR3, TLR4, TLR7 and TLR9, respectively [11–18].

TLRs recognize pathogens at either the cell surface or lysosome/endosome membranes, indicating that this system might be invalid for the detection of pathogens that have invaded the cytosol. Recent studies have revealed that such pathogens already present in the cytoplasm are detected by various cytoplasmic receptors without a transmembrane domain.

Synthesis of dsRNA in the infected cells is required for the replication of ssRNA viruses, and such viral dsRNA is believed to be a virus-specific molecular structure recognized by hosts. Most virus-infected cells produce type I IFNs in a TLR3-independent manner, implying that the mechanism for dsRNA recognition in the cytoplasm plays an important role in the IFN response. Protein kinase R (PKR) has been implicated in viral dsRNA recognition. PKR belongs to a family of proteins containing dsRNA-binding domains, and is induced in response to stimulation with IFNs. Activation of PKR results in growth arrest of the cells via eIF2α phosphorylation. Several reports have demonstrated that virus-induced type I IFN production is modestly impaired in PKR$^{-/-}$ mice [19]. Furthermore, PKR$^{-/-}$ mice showed defective induction of apoptosis in response to poly I:C and bacterial burdens. However, PKR$^{-/-}$ mice have also been reported to show no alterations in IFN production to viral exposure [20].

Recently, retinoic acid-inducible protein-I (RIG-I), an IFN-inducible protein containing caspase recruitment domains (CARDs) and a helicase domain, has been identified as a cytoplasmic dsRNA detector. RIG-I also interacts with poly I:C [21]. RIG-I overexpression leads to the activation of IFN-beta promoter in the infection of Newcastle Disease virus (NDV) and transfection of poly I:C. Mda-5, a molecule showing homology to RIG-I, has also been implicated in the recognition of viral dsRNA [22]. Most of RIG-I$^{-/-}$ mice showed embryonic lethality due to liver degeneration, although a few were born alive. RIG-I$^{-/-}$ MEFs did not produce IFNβ, activate IFN-inducible genes or induce proinflammatory cytokines in response to infections with several RNA viruses including NDV, Sendai virus and Vesicular Stomatitis virus (VSV) [23]. NDV-induced activation of NF-κB and ISRE-containing genes was abrogated in RIG-I$^{-/-}$ cells. RIG-I overexpression in TBK1/IKK-i double-deficient cells failed to activate the IFNβ promoter, indicating that RIG-I acts upstream of TBK1/IKK-i and governs both NF-κB and IRFs.

In MEFs, FADD and RIP1 are required for type I IFN responses to stimulation with dsRNA, and FADD$^{-/-}$ or RIP1$^{-/-}$ MEFs were highly susceptible to VSV infection [24]. FADD and RIP1 act upstream of TBK1/IKK-i, suggesting that these molecules transduce signals from RIG-I to TBK1. However, the cited report [24] only described the response to poly I:C, and not that against viral infection. Further analyses are therefore required to clarify the roles of FADD and RIP1 in the IFN response to viral infection.

Furthermore, cDCs derived from the RIG-I$^{-/-}$ mice also failed to induce type I IFNs and cytokines upon exposure to NDV. Interestingly, pDCs from RIG-I$^{-/-}$ mice produced a comparable amount of IFNα with pDCs from wild-type mice upon NDV stimulation; furthermore, the NDV-induced IFNα from pDCs are mainly TLR7-dependent. These indicate that induction of type I IFNs in RNA viral infection would be triggered by either RIG-I or the TLR system in a cell type specific manner [23].

The mechanism of RIG-I-induced signaling as well as the relationships among RIG-I, Mda-5 and TLR signaling will be extremely interesting to explore.

References

[1] S. Akira, K. Takeda, Toll-like receptor signalling, Nat. Rev., Immunol. 4 (2004) 499–511.

[2] B. Beutler, Inferences, questions and possibilities in Toll-like receptor signalling, Nature 430 (2004) 257–263.

[3] C.A. Biron, Initial and innate responses to viral infections: pattern setting in immunity or disease, Curr. Opin. Microbiol. 2 (1999) 374–381.

[4] A. Le Bon, D.F. Tough, Links between innate and adaptive immunity via type I interferon, Curr. Opin. Immunol. 14 (2002) 432–436.

[5] M. Cella, et al., Plasmacytoid monocytes migrate to inflamed lymph nodes and produce large amounts of type I interferon, Nat. Med. 5 (1999) 919–923.

[6] M. Colonna, A. Krug, M. Cella, Interferon-producing cells: on the front line in immune responses against pathogens, Curr. Opin. Immunol. 14 (2002) 373–379.

[7] H. Hemmi, et al., The roles of Toll-like receptor 9, MyD88, and DNA-dependent protein kinase catalytic subunit in the effects of two distinct CpG DNAs on dendritic cell subsets, J. Immunol. 170 (2003) 3059–3064.

[8] T. Kawai, et al., Interferon-alpha induction through Toll-like receptors involves a direct interaction of IRF7 with MyD88 and TRAF6, Nat. Immunol. 5 (2004) 1061–1068.

[9] K. Honda, et al., Role of a transductional-transcriptional processor complex involving MyD88 and IRF-7 in Toll-like receptor signaling, Proc. Natl. Acad. Sci. U. S. A. 101 (2004) 15416–15421.

[10] S. Uematsu, et al., Interleukin-1 receptor-associated kinase-1 plays an essential role for Toll-like receptor (TLR)7- and TLR9-mediated interferon-{alpha} induction, J. Exp. Med. 201 (2005) 915–923.

[11] L. Alexopoulou, et al., Recognition of double-stranded RNA and activation of NF-kappaB by Toll-like receptor 3, Nature 413 (2001) 732–738.

[12] E.A. Kurt-Jones, et al., Pattern recognition receptors TLR4 and CD14 mediate response to respiratory syncytial virus, Nat. Immunol. 1 (2000) 398–401.

[13] F. Heil, et al., Species-specific recognition of single-stranded RNA via toll-like receptor 7 and 8, Science 303 (2004) 1526–1529.

[14] S.S. Diebold, et al., Innate antiviral responses by means of TLR7-mediated recognition of single-stranded RNA, Science 303 (2004) 1529–1531.

[15] J.M. Lund, et al., Recognition of single-stranded RNA viruses by Toll-like receptor 7, Proc. Natl. Acad. Sci. 101 (2004) 5598–5603.

[16] J. Lund, et al., Toll-like receptor 9-mediated recognition of Herpes simplex virus-2 by plasmacytoid dendritic cells, J. Exp. Med. 198 (2003) 513–520.

[17] A. Krug, et al., Herpes simplex virus type 1 activates murine natural interferon-producing cells through toll-like receptor 9, Blood 103 (2004) 1433–1437.

[18] A. Krug, et al., TLR9-dependent recognition of MCMV by IPC and DC generates coordinated cytokine responses that activate antiviral NK cell function, Immunity 21 (2004) 107–119.

[19] S.S. Diebold, et al., Viral infection switches non-plasmacytoid dendritic cells into high interferon producers, Nature 424 (2003) 324–328.

[20] E.J. Smith, et al., IRF3 and IRF7 phosphorylation in virus-infected cells does not require double-stranded RNA-dependent protein kinase R or Ikappa B kinase but is blocked by Vaccinia virus E3L protein, J. Biol. Chem. 276 (2001) 8951–8957.

[21] M. Yoneyama, et al., The RNA helicase RIG-I has an essential function in double-stranded RNA-induced innate antiviral responses, Nat. Immunol. 5 (2004) 730–737.

[22] J. Andrejeva, et al., The V proteins of paramyxoviruses bind the IFN-inducible RNA helicase, mda-5, and inhibit its activation of the IFN-beta promoter, Proc. Natl. Acad. Sci. U. S. A. 101 (2004) 17264–17269.
[23] Kato, H., et al., Cell type specific involvement of retinoicacid inducible gene-I and Toll-like receptors in antiviral response, Immunity 23 (2005) 19–28.
[24] S. Balachandran, E. Thomas, G.N. Barber, A FADD-dependent innate immune mechanism in mammalian cells, Nature 432 (2004) 401–405.

ELSEVIER

International Congress Series 1285 (2005) 15–18

www.ics-elsevier.com

Molecular mechanism for innate recognition of microbial products by toll-like receptors

Kensuke Miyake *

Division of Infectious Genetics, The Institute of Medical Science, The University of Tokyo, Tokyo, Japan
CREST, Japan Science and Technology Corporation, Tokyo, Japan

Abstract. The Toll family of receptors (Toll-like receptor, TLR) plays an essential role in innate recognition of microbial products. TLR is a type I transmembrane protein that contains a large, leucine-rich repeats in the extracellular region and a Toll/IL-1 receptor homology (TIR) domain in the cytoplasmic region. Microbial membranes are recognized by TLR4, TLR2, TLR1, and TLR6, whereas DNA or RNA derived from pathogens are sensed by TLR3, TLR7, TLR8 and TLR9. Despite identification of microbial ligands for TLRs, molecular mechanisms underlying microbial recognition by Toll-like receptors remain enigmatic. Lipopolysaccharide (LPS) is one of the most immunostimulatory glycolipids constituting the outer membrane of the Gram-negative bacteria. LPS in the membrane is transferred to CD14 by LPS-binding protein (LBP). CD14 then transfers LPS to the receptor complex consisting of TLR4 and MD-2. MD-2 is an extracellular molecule that is associated with the extracellular domain of TLR4 and essential for LPS responses, since mice lacking MD-2 are hyporesponsive to LPS. LPS directly interacts with cell surface TLR4/MD-2, which leads to ligand-dependent oligomerization of TLR4 and subsequent signaling. Soluble MD-2 as well as TLR4/MD-2 was reported to bind to LPS, and subsequent ligand-induced oligomerization of TLR4 was regulated by MD-2. These results demonstrate roles for MD-2 as a coreceptor in microbial recognition of LPS. TLR4, therefore, requires additional molecules such as MD-2, CD14, and LBP for processing and recognizing LPS. It is well possible for other TLRs to require similar molecules in microbial recognition. © 2005 Published by Elsevier B.V.

Keywords: Lipopolysaccharide; Toll-like receptor

* Division of Infectious Genetics, The Institute of Medical Science, The University of Tokyo, Tokyo, Japan.
E-mail address: kmiyake@ims.u-tokyo.ac.jp.

0531-5131/ © 2005 Published by Elsevier B.V.
doi:10.1016/j.ics.2005.07.027

1. Introduction

Innate immunity is the first line of defense against bacterial infection [1]. The Toll family of receptors plays an essential role in innate recognition of microbial products [2]. TLR4 recognizes lipopolysaccharide (LPS), one of the most immunostimulatory glycolipids constituting the outer membrane of the Gram-negative bacteria [3–7]. LPS consists of lipid A, core oligosaccharide, and an O side chain [8]. Lipid A is responsible for immunostimulating activity of LPS. Because of its potent activity, LPS has been implicated in a variety of diseases, such as septic shock [9].

LPS in the membrane poorly activates the immune system. LPS is transferred to CD14 by a lipid transferase LPS-binding protein (LBP) [10,11]. LPS/CD14 stimulates TLR4/MD-2 on the cell surface [12]. TLR4 is a type I transmembrane protein that contains leucine-rich repeats in the extracellular region and a Toll/IL-1 receptor homology (TIR) domain in the cytoplasmic region [3]. MD-2 is an extracellular molecule that is associated with the extracellular domain of TLR4 and is indispensable for cell surface expression of and LPS recognition by TLR4 [12–15]. LPS recognition begins with LPS interaction with TLR4/MD-2, followed by homotypic interaction of TLR4, and ends with an activation signal from TLR4 [16].

2. A role for MD-2 in cell surface expression of TLR4

We demonstrated that TLR4 alone is little expressed on the cell surface and most TLR4 reside in ER or the Golgi apparatus without mature glycosylation, revealing an essential role for MD-2 in cell surface expression of TLR4 [13]. A role for MD-2 in cell surface expression of TLR4 was confirmed by an independent study with a B cell line deficient in gp96, in which TLR4 failed to associate with MD-2. TLR4 was little expressed on the cell surface and LPS responses were severely impaired in the gp96-deficient B cell line [17]. Despite these results, several studies claimed that TLR4 alone is expressed on the cell surface and respond to the LPS/MD-2 complex [18–20]. These functional results raise a possibility that a trace amount of TLR4 is expressed on the cell surface without MD-2. Whereas requirement for MD-2 in LPS recognition is well documented, molecular mechanisms underlying cell surface expression of TLR4 are not completely understood. Further study needs to focus on this issue.

3. A role for MD-2 in ligand interaction

A number of studies clearly demonstrated the direct interaction between LPS and MD-2. Mancek et al. [21] searched LPS binding motif of MD-2 by comparing MD-2 with other LPS binding proteins, and found high amphipathicity and high content of positively charged residues at the region from aa119 to 132 in human MD-2. The importance of this region (aa119–132) was underscored by the studies using MD-2 mutants. Visintin et al. reported that human MD-2 mutants, K128E or K132E, normally associated with TLR4 but were impaired in interaction with LPS [22]. Re et al. focused especially basic aromatic residues around LPS binding motif of human MD-2 [23]. Human MD-2 with 2–4 amino acid substitution, such as K125A and F126A, was not impaired in association with TLR4 but impaired in LPS responses. Mouse MD-2 mutants, F119A or F121A, did not bind to

LPS when prepared as recombinant soluble MD-2 [24]. In contrast to MD-2, the extracellular domain of TLR4 has never been shown to bind to LPS. MD-2 seems to have a principal role in interaction with LPS, whereas TLR4 augments the interaction between LPS and MD-2 [25].

4. The role for MD-2 in ligand-induced receptor clustering

The interaction between LPS and TLR4/MD-2 induces homotypic interaction of TLR4, which is thought to deliver a signal via the cytoplasmic TIR domain of TLR4 [16]. Receptor clustering does not always occur after ligand-binding, since a lipid A antagonist, lipid IVa, binds to human TLR4/MD-2 but does not induce receptor clustering. TLR4-oligomerization seems to be regulated differently from LPS-binding and molecular mechanism regulating TLR4-oligomerization would have a role in discrimination of the fine structure of LPS. The fine structure of LPS varies among a variety of Gram-negative bacteria and changes with their response to environmental changes. TLR4/MD-2 is able to discriminate such fine differences. Whereas LPS from *Escherichia coli* is a full agonist, LPS from *Rhodobacter sphaeroides* is antagonistic on human TLR4/MD-2 [26]. One opportunistic bacterium, *Pseudomonas aeruginosa*, synthesizes more highly acylated (hexa-acylated) LPS structures during adaptation to the cystic fibrosis airway. Human, but not murine, TLR4/MD-2 recognizes this adaptation and transmits robust proinflammatory signals in response to hexa-acylated but not penta-acylated LPS from *P. aeruginosa*, suggesting that *P. aeruginosa* control host responses by changing their fine structure of LPS [27]. It seems to be important to understand molecular mechanism by which TLR4/MD-2 discriminate the fine structure of LPS for understanding host–pathogen relationship during infection. Considering discrimination between lipid A and lipid A antagonist, a link between ligand binding and receptor clustering should be a critical step for recognition of the fine structures of LPS [16,28]. It is important to understand how receptor clustering is initiated and terminated. Whereas mouse TLR4 clustering upon lipid A stimulation was triggered by both mouse and human MD-2 that upon lipid IVa stimulation was triggered by mouse MD-2 but not by human MD-2 [16]. MD-2 seems to have an important role in triggering receptor clustering after ligand binding.

In contrast to a number of structure–function studies on the interaction between LPS and MD-2 as mentioned above, little is known about the structure–function relationship for MD-2 in a link between ligand binding and receptor clustering. Future study has to focus on a role for MD-2 in the link.

References

[1] C.A. Janeway Jr., R. Medzhitov, Innate immune recognition, Annu. Rev. Immunol. 20 (2002) 197.

[2] K. Takeda, T. Kaisho, S. Akira, Toll-like receptors, Annu. Rev. Immunol. 21 (2003) 335.

[3] R. Medzhitov, P. Preston-Hurlburt, C.A. Janeway Jr., A human homologue of the *Drosophila* Toll protein signals activation of adaptive immunity, Nature 388 (1997) 394.

[4] A. Poltorak, et al., Defective LPS signaling in C3H/HeJ and C57BL/10ScCr mice: mutations in Tlr4 gene, Science 282 (1998) 2085.

[5] S.T. Qureshi, et al., Endotoxin-tolerant mice have mutations in Toll-like receptor 4 (Tlr4), J. Exp. Med. 189 (1999) 615.

[6] K. Hoshino, et al., Cutting edge: toll-like receptor 4 (TLR4)-deficient mice are hyporesponsive to lipopolysaccharide: evidence for TLR4 as the Lps gene product, J. Immunol. 162 (1999) 3749.

[7] J.C. Chow, et al., Toll-like receptor-4 mediates lipopolysaccharide-induced signal transduction, J. Biol. Chem. 274 (1999) 10689.

[8] C.R. Raetz, C. Whitfield, Lipopolysaccharide endotoxins, Annu. Rev. Biochem. 71 (2002) 635.

[9] J. Cohen, The immunopathogenesis of sepsis, Nature 420 (2002) 885.

[10] R.R. Schumann, et al., Structure and function of lipopolysaccharide binding protein, Science 249 (1990) 1429.

[11] R.J. Ulevitch, P.S. Tobias, Receptor-dependent mechanisms of cell stimulation by bacterial endotoxin, Annu. Rev. Immunol. 13 (1995) 437.

[12] R. Shimazu, et al., MD-2, a molecule that confers lipopolysaccharide responsiveness on Toll-like receptor 4, J. Exp. Med. 189 (1999) 1777.

[13] Y. Nagai, et al., Essential role of MD-2 in LPS responsiveness and TLR4 distribution, Nat. Immunol. 3 (2002) 667.

[14] A.B. Schromm, et al., Molecular genetic analysis of an endotoxin nonresponder mutant cell line: a point mutation in a conserved region of MD-2 abolishes endotoxin-induced signaling, J. Exp. Med. 194 (2001) 79.

[15] K. Miyake, et al., Innate recognition of lipopolysaccharide by Toll-like receptor 4/MD-2 and RP105/MD-1, J. Endotoxin Res. 6 (2000) 389.

[16] S. Saitoh, et al., Lipid A antagonist, lipid IVa, is distinct from lipid A in interaction with Toll-like receptor 4 (TLR4)-MD-2 and ligand-induced TLR4 oligomerization, Int. Immunol. 16 (2004) 961.

[17] F. Randow, B. Seed, Endoplasmic reticulum chaperone gp96 is required for innate immunity but not cell viability, Nat. Cell Biol. 3 (2001) 891.

[18] H.P. Jia, et al., Endotoxin responsiveness of human airway epithelia is limited by low expression of MD-2, Am. J. Physiol., Lung Cell. Mol. Physiol. 287 (2004) L428.

[19] T.L. Gioannini, et al., Isolation of an endotoxin-MD-2 complex that produces Toll-like receptor 4-dependent cell activation at picomolar concentrations, Proc. Natl. Acad. Sci. U. S. A. 101 (2004) 4186.

[20] M.N. Kennedy, et al., A complex of soluble MD-2 and lipopolysaccharide serves as an activating ligand for Toll-like receptor 4, J. Biol. Chem. 279 (2004) 34698.

[21] M. Mancek, P. Pristovsek, R. Jerala, Identification of LPS-binding peptide fragment of MD-2, a toll-receptor accessory protein, Biochem. Biophys. Res. Commun. 292 (2002) 880.

[22] A. Visintin, et al., Lysines 128 and 132 enable lipopolysaccharide binding to MD-2, leading to Toll-like receptor-4 aggregation and signal transduction, J. Biol. Chem. 278 (2003) 48313.

[23] F. Re, J.L. Strominger, Separate functional domains of human MD-2 mediate Toll-like receptor 4-binding and lipopolysaccharide responsiveness, J. Immunol. 171 (2003) 5272.

[24] N. Tsuneyoshi, et al., The functional and structural properties of MD-2 required for lipopolysaccharide binding are absent in MD-1, J. Immunol. 174 (2005) 340.

[25] N. Hyakushima, et al., Interaction of soluble form of recombinant extracellular TLR4 domain with MD-2 enables lipopolysaccharide binding and attenuates TLR4-mediated signaling, J. Immunol. 173 (2004) 6949.

[26] G.D. Kutuzova, et al., Diphosphoryl lipid A from *Rhodobacter sphaeroides* blocks the binding and internalization of lipopolysaccharide in RAW 264.7 cells, J. Immunol. 167 (2001) 482.

[27] A.M. Hajjar, et al., Human Toll-like receptor 4 recognizes host-specific LPS modifications, Nat. Immunol. 3 (2002) 354.

[28] S. Akashi, et al., Lipopolysaccharide interaction with cell surface Toll-like receptor 4-MD-2: higher affinity than that with MD-2 or CD14, J. Exp. Med. 198 (2003) 1035.

ELSEVIER

International Congress Series 1285 (2005) 19–27

www.ics-elsevier.com

Initiating protective T cell immunity by targeting antigens directly to maturing dendritic cells in lymphoid tissues

Ralph M. Steinman [a,*], Christine Trumpfheller [a], Kang Liu [a,b], Laura Bonifaz [a], Jennifer Finke [a], Angela Granelli-Piperno [a], Michel C. Nussenzweig [b]

[a] *Laboratory of Cellular Physiology and Immunology, New York, NY 10021-6399, USA*

[b] *Laboratory of Molecular Immunology in the Howard Hughes Medical Institute, The Rockefeller University, New York, NY 10021-6399, USA*

Abstract. To initiate immunity, dendritic cells (DCs) must capture antigens and respond to additional stimuli that induce their differentiation or maturation. Maturation allows DCs to switch from their steady state function of tolerance to the induction of different types of immune responses, such as the formation of effector T cells and memory. To understand the control of immunity, particularly protective immunity, and to better harness immunology during vaccine design, we directly targeted antigens to DCs in vivo and manipulated their state of maturation. For tumors, we studied irradiated plasmacytoma cells, which best target DCs when the tumor cells are injected i.v. rather than s.c. The $CD8^+$ $CD205^+$ splenic DC subset selectively took up fragments of the tumor cells. When the CD1d binding glycolipid, α-galactosyl ceramide, was injected together with the tumor cells to engage NKT lymphocytes, DCs displayed many of the cardinal features of maturation. In particular, mice developed protective immunity that was long lived (>2 months after a single vaccination), specific for J558 and not for other tumors, and required both $CD4^+$ and $CD8^+$ T cells. In the case of immunity to defined antigens, we engineered proteins into monoclonal antibodies that targeted to DCs in vivo. Following initial proof of concept studies to elicit protective immunity with ovalbumin as a model antigen, we inserted the HIV gag p24 protein in frame at the C-terminus of the heavy chain of antibodies to DEC-205 (anti-DEC-p24), an abundant endocytic receptor on DCs in lymphoid tissues. Targeting of antigens with this anti-DC monoclonal antibody increased the efficiency of immunization ~100 fold relative to non-targeted p24 protein. Administration of anti-DEC-p24 with a maturation stimulus produced strong $CD4^+$ T cell immunity to six different

* Corresponding author. Tel.: +1 212 327 8106; fax: +1 212 327 8875.
E-mail address: steinma@mail.rockefeller.edu (R.M. Steinman).

doi:10.1016/j.ics.2005.07.095

immunogenic peptides in three separate MHC backgrounds. Immunity was associated with protection against challenge with recombinant vaccinia gag at an airway surface. We propose that significant improvements in vaccine efficacy can be obtained by controlling two fundamental principles of immune function, i.e., antigen uptake by DCs and control of DC maturation.

Keywords: Dendritic cells; Vaccines; Immune therapy; DEC-205; HIV; Tumors

1. Introduction

Immunology interfaces with medicine at many points, the most prominent currently being infectious diseases, cancer, transplantation, allergy, and autoimmunity. In each of these instances, there is a need for treatments that increase (immunize) or decrease (tolerize) the immune response to the disease causing antigens. For example, in infectious diseases and cancer, many antigens are known but it remains difficult to achieve protective immunization in both mice and humans. In other clinical conditions, it will be valuable to silence the patient's response to disease causing antigens. For example, in transplantation and in inflammatory diseases, it is possible to block graft rejection and arthritis with cyclosporine and TNF antagonists respectively, but these do not eliminate the stimuli that initiate the disease, which returns when the therapy ceases. The ultimate goal of our current research is to both unravel and harness dendritic cell (DC) biology to gain improved antigen specific control of the immune system. In this article we will summarize approaches to increase protective immunity, i.e., resistance to cancer and to infectious agents.

2. Some features of dendritic cells that are pertinent to vaccine design

DCs guide critical decisions of lymphocytes, particularly T cells, involving tolerance, differentiation into different types of helper and killer cells, and memory. DCs are sentinels (Fig. 1), positioned at body surfaces and able to pick up and process antigens for presentation to different classes of lymphocytes. This antigen uptake step is a first and essential step in inducing immune responses, but by and large, it has been taken for granted in most vaccine approaches. Antigens or vaccines are injected, and it is assumed that these will be captured by DCs, as is indeed the case to some extent. However, it has

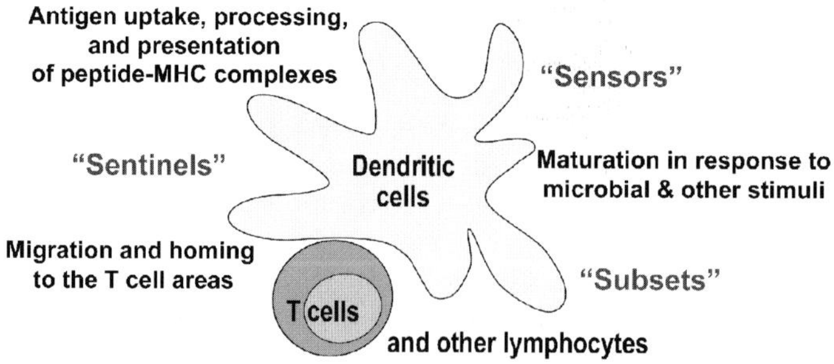

Fig. 1. Some valuable features of dendritic cells for vaccine design.

become evident that DCs express a number of potential receptors for antigen uptake [1], and that these improve antigen capture and presentation to a large extent, more than 100 fold [2,3]. Another component of the sentinel function of DCs is that they are able to migrate and home with precision to the T cell areas of lymphoid tissues (Fig. 1). The DCs are thereby positioned to identify antigen-specific T cells from the recirculating pool of lymphocytes, which move continuously into and through the T cell area, entering via high endothelial venules and leaving via efferent lymphatics. The positioning of DCs has now been visualized in living lymph nodes with two photon microscopy [4–8]. A vast and vibrant DC network is evident in the T cell areas, and the binding of antigen-specific T cells for prolonged periods has been followed [7,8]. A third area of DC function relevant to vaccine design is that DCs are sensors (Fig. 1). They respond quickly and extensively to a number of different stimuli ranging from microbial ligands for toll like receptors (TLR), TNF family members like TNF itself and CD40L, the different types of innate lymphocytes (NK, NKT, $\gamma\delta$), immune complexes, and many more. These stimuli induce the differentiation or maturation of the DCs, and the type of differentiation allows the DCs to determine the subsequent T cell outcome. For example, CD40 ligation of human blood DCs allows the DCs to differentiate T cells along a Th1 pathway, whereas exposure of DCs to the epithelial derived cytokine, thymic stromal lymphopoietin (TSLP) generates a DC that induces “inflammatory Th2 cells”, able to produce IL-4, 5, 13 and TNF [9]. CD40L and TSLP treated DCs are similar in being highly dendritic and rich in MHC II and CD86 stimulatory molecules. However, they show numerous differences in cytokine and chemokine production, and as mentioned, the functional consequences for T cells differ dramatically depending on the maturation stimuli that are sensed by the DCs.

As indicated in Fig. 1, each area of DC function (antigen uptake, positioning, maturation) is relevant to different DC subsets, of which there are several. Interestingly, different DC subsets can have different receptors for antigen uptake and different toll like receptors for sensing microbes. Therefore if one wants to harness the biology of DCs in the design of antigen specific therapies, there are some rules to pursue including: getting the antigen to the DC, ensuring that the DC positions itself in the T cell areas, selecting the appropriate DC subset, and applying a maturation stimulus appropriate to the targeted DC subset and the desired T cell response.

3. Combined CD4$^+$ Th1 type and CD8$^+$ cytolytic type immunity to whole tumor cells

The changes that drive the development of malignancy, or are associated with it, provide potential antigens to be recognized by the immune system. Lymphocytes comprise a vast repertoire of clones, including those specific for tumor associated antigens. The challenge is to learn to expand and differentiate these tumor-specific lymphocytes to attack the tumor. Of course there are other obstacles to successful immune therapy. Tumors have the capacity to evade or block immunity, and tumor antigens may be regarded as self and induce tolerance. Interestingly, tolerance does not seem to represent an insurmountable obstacle, because patients with tumors, e.g., melanoma [10,11], myeloma [12], and breast cancer [13] can mount T cell responses to tumor antigens, particularly when provoked by DCs. Since it is difficult to assess the various obstacles to vaccination and therapy of tumors, and to try to overcome them, one needs to understand how to induce strong immunity in the first place. This remains a major issue. Just consider the inability to immunize the T cells of healthy individuals in a reliable way to foreign HIV proteins.

In the case of experimental tumor immunology, several approaches have dominated efforts to learn how to induce immunity. One is to transduce the gene for a foreign protein into the tumor, such as ovalbumin, influenza hemagglutinin, or beta galactosidase. This allows one to induce immunity to the surrogate foreign antigen and to take advantage of the elegant reagents that are available to study immunity to these proteins, particularly TCR transgenic T cells. However, immunity to authentic tumor antigens is not induced. A second method also involves genetic modification of the tumor, but this time with different cytokine or costimulatory molecules to try to improve immunity. This method is being approached using allogeneic tumor cell lines transduced to produce high levels of GM-CSF [14]. Thirdly, it is now possible to ablate some of the regulatory circuits that can limit T cell mediated immunity, such as CTLA-4 signaling and $CD25^{+}$ $CD4^{+}$ suppressor T cells [15,16]. These approaches hold promise, although they do not target tumor antigen-specific T cells and therefore run a risk of inducing autoimmunity [17], which is normally controlled by these regulatory pathways.

We wanted to find out if DCs could elicit strong T cell immunity to tumor cells by following some of the rules that were outlined above. To target tumor cells to DCs in situ in lymphoid organs, we took advantage of a fascinating discovery by Iyoda et al. that splenic DCs take up many different forms of dying cells such as freshly irradiated tumor cells, targets killed by NK cells, and even autologous lymphocytes induced to die by osmotic shock or irradiation [18]. The uptake of cells is restricted to the CD8α positive subset of DCs, which is also the subset that seems specialized for cross presentation onto MHC class I [19]. CD8α positive DCs (which typically also express a distinct uptake receptor called DEC-205 or CD205, below) present peptides on MHC class II as well, and this can be established directly in vivo with a monoclonal antibody that identifies a specific peptide-MHC class II complex. The antibody stains all the DCs that take up dying cells, the latter labeled with CFSE [18]. Therefore cell-associated antigens can be targeted for uptake and processing to DCs, but the CD8α positive subset is preferentially involved.

When we administered dying cells in the steady state, we found that peripheral T cell tolerance developed [20]. An important feature was that tolerance was able to be induced with small amounts of antigen. Less than 1 μg of cell-associated ovalbumin led to tolerance as opposed to 100s of micrograms if targeting was not utilized. However, if we administered a maturation stimulus, such as agonistic CD40 mAb, immunity ensued [20].

We set out to pursue this strategy with MHC negative, J558 plasmacytoma cells. Plasmacytomas do not express MHC class II, and an MHC I negative variant of J558 had been isolated by Dr. Yang Liu, who also prepared a $CD8^{+}$ TCR transgenic mouse specific for the classical P1A peptide found in this tumor. We found that irradiated J558 cells were taken up by splenic DCs and cross presented to the P1A specific T cell line [18]. Importantly, we only saw good uptake by DCs (again the CD8α positive subset) when we injected tumor cells i.v. Minimal uptake took place in lymph node DCs when the s.c. route was used. Therefore, the frequent use of the s.c. or i.m. route for tumor cell vaccines may be suboptimal if one wants to follow the rule of getting the tumor cell to the DCs.

When we evaluated maturation stimuli, we found that we could not induce resistance to MHC I bearing J558 tumor cells if we used some common stimuli such as LPS, poly IC, or anti-CD40. These stimuli induce some components of DC maturation, such as increased cell surface expression of CD40, CD86 and MHC class II, but not the cardinal one, the ability to elicit protective immunity [21]. In contrast, when the NKT cell ligand, α-galactosyl ceramide, was tested, protective immunity was induced. The immunity required both $CD4^+$ and $CD8^+$ T cells, and was long lived, 2 months or more, after a single dose of tumor cell vaccine. We showed that mature DCs, taken from mice injected with tumor cells and α-Gal Cer, were able to transfer immunity to a naïve animal. The use of α-Gal Cer as an inducer of the full maturation of DCs was revealed by Fujii et al. [22] and Hermans et al. [23]. Fujii also showed that maturation entailed more than the presentation of MHC peptide and upregulation of CD86 costimulatory molecules. The latter was induced by inflammatory cytokines like TNF, but was insufficient to yield $CD4^+$ and $CD8^+$ T cell immunity in the absence of additional CD40 based signals [24]. These findings were extended by Sporri et al. who also concluded that inflammatory mediators could activate bystander DCs, as manifest by CD86 upregulation, but these bystander DCs did not induce immunity. Instead, direct contact with the TLR ligand was needed for the full maturation of DCs, as reflected by T cell immunization [25], much like CD40 was required for DCs to induce immunity in the studies of Fujii et al. In the latter experiments, CD40 negative DCs were comparable with wild-type DCs in the efficiency of antigen presentation and in the expression of high levels of costimulatory molecules, so that CD40 ligation was not required for the assembly of so called “signals one and two” on the DCs [24]. It is not yet clear why NKT lymphocytes are superior as a DC maturation stimulus for tumor immunity, although it is evident that these innate cells release high levels of IFNγ and seem capable of delivering a CD40 signal.

These experiments show that strong, combined $CD4^+$ and $CD8^+$ T cell immunity can be induced to tumor cells without having to modify them genetically. The biology entails uptake of tumor cells by DCs, possibly a requisite CD8α positive subset for cross presentation to $CD8^+$ T cells, and their “appropriate” maturation via NKT lymphocytes.

4. Induction of strong T cell mediated immunity to model antigens using fusion monoclonal antibodies

Another approach to harnessing the tolerizing and immunizing roles of DCs in vivo in intact lymphoid tissues is to directly target antigens to DCs by incorporating them into monoclonal antibodies (mAbs) to DC receptors, with DEC-205/CD205 being the prototype. DEC-205, formerly called NLDC-145, is a type I transmembrane protein with 10 putative, external, C-type lectin domains and a cytosolic region that has coated pit and endocytic targeting sequences [26]. DEC-205 mediates efficient presentation of ligands, in this case peptides carried within rabbit antibodies to mouse DEC-205 [26,27]. Importantly, when anti-DEC mAb is injected in vivo, it selectively targets to DCs in the T cell areas of lymphoid tissues, i.e., we can visualize the injected mAb in the DCs in sections, and when we prepare cell suspensions, it is the CD11c integrin positive DCs that have captured the mAb [2].

Targeting antigens to DCs in vivo with monoclonal antibodies provides a means to analyze DC function in intact lymphoid organs without having to isolate the DCs or generate them ex vivo from progenitors. Initially, we engineered sequences for antigenic peptides into the carboxy terminus of the heavy chain of the DEC-205 antibody [2,28]. We also introduced an entire protein, ovalbumin (OVA), by chemically cross linking OVA to inter-heavy chain thiols exposed by reduction [29]. In these instances, the anti-DEC-205 antibody efficiently targeted the antigens for presentation on MHC class I and II in vivo. In the steady state, the T cells proliferated and then were deleted or anergized. However, in the case of OVA, less than 1 μg of protein was sufficient to induce tolerance, as opposed to 400 μg of soluble nontargeted OVA. If agonistic anti-CD40 mAb was also administered, then antigen presentation led to immunity, i.e., the T cells produced large amounts of cytokines, developed cytolytic activity in the case of $CD8^+$ T cells, and showed a strong recall response. Thus, antigen targeting via DEC-205 greatly enhanced the efficiency of antigen presentation in vivo, and the approach showed that DCs are a major cell type involved in peripheral tolerance and immunity within intact lymphoid organs.

We then studied the immunization of naïve mice to OVA. We were able to induce primary $CD4^+$ and $CD8^+$ immune responses, again with low doses of OVA coupled to the anti-DEC mAb [3]. Several interesting features were noted beyond the increase in the efficiency of antigen presentation. The immune responses were much stronger than other means of immunization, such as OVA pulsed onto DCs ex vivo, or OVA given together with either anti-CD40 or complete Freund's adjuvant. Therapeutic resistance to an OVA-transduced tumor could be induced, and the resistance was again stronger with anti-DEC:OVA plus anti-CD40 than with other modes of immunization. Also, vaccination with anti-DEC:OVA s.c. led to protective immunity in the lung to a challenge with recombinant vaccinia:OVA. This protection at a mucosal surface was ascribed to the fact that the antibody was targeting systemically to DCs in lymphoid organs, including DCs in lymph nodes that drain the airway and intestine. These findings suggest that anti-DEC-205 mAb targeting should be explored for vaccination against clinically relevant antigens.

5. Induction of strong T cell mediated immunity to HIV gag using fusion monoclonal antibodies

After introducing antigenic peptides into the heavy chain of anti-DEC-205 mAb [2,28], we turned to full length proteins, which were also cloned in frame at the carboxy terminus of the heavy chain. The anti-DEC-205 fusion heavy chain and light chains and controls were expressed by cotransfection in 293T cells. Antibody produced by transfection was shown to bind normally to DEC-205 expressing cells. In Fig. 2 we show an experiment in which naïve mice were vaccinated with graded doses of fusion mAb carrying HIV gag p24 protein (1, 5 and 20 μg of mAb). The maturation stimulus was a combination of anti-CD40 and poly IC. 3 weeks after immunization, we monitored T cell responses by staining for intracellular IFN-γ and IL-2. Because relatively little is known about gag peptides that are presented on mouse MHC molecules, we used overlapping peptide pools (15 mers staggered every 4 amino acids) along the length of the gag p24 protein [30,31] for the immune assays. We observed a strong IFNγ producing, $CD4^+$ T cell response, as shown in Fig. 2 for Balb/c mice. The two peptide pools for most of the recognition are shown in Fig. 2, which also indicates that anti-DEC:p24 immunizes mice much better than control Ig:p24 (100 times or more in multiple experiments).

When we examine the literature, we cannot find an instance in which $CD4^+$ T cell responses of comparable magnitude have been induced with safe vaccines in mice, and

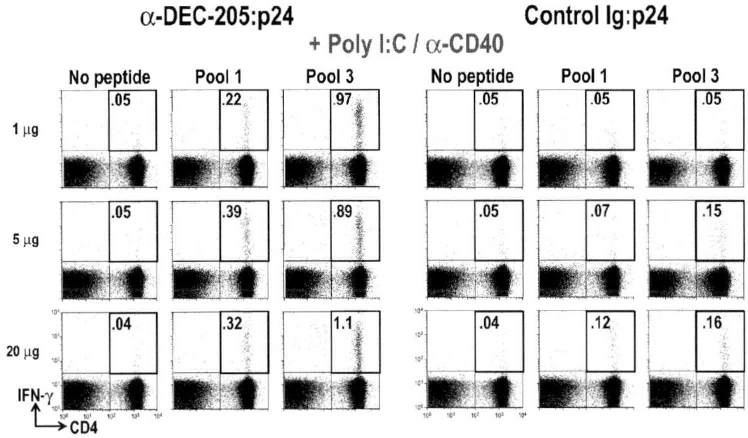

Fig. 2. Induction of HIV-specific CD4$^+$ T cells in BALB mice by a single dose of anti-DEC-205:HIV-*gag* p24 vaccine. Mice were injected i.p. with graded doses (*y*-axis) of HIV gag p24 fusion mAbs, either anti-DEC-205 (left) or control Ig (right) together with stimuli for DC maturation, which were poly IC and anti-CD40. 3 weeks later, spleen cells were assayed for production of IFN-γ by CD4$^+$ T cells (similar results were obtained for IL-2 production) with either no peptide or 5 different pools of peptides covering the full p24 sequence. Only the reactive pools 1 and 3 for BALB mice are shown. The numbers in the boxes are the frequencies of CD4$^+$ T cells making IFN-γ.

with a single dose. Importantly the response was broad. When we studied different MHC haplotypes, three different mouse stains presented at least two different gag peptides (six in all) from this small protein.

To assess protective immunity, we collaborated with Carolina Lopez and Tom Moran at the Mt. Sinai School of Medicine to challenge mice with recombinant vaccinia gag via the airway. Even though the mice were immunized with anti-DEC:gag s.c., they showed good protection at a mucosal surface. We are finding that this CD4$^+$ T cell immunity is long-lived, at least 20 weeks after a single dose of the DC targeted vaccine.

6. Discussion

The immune system has almost limitless potential to respond to vaccines, but effective vaccination with protein antigens has been difficult. Given the central role of DCs in controlling tolerance and immunity, some principles can be suggested to harness immune system to improve vaccination. One is to ensure that vaccines gain access to DCs, something that is best achieved through specific receptor mediated routes. However, there is much to be learned in terms of which receptor is optimal, the antigen processing pathways, and the role of DC subsets. A second rule is that DCs must be switched from their normal tolerogenic function to immunity. Here too, much needs to be learned concerning the types of maturation stimuli that are functional in vivo and the immune responses elicited under different DC maturation conditions. At this point, it is apparent that antigen targeting to maturing DCs in mice is an effective new method to elicit long lived and protective immunity to tumor cells and microbial proteins.

Acknowledgements

This work was supported by grants AI13013 and AI40874, as well as a training fellowship to K. Liu. Dr. Yang Liu developed the J558 system for studying tumor immunity, while Dr. Tom Moran and Carolina Lopez collaborated with the vaccinia challenge system for studying HIV gag immunity.

References

[1] I. Mellman, R.M. Steinman, Dendritic cells: specialized and regulated antigen processing machines, Cell 106 (2001) 255–258.
[2] D. Hawiger, et al., Dendritic cells induce peripheral T cell unresponsiveness under steady state conditions in vivo, J. Exp. Med. 194 (2001) 769–780.
[3] L.C. Bonifaz, et al., In vivo targeting of antigens to the DEC-205 receptor on maturing dendritic cells improves T cell vaccination, J. Exp. Med. 199 (2004) 815–824.
[4] P. Bousso, E. Robey, Dynamics of $CD8^+$ T cell priming by dendritic cells in intact lymph nodes, Nat. Immunol. 4 (2003) 579–585.
[5] M.J. Miller, et al., Imaging the single cell dynamics of $CD4^+$ T cell activation by dendritic cells in lymph nodes, J. Exp. Med. 200 (2004) 847–856.
[6] T.R. Mempel, S.E. Henrickson, U.H. Von Andrian, T-cell priming by dendritic cells in lymph nodes occurs in three distinct phases, Nature 427 (2004) 154–159.
[7] R.L. Lindquist, et al., Visualizing dendritic cell networks in vivo, Nat. Immunol. 5 (2004) 1243–1250.
[8] G. Shakhar, et al., Stable T cell-dendritic cell interactions precede the development of both tolerance and immunity in vivo, Nat. Immunol. 6 (2005) 707–714.
[9] V. Soumelis, et al., Human epithelial cells trigger dendritic cell-mediated allergic inflammation by producing TSLP, Nat. Immunol. 3 (2002) 673–680.
[10] J. Banchereau, et al., Immune and clinical responses in patients with metastatic melanoma to $CD34^+$ progenitor-derived dendritic cell vaccine, Cancer Res. 61 (2001) 6451–6458.
[11] B. Schuler-Thurner, et al., Rapid induction of tumor-specific type 1 T helper cells in metastatic melanoma patients by vaccination with mature, cryopreserved, peptide-loaded monocyte-derived dendritic cells, J. Exp. Med. 195 (2002) 1279–1288.
[12] M.V. Dhodapkar, J. Krasovsky, K. Olson, T cells from the tumor microenvironment of patients with progressive myeloma can generate strong, tumor-specific cytolytic responses to autologous, tumor-loaded dendritic cells, Proc. Natl. Acad. Sci. U. S. A. 99 (2002) 13009–13013.
[13] H. Kao, et al., Identification of cyclin B1 as a shared human epithelial tumor-associated antigen recognized by T cells, J. Exp. Med. 194 (2001) 1313–1323.
[14] A.M. Thomas, et al., Mesothelin-specific $CD8^+$ T cell responses provide evidence of in vivo cross-priming by antigen-presenting cells in vaccinated pancreatic cancer patients, J. Exp. Med. 200 (2004) 297–306.
[15] R.P. Sutmuller, et al., Synergism of cytotoxic T lymphocyte-associated antigen 4 blockade and depletion of $CD25^+$ regulatory T cells in antitumor therapy reveals alternative pathways for suppression of autoreactive cytotoxic T lymphocyte responses, J. Exp. Med. 194 (2001) 823–832.
[16] S. Sakaguchi, Naturally arising $CD4^+$ regulatory T cells for immunologic self-tolerance and negative control of immune responses, Annu. Rev. Immunol. 22 (2004) 531–562.
[17] G.Q. Phan, et al., Cancer regression and autoimmunity induced by cytotoxic T lymphocyte-associated antigen 4 blockade in patients with metastatic melanoma, Proc. Natl. Acad. Sci. U. S. A. 100 (2003) 8372–8377.
[18] T. Iyoda, et al., The $CD8^+$ dendritic cell subset selectively endocytoses dying cells in culture and in vivo, J. Exp. Med. 195 (2002) 1289–1302.
[19] G.T. Belz, et al., The $CD8\alpha^+$ dendritic cell is responsible for inducing peripheral self-tolerance to tissue-associated antigens, J. Exp. Med. 196 (2002) 1099–1104.
[20] K. Liu, et al., Immune tolerance after delivery of dying cells to dendritic cells in situ, J. Exp. Med. 196 (2002) 1091–1097.

[21] K. Liu, et al., Innate NKT lymphocytes confer superior adaptive immunity via tumor capturing dendritic cells (submitted for publication).
[22] S. Fujii, et al., Activation of natural killer T cells by α-galactosylceramide rapidly induces the full maturation of dendritic cells in vivo and thereby acts as an adjuvant for combined CD4 and CD8 T cell immunity to a co-administered protein, J. Exp. Med. 198 (2003) 267–279.
[23] I.F. Hermans, et al., NKT cells enhance $CD4^+$ and $CD8^+$ T cell responses to soluble antigen in vivo through direct interaction with dendritic cells, J. Immunol. 171 (2003) 5140–5147.
[24] S. Fujii, et al., The linkage of innate to adaptive immunity via maturing dendritic cells in vivo requires CD40 ligation in addition to antigen presentation and CD80/86 costimulation, J. Exp. Med. 199 (2004) 1607–1618.
[25] R. Sporri, C. Reis e Sousa, Inflammatory mediators are insufficient for full dendritic cell activation and promote expansion of $CD4^+$ T cell populations lacking helper function, Nat. Immunol. 6 (2005) 163–170.
[26] W. Jiang, et al., The receptor DEC-205 expressed by dendritic cells and thymic epithelial cells is involved in antigen processing, Nature 375 (1995) 151–155.
[27] K. Mahnke, et al., The dendritic cell receptor for endocytosis, DEC-205, can recycle and enhance antigen presentation via major histocompatibility complex class II-positive lysosomal compartments, J. Cell Biol. 151 (2000) 673–683.
[28] D. Hawiger, et al., Immunological unresponsiveness characterized by increased expression of CD5 on peripheral T cells induced by dendritic cells in vivo, Immunity 20 (2004) 695–705.
[29] L. Bonifaz, et al., Efficient targeting of protein antigen to the dendritic cell receptor DEC-205 in the steady state leads to antigen presentation on major histocompatibility complex class I products and peripheral $CD8^+$ T cell tolerance, J. Exp. Med. 196 (2002) 1627–1638.
[30] F. Kern, et al., Analysis of CD8 T cell reactivity to cytomegalovirus using protein-spanning pools of overlapping pentadecapeptides, Eur. J. Immunol. 30 (2000) 1676–1682.
[31] H.T. Maecker, et al., Use of overlapping peptide mixtures as antigens for cytokine flow cytometry, J. Immunol. Methods 255 (2001) 27–40.

ELSEVIER

International Congress Series 1285 (2005) 28–33

www.ics-elsevier.com

Maturation and function of plasmacytoid dendritic cells

Yoshiki Omatsu [a], Tomonori Iyoda [a], Akiko Maki [b], Tomoki Ito [c], Shiro Fukuhara [c], Noriko Toyama-Sorimachi [b], Kayo Inaba [a,*]

[a] *Department of Animal Development and Physiology, Graduate School of Biostudies, Kyoto University, Bldg G, Rm 509, Yoshida-Konoe-cho, Sakyo, Kyoto 606-8501, Japan*

[b] *Department of Gastroenterology, Research Institute, International Medical Center of Japan, Japan*

[c] *First Department of Internal Medicine, Kansai Medical University, Japan*

Abstract. Dendritic cells (DCs) are comprised of a number of subsets with distinct functions. An example is plasmacytoid DCs (PDCs), also known as type I interferon-producing cells. Other studies have demonstrated some heterogeneity in PDCs. While it is known that proliferating progenitors exist in the bone marrow, little attention has been paid to intermediate stages of PDC development. Here we show PDCs express. We here show that Ly49Q, a lectin-type natural killer cell inhibitory receptor, is expressed on Gr-1^+ cells including PDCs in spleen and bone marrow. It is found that different expression levels of Ly49Q define sequential developmental stages of PDCs in bone marrow. Functional roles of PDC subsets in T cell activation are also investigated in reference to human PDCs. © 2005 Published by Elsevier B.V.

Keywords: Plasmacytoid; Dendritic cells; Differentiation; Maturation; IFN-α; IL-12; T cell activation

1. Introduction

Dendritic cells (DCs) undergo phenotypic and functional changes that characterize their transition from immature to mature DCs exhibiting a strong capability to initiate an immune response [1]. However, it is also known to be comprised of a number of subsets with distinct functions. DC subpopulations are characterized by expression of different surface markers and ability to produce cytokines that modulate both innate resistance and

* Corresponding author. Tel.: +81 75 753 4088; fax: +81 75 753 4112.
E-mail address: kayo@lif.kyoto-u.ac.jp (K. Inaba).

0531-5131/
doi:10.1016/j.ics.2005.08.004

adaptive immune response [2]. In human, CD11c^{-} IL-3R^{hi} plasmacytoid pre-DCs (PDCs) are distinguished from CD11c^{+} GM-CSFG^{+} conventional DCs by not only their phenotype but also cytokine producing abilities, especially high levels of type I interferons (IFN-α/β) in response to virus stimulation or unmethylated oligodeoxynucleotide containing CpG-motif (CpG-ODN) [3,4]. Murine PDCs were also identified in lymphoid tissues, including spleen, LNs, thymus, bone marrow (BM), and even liver, as CD11c^{+} B220^{+} Gr-1^{+} CD45Rb^{high} CD11b^{-} cells [5–10].

Recently, murine PDCs have been identified with a new mAb 120G8 [11]. The 120G8 mAb displayed a high specificity against both activated and resting PDCs, reacting with most of the PDC population in various tissues. Other studies have demonstrated some heterogeneity in PDCs, involving CD4 and CD8 expression and turnover rate [8,10,12]. While it is known that proliferating progenitors exist in the bone marrow [13–16], little attention has been paid to intermediate stages of PDC development. Here, we will show that sequential maturational stages of PDCs can be identified in the marrow on the basis of expression levels of Ly49Q.

2. NK receptor in Ly49 family and Ly49Q molecule

Ly49 family members are expressed on subsets of NK and NKT cells as disulfide-linked dimmers. The Ly-49 family belongs to a group of type II integral membrane protein that contains external domains homologous to the superfamily of Ca^{2+}-dependent lectins. In the cytoplasmic domains, they contain an ITIM that engages the intracellular tyrosine phosphatases, SHP-1 or SHP-2. However, not all Ly-49 molecules contain an ITIM. Some Ly49 family members have related isoforms that do not display ITIMs, but instead, activate NK cells. Ly49 genes are highly polymorphic and located within the NK complex, a stretch of 2-Mb on mouse chromosome 6 as a complex multigene family. This NK complex region is conserved among species, having been identified on syntenic regions of rat and human chromosomes.

Ly49Q, an ITIM-bearing inhibitory receptor, is a member of the Ly49 family of murine NK receptors, but it is unusual in several respects [17]. First, it is not expressed on NK or NKT cells, but instead on Gr-1^{+} myeloid lineage cells. Second, the expression on macrophages is regulated during development and activation, and is greatly enhanced by IFN-γ. Third, signals via Ly49Q rapidly induce morphological changes in macrophages including formation of polarized actin structures with filopodia-like structure on the one side and lamellipodia-like structure on the other side. In addition, we recently found that Ly49Q is expressed on PDCs in spleen and a portion of cultured DCs generated from bone marrow using cytokines such as Flt3-ligand and GM-CSF [18].

2.1. Heterogeneous expression of Ly49Q in marrow and nonlymphoid tissues

Since the expression of surface molecules on DCs varies with their tissue localization and maturational state [8,12,19], we studied Ly49Q expression on PDCs and conventional DCs from various lymphoid and nonlymphoid organs of BALB/c mice. Ly49Q was highly expressed on most PDCs in subcutaneous LNs as well as spleen, whereas in thymus, BM, blood, lung, and liver, a significant portion of PDCs was negative or low for Ly49Q. In contrast, the conventional DCs failed to express Ly49Q.

Regarding Ly49Q$^-$ cells in CD11c$^+$ B220$^+$ population, there was the possibility that cell types other than PDCs could be expressing CD11c and B220, especially NK cells. However, the Gr-1$^+$ Ly49Q$^-$ cells in the B220$^+$ CD11c$^+$ population from bone marrow (i.e., presumptive PDCs) had high levels of Ly6C and lacked the NK marker DX5, indicating that there is a Ly49Q$^-$ population in the CD11c$^+$ B220$^+$ presumptive PDC fraction of many tissues.

2.2. PDC differentiation revealed by the expression pattern of Ly49Q

When bone marrow and splenic B220$^+$ PDCs were compared for the expression of CD11c and Ly49Q, splenic PDCs were Ly49Q$^+$ with intermediate expression of CD11c as reported previously [5,12], while PDCs in bone marrow were high in CD11c expression relative to those in spleen and heterogeneous in Ly49Q expression. To further characterize PDCs in BM, we arbitrarily divided the cells into 6 populations based on the expression levels of CD11c and Ly49Q. As the subsets expressed more Ly49Q, they also acquired increased levels of CD4 and MHC II. Likewise, if we double labeled these subsets for CD4 and CD8, we found progressive upregulation of both markers concomitant with increasing Ly49Q expression, eventually resembling the PDCs in spleen [8].

2.3. Ly49Q$^-$ PDCs differentiate to express Ly49Q

To assess the possibility that Ly49Q$^-$ cells are precursor PDCs (pre-PDCs) at earlier developmental stage, we cultured the purified Ly49Q$^-$ (presumptive BM pre-PDCs) and Ly49Q$^+$ PDCs. Results clearly showed that the Ly49Q$^-$ cells spontaneously and gradually increased Ly49Q expression following overnight culture in medium without any cell proliferation. In addition, when stimulated with CpG-ODN or HVJ virus, both Ly49Q$^-$ and Ly49Q$^+$ PDCs populations upregulated the expression of MHC II and CD86.

2.4. Difference in cytokine producing abilities between Ly49Q$^-$ and Ly49Q$^+$ PDCs

When cytokine producing abilities were examined in Ly49Q$^-$ and Ly49Q$^+$ PDCs, we found that Ly49Q$^+$ PDCs produced about twice the level of IFN-α/β with either stimulus. Results of intracellular staining for IFN-α also confirmed that Ly49Q$^+$ PDCs were much better at producing IFN-α in response to CpG-ODN than Ly49Q$^-$ pre-PDCs. Similar observation was recently reported by Olweus et al. [19]. As in the case of IFN-α/β, higher amounts of IL-12p70 and IL-6 were produced from Ly49Q$^+$ PDCs than Ly49Q$^-$ pre-PDCs, but TNF-α production was nearly comparable between them. Interestingly, when Ly49$^+$ PDC and Ly49Q$^-$ pre-PDC populations were stimulated with Pam3CSK$_4$, TLR2 ligand, Ly49Q$^+$ marrow PDCs produced much larger amounts of TNF-α than Ly49Q$^-$ pre-PDCs. However, all PDC populations from bone marrow and spleen produced no IL-6, IL-12p70 and IFN-α/β in response to Pam3CSK$_4$.

2.5. T cell activation by human PDCs

In vitro studies suggest that PDCs are incapable of stimulating allogeneic T cells because of low levels of costimulatory molecules, but that they differentiate into mature DCs and acquired the capacity to directly activate T cells. In human, PDCs express high levels of IL-3 receptors [20] and differentiated into mature DCs with IL-3 or IL-3+ CD40L [21,22] to preferentially prime Th2 response. On the other hand, PDCs stimulated with signaling through TLR7 and TLR9 by viruses or by synthetic CpG-ODN preferentially prime naive $CD4^+$ T cells to produce IFN-γ and IL-10 by producing IFN-α and TNF-β [23]. Therefore, we have investigated the Th-polarizing capacity of human PDCs after short (24 h) or long (72 h) culture with stimuli and have assessed the expression and function of OX40 ligand (OX40L) in PDC-mediated Th polarization in addition to type I IFN-α-dependent responses. IL-3-treated PDCs expressed OX40L, but produced almost no IFN-α in response to T cell stimulation (CD40 ligand or T cell interaction), resulting in the preferential priming of Th2 cells through OX40L-dependent mechanisms. Meanwhile, PDCs were rapidly endowed by viral infection with a high potency to develop IFN-γ-producing Th cells depending on their capacity to residually produce IFN-α. Although virus-stimulated PDCs simultaneously expressed OX40L in their maturational process, the Th1-inducing effect of endogenous type I IFNs may overcome and thus conceal the OX40L-dependent Th2 responses. However, during maturation in response to virus over the longer 72-h period, the expression level of OX40L was upregulated, whereas the residual IFN α producing ability was downregulated, and consequently, the PDCs with prolonged Sendai virus stimulation induced Th2 responses to some extent [24]. Thus, PDCs have the distinct means to dictate an appropriate response to environmental stimuli.

2.6. T cell activation by murine PDC subsets

Unlike conventional DCs, PDCs are poor in phagocytosis and macropinocytosis [21]. Although immature PDCs do not have the capacity to induce strong T cell proliferation, they appear to prime naïve $CD4^+$ T cells to differentiate into IL-10-producing Tr1 cells in culture [12,25]. A recent study also demonstrated that mature PDCs activated by CpG-ODN were capable of priming $CD8^+$ T cell responses to endogenous antigens or peptides, but not those to exogenous antigens [26]. Furthermore, unlike mature conventional DCs, the PDCs can prime T cells to produce IL-10 even after maturation [26]. Thus, we compared T cell stimulating activity of Ly49Q subsets obtained from mice that had been injected with PBS or CpG-ODN 3d previously. As previously reported, immature PDC subsets induced little proliferation in both $CD4^+$ and $CD8^+$ T cells. However, PDCs from CpG-injected mice, especially $Ly49Q^-$ subset, induced significant T cell proliferation. This is also the case in peptide presentation to specific T cells. Although CpG injection upregulated the expression of MHC class II, CD40 and CD86 in both $Ly49Q^+$ and $Ly49Q^-$ PDCs, cytokine producing abilities, especially IL-6 and IFN-α/β, were much less in $Ly49Q^-$ than $Ly49Q^+$ subsets as PDC subsets in steady state. Interestingly, Ly49Q-PDCs from CpG-induced mice were the most potent to prime antigen-specific $CD4^+$ T cells to secrete IL-10. Yang et al. have recently reported that $CD4^-$ PDCs activated with CpG-ODN 16 h before produced larger amounts of IL-6, IL-12p40 as well as IFN-α and stronger T cells proliferation than $CD4^+$ PDCs [27]. Although $CD4^-$ PDCs has been shown as an immediate precursor of $CD4^+$ PDCs and to produce less amounts of IFN-α than $CD4^+$ PDCs [8], PDCs that have been exposed to virus in vivo for 24 h were unable to respond to a rechallenge with the same virus in vitro to produce IFN-α [28] as in the case of human PDCs [24]. Therefore, the discrepancy in the results of Yang's and ours is possibly due to the differences in differentiation/maturation and developing stages.

3. Conclusion

We showed sequential developmental stages of PDCs in mouse BM by the different expression levels of an inhibitory NK receptor, Ly49Q. Ly49Q$^+$ cells are differentiated PDC distributed in peripheral lymphoid organs, such as spleen and nodes, to produce large amounts of IL-6, IL-12p70 as well as IFN-α, but newly generated PDCs that had been proliferated from bone marrow precursor cells during inflammatory response showed remarkably different immunological features.

References

[1] J. Banchereau, R.M. Steinman, Dendritic cells and the control of immunity, Nature 392 (6673) (1998) 245–252.
[2] K. Shortman, Y.J. Liu, Mouse and human dendritic cell subtypes, Nat. Rev., Immunol. 2 (3) (2002) 151–161.
[3] F.P. Siegal, et al., The nature of the principal type 1 interferon-producing cells in human blood, Science 284 (5421) (1999) 1835–1837.
[4] N. Kadowaki, S. Antonenko, Y.J. Liu, Distinct CpG DNA and polyinosinic–polycytidylic acid double-stranded RNA, respectively, stimulate CD11c-type 2 dendritic cell precursors and CD11c+ dendritic cells to produce type I IFN, J. Immunol. 166 (4) (2001) 2291–2295.
[5] H. Nakano, M. Yanagita, M.D. Gunn, CD11c$^+$ B220$^+$ Gr-1$^+$ cells in mouse lymph nodes and spleen display characteristics of plasmacytoid dendritic cells, J. Exp. Med. 194 (2001) 1171–1178.
[6] C. Asselin-Paturel, et al., Mouse type I IFN-producing cells are immature APCs with plasmacytoid morphology, Nat. Immunol. 2 (12) (2001) 1144–1150.
[7] P. Bjorck, Isolation and characterization of plasmacytoid dendritic cells from Flt3 ligand and granulocyte–macrophage colony-stimulating factor-treated mice, Blood 98 (13) (2001) 3520–3526.
[8] M. O'Keeffe, et al., Mouse plasmacytoid cells: long-lived cells, heterogeneous in surface phenotype and function, that differentiate into CD8$^+$ dendritic cells only after microbial stimulus, J. Exp. Med. 196 (10) (2002) 1307–1319.
[9] T. Okada, et al., Murine thymic plasmacytoid dendritic cells, Eur. J. Immunol. 33 (4) (2003) 1012–1019.
[10] Z.X. Lian, et al., Heterogeneity of dendritic cells in the mouse liver: identification and characterization of four distinct populations, J. Immunol. 170 (5) (2003) 2323–2330.
[11] C. Asselin-Paturel, et al., Mouse strain differences in plasmacytoid dendritic cell frequency and function revealed by a novel monoclonal antibody, J. Immunol. 171 (12) (2003) 6466–6477.
[12] P. Martin, et al., Characterization of a new subpopulation of mouse CD8α^+ B220$^+$ dendritic cells endowed with type 1 interferon production capacity and tolerogenic potential, Blood 100 (2) (2002) 383–390.
[13] B. Blom, et al., Generation of interferon alpha-producing predendritic cell (pre-DC)2 from human CD34$^+$ hematopoietic stem cells, J. Exp. Med. 192 (12) (2000) 1785–1796.
[14] R. Schotte, et al., The transcription factor Spi-B is expressed in plasmacytoid DC precursors and inhibits T-, B-, and NK-cell development, Blood 101 (3) (2003) 1015–1023.
[15] A. D'Amico, L. Wu, The early progenitors of mouse dendritic cells and plasmacytoid predendritic cells are within the bone marrow hemopoietic precursors expressing Flt3, J. Exp. Med. 198 (2) (2003) 293–303.
[16] J. Diao, et al., Characterization of distinct conventional and plasmacytoid dendritic cell-committed precursors in murine bone marrow, J. Immunol. 173 (3) (2004) 1826–1833.
[17] N. Toyama-Sorimachi, et al., Ly49Q, a member of the Ly49 family that is selectively expressed on myeloid lineage cells and involved in regulation of cytoskeletal architecture, Proc. Natl. Acad. Sci. U. S. A. 101 (4) (2004) 1016–1021.
[18] N. Toyama-Sorimachi, et al., Inhibitory NK receptor Ly49Q is expressed on subsets of dendritic cells in a cellular maturation- and cytokine stimulation-dependent manner, J. Immunol. 174 (8) (2005) 4621–4629.
[19] Y. Kamogawa-Schifter, et al., Ly49Q defines 2 pDC subsets in mice, Blood 105 (7) (2005) 2787–2792.
[20] J. Olweus, et al., Dendritic cell ontogeny: a human dendritic cell lineage of myeloid origin, Proc. Natl. Acad. Sci. U. S. A. 94 (23) (1997) 12551–12556.

[21] G. Grouard, et al., The enigmatic plasmacytoid T cells develop into dendritic cells with interleukin (IL)-3 and CD40-ligand, J. Exp. Med. 185 (6) (1997) 1101–1111.

[22] T. Ito, et al., Differential regulation of human blood dendritic cell subsets by IFNs, J. Immunol. 166 (5) (2001) 2961–2969.

[23] N. Kadowaki, et al., Natural interferon alpha/beta-producing cells link innate and adaptive immunity, J. Exp. Med. 192 (2) (2000) 219–226.

[24] T. Ito, et al., Plasmacytoid dendritic cells regulate Th cell responses through OX40 ligand and type I IFNs, J. Immunol. 172 (7) (2004) 4253–4259.

[25] J. Bilsborough, et al., Mucosal $CD8\alpha^{+}$ DC, with a plasmacytoid phenotype, induce differentiation and support function of T cells with regulatory properties, Immunology 108 (4) (2003) 481–492.

[26] M. Salio, et al., CpG-matured murine plasmacytoid dendritic cells are capable of in vivo priming of functional CD8 T cell responses to endogenous but not exogenous antigens, J. Exp. Med. 199 (4) (2004) 567–579.

[27] G.X. Yang, et al., $CD4^{-}$ plasmacytoid dendritic cells (pDCs) migrate in lymph nodes by CpG inoculation and represent a potent functional subset of pDCs, J. Immunol. 174 (6) (2005) 3197–3203.

[28] P. Björck, Dendritic cells exposed to herpes simplex virus in vivo do not produce IFN-alpha after rechallenge with virus in vitro and exhibit decreased T cell alloreactivity, J. Immunol. 172 (9) (2004) 5396–5404.

International Congress Series 1285 (2005) 34–41

www.ics-elsevier.com

Characteristics of nucleic acid TLR ligands

Tsuneyasu Kaisho *

Laboratory for Host Defense, RIKEN Research Institute for Allergy and Immunology, Suehiro-cho 1-7-22, Tsurumi-ku, Yokohama city, Kanagawa 230-0045, Japan

Abstract. Dendritic cells (DCs) play critical roles as sentinels in host defense and can activate naïve T cells. DC activation and maturation are induced by signaling through a group of type I transmembrane proteins, Toll-like receptors (TLRs), which can discriminate various microorganism-associated molecular structures. TLR ligands include lipid, protein, and nucleic acid components, all of which function as immune adjuvants. Each TLR function is common, but nucleic acid-recognizing TLRs are distinct from other TLRs in several aspects. Here I focus on the characteristics of nucleic acid TLR ligand system and describe how nucleic acids are recognized and processed by DCs. Clarification on diversified function of TLRs should provide us with critical information for manipulating the host defense mechanism.

Keywords: Dendritic cell; Toll-like receptor; Type I interferon; CpG DNA; Plasmacytoid dendritic cells

1. TLR ligands

Toll-like receptors (TLRs) are involved in recognizing a variety of microorganism-derived molecular structures (Fig. 1) [1,2]. According to the molecular characteristics, TLR ligands can be roughly divided into three categories: lipid, protein, and nucleic acids. For example, bacterial wall components such as lipopolysaccharides (LPS) or lipoproteins are recognized by TLR4 or TLR2. TLR2 heterodimerizes with TLR1 or TLR6, which is a close relative to TLR2, and this heterodimerization contributes to discriminating fine lipid and peptide structures. TLR5 is involved in recognizing a flagellin, a protein component

Abbreviations: DC, dendritic cell; TLR, Toll-like receptor; LPS, Lipopolysaccharides; PAMPs, pathogen-associated molecular patterns; APC, Ag presenting cell; IFN, interferon; PDC, plasmacytoid DC; dsRNA, double-stranded RNA; SLE, systemic lupus erythematosus; RF, rheumatoid factor; Ig, immunoglobulin; polyuridylic acid, (polyU); polyinosinic–polycytidylic acid, (poly(I:C)); bone marrow, (BM); polyadenylic–polyuridylic acid, (polyA:U).

* Tel.: +81 45 503 7065; fax: +81 45 503 7064.
E-mail address: tkaisho@rcai.riken.jp.

0531-5131/
doi:10.1016/j.ics.2005.08.003

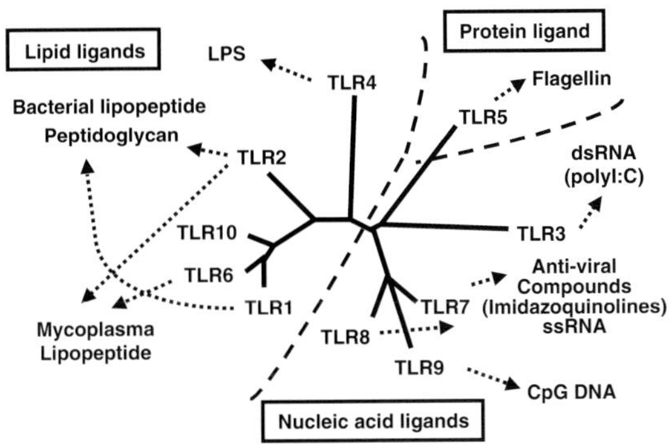

Fig. 1. Phylogenetic tree of human TLRs and their representative ligands. TLRs and their representative ligands are indicated by dotted arrows. As shown by dotted lines, TLRs can be subdivided according to their ligand characteristics.

from bacterial flagella. Murine TLR11, although its human counterpart is not present, shows similar structure to murine TLR5 and is critical for immune responses induced by a protozoan profilin-like protein. Furthermore, nucleic acids are recognized by TLR3, TLR7, TLR8 and TLR9, all of which are also similar in amino acid structures. Thus, structurally similar molecules are recognized by phylogenetically related TLRs (Fig. 1).

These TLR ligands are characterized as exogenous molecules not derived from the host and are regarded as non-self-components. They are often referred to as pathogen-associated molecular patterns (PAMPs), but this term is somewhat misleading since these structures are expressed in both pathogenic and nonpathogenic microorganisms.

TLR ligands are required for the survival of microorganisms and therefore are highly conserved over the course of evolution. This is typified by bacterial cell wall constituents, which are TLR2/4 ligands. Proteins do not usually function as TLR ligands, because they are far too diverse for recognition through a limited repertoire of receptors. For example, viruses change the structures of many proteins very rapidly in order to escape from host immune surveillance. Thus, the recognition of viral proteins requires a large repertoire of Ag receptors in the adaptive immune system. The ligands for TLR5 or TLR11 are exceptionally proteins, but these are highly conserved and not so diverse.

All of these TLR ligands have common immunostimulatory function. Firstly, they can induce inflammatory cytokines such as IL-6 or TNF-α, thereby inducing inflammatory reactions. An excess of this reaction can lead to shock status such as endotoxin shock. Secondly, the ligands can activate Ag presenting cells (APCs) to upregulate costimulatory molecule expression and to produce Th1-inducing cytokines including IL-12. This APC activation can lead to clonal T cell expansion and Th1 cell differentiation. Based on these activities, TLRs can be regarded as adjuvant receptors [3].

2. Characteristics of nucleic acid TLR ligands

Although TLRs have similar and overlapping function, they still exhibit their own characteristics. Notably, nucleic acid-recognizing TLRs possess distinct characteristics from other TLRs.

Lipid or protein TLR ligands are recognized by respective TLRs on the plasma membrane. Meanwhile, nucleic acid-recognizing TLRs are not expressed on the membrane, but in the endosome. The nucleic acid TLR ligands are incorporated into the cells, independent of nucleic acid sequences. Then TLR ligands are recognized by respective TLRs in the endosome and trigger the signaling pathway.

Another feature of nucleic acid ligands is the ability to induce type I interferons (IFNs). Type I IFNs consist of more than 10 IFN-αs and a single IFN-β [4]. Type I IFNs can induce expression of several antiviral proteins and MHC, and induce DC maturation, thereby exerting critical function in antiviral immunity. Nucleic acid TLR ligands can induce both IFN-α and IFN-β. The other TLR ligands fail to induce type I IFNs, although LPS is exceptional in that it can induce only IFN-β, but not IFN-α. This type I IFN-inducing ability greatly contributes to antiviral function in nucleic acid-recognizing TLRs.

Notably, expression of nucleic acid-recognizing TLRs is confined to certain types of cells. Plasmacytoid DC (PDC) is a discrete DC subset from conventional DC and also known as IFN-α producing cells [5]. PDC expresses TLR7 and TLR9 exclusively among TLRs and secretes vigorous amounts of type I IFN, especially IFN-α, in a TLR7/9-dependent manner. PDC plays critical roles in antiviral immune responses. However, PDC does not express TLR3 and fail to respond to double stranded RNA (dsRNA). TLR3-induced type I IFN production depends on other types of cells (see below).

Furthermore, nucleic acid TLR ligands are featured by their similarity to host-derived components. Protein or lipid TLR ligands are absent in the host; they are principally non-self-components. However, compared with these substances, the structural difference between pathogen and host nucleic acid TLR ligands is not very prominent. For example, unmethylated CpG motifs are still found in mammals although their frequency is very low. Furthermore, ssRNAs irrelevant to viruses also behave as TLR7 agonists. Host cells are phagocytosed after they die and nucleic acids from ingested cells are then released into endosomes or phagosomes. Thus, hosts potentially expose themselves to the risk of an autoimmune response. However, this risk is contained by several factors. Firstly, these nucleic acids are unstable and easily degraded. Secondly, TLR7 expression is very low in cells with high phagocytic activity. Thirdly, TLR7/9 expression and released nucleic acids are localized in different cell compartments. Furthermore, the host possesses certain DNA sequences which can inhibit TLR9 signaling [6]. In fact, such sequences can be found in the telomere. Thus, several fail-safe mechanisms prevent an autoimmune reaction. Still, it remains unclear how the host tolerates adjuvant effects of self-nucleic acids.

3. Pathological roles of TLR7 and TLR9

The break of this tolerance seems to contribute to the pathogenesis of autoimmune diseases, such as systemic lupus erythematosus (SLE) [5]. In SLE, antinuclear antibodies are produced and nuclear proteins are released from damaged or inflamed tissues. These proteins stabilize nucleic acids, thus creating efficient TLR agonists for PDC stimulation. Nucleic acid-containing complexes can activate PDC to produce IFN-α by co-engaging TLR and FcR. Notably, serum IFN-α levels are often increased in SLE patients and correlate with the severity of the disease (Fig. 2). Furthermore, the number of activated

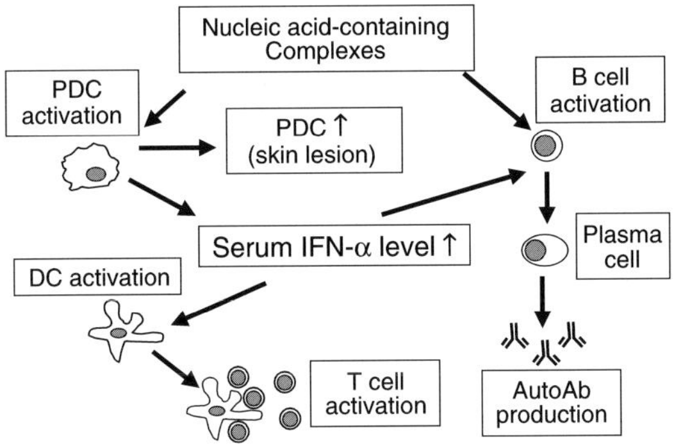

Fig. 2. Pathological roles of PDC-derived IFN-α in autoimmunity.

PDCs is increased in skin lesions in SLE. It can thus be assumed that prolonged activation of PDCs is involved in elevated production of IFN-α, leading to clinical manifestations. TLR7- and TLR9-mediated signaling should be quite important, because these TLRs are only TLRs expressed on PDC.

Autoreactive B cells can also be activated by nucleic acid–Ab complexes (Fig. 3) [7]. Rheumatoid factor (RF) is an immunoglobulin (Ig) that can bind to certain types of IgG and is often found in the sera of patients with autoimmune disorder. DNA–anti-DNA complexes are recognized by RF on the B cell surface. RF BCR mediates internalization and transport of these complexes into the endosome where TLR9 is expressed. Then CpG DNA in the complex stimulates TLR9 and, in turn, activates B cells to produce RF. Dual engagement of both BCR and TLR9 is mandatory for this type of autoreactive B cell activation. Thus, TLR signaling is critically involved in autoimmunity in both PDC and B cells.

4. Differential effects of two types of TLR7/9 ligands

TLR9 signaling is peculiar in that its effects depend on the ligands [8]. Through the screening of a variety of CpG DNAs, another type of CpG DNAs, called also as D-type

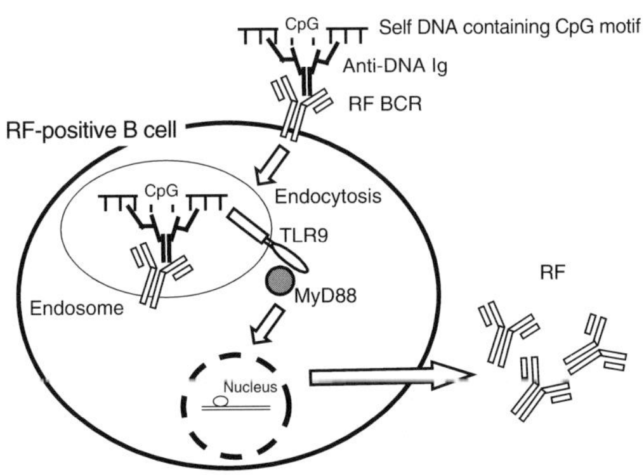

Fig. 3. Mechanism for RF B cell activation.

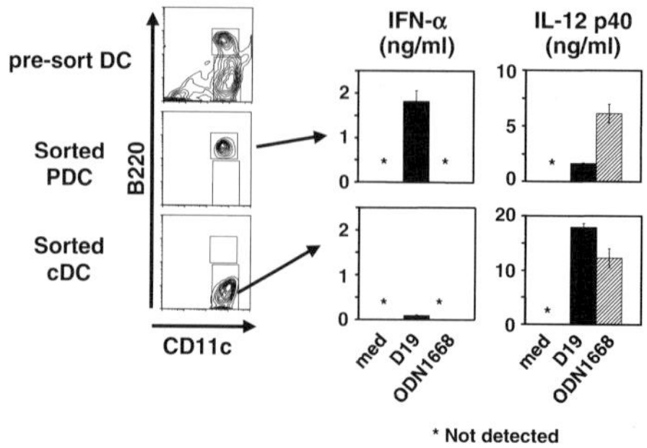

Fig. 4. PDC differentially responds to two types of CpG DNAs. Flt3L-induced BM DCs were sorted into PDC ($CD11c^+B220^+$) and conventional DC ($CD11c^+B220^-$). Classical CpG DNA (ODN1668) can induce IL-12p40 from both DCs, while A/D-type CpG DNA (D19) can dominantly induce IFN-α and IL-12p40 from PDC and conventional DC, respectively.

CpG DNAs or CpG-A, were found. A/D-type CpG DNAs have a potent ability to induce IFN-α production, but are weaker at activating B cells and require higher concentrations for inducing comparable amounts of IL-12 than classical CpG DNAs. A/D-type CpG DNAs are featured by central palindromic CpG motif-containing sequences with phosphodiester linkages and by the 3′ phosphorothioated polyG stretch, while classical CpG DNAs have a phosphorothioate backbone and lack polyG tails. Despite a variety of effects, they all depend on the TLR9-MyD88-mediated pathway [9].

In mice, both PDC and conventional DC express TLR9. cDC can secrete IL-12, but not IFN-α, in response to both CpG DNAs, whereas PDC can produce IL-12 and IFN-α in response to classical and A/D-type CpG DNAs, respectively (Fig. 4). Thus, two types of CpG DNAs differentially activate PDC to induce distinct cytokines [9]. After incorporated into cells, classical CpG DNA is destined to the lysosome, while A/D-type CpG DNA is delivered to the endosome. This intracellular localization of these two types of CpG DNAs seems critical for their differential activity. Notably, A/D-type CpG DNA tends to form virus-like nanoparticles and can stay long in a endosomal vesicle [10]. It remains unknown how this differential property leads to distinct pattern of cytokine induction.

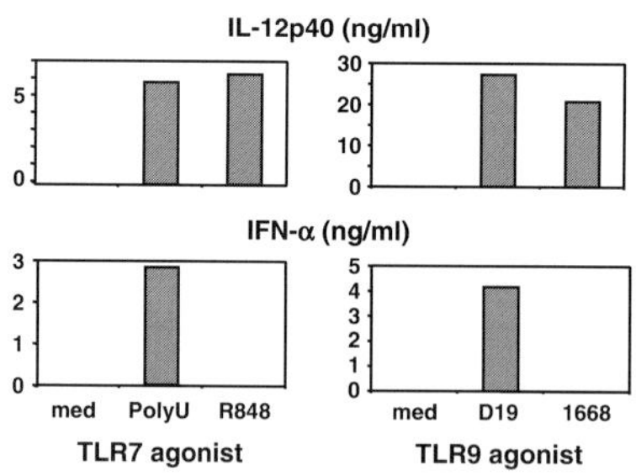

Fig. 5. Effects of various TLR7/9 agonists on Flt3L-induced BM DCs. Flt3L-induced BM DCs can produce IL-12p40 in response to all TLR7/9 agonists. However, IFN-α production was observed only in polyU- or D19-stimulated DCs.

Several TLR7 agonists have been so far identified. Small synthetic antiviral compounds, called imidazoquinoline derivatives, are the first clarified TLR7 ligands [11]. The derivatives include imiquimod or resiquimod (R848) and the latter is 100 times more active than the former. R848 can activate in vitro PDC to produce IL-12p40. However, it fails to activate in vitro PDC to produce IFN-α (Fig. 5), although it can increase serum IFN-α levels after injection into mice [11]. In addition to imidazoquinolines, polyuridylic acids (polyU) can also activate DCs in a TLR7-dependent manner. PolyU-stimulated in vitro PDC can produce IFN-α (Fig. 5). Thus, TLR7 agonists can also be divided into two categories, IFN-α-inducing or IFN-α-noninducing, as in the case of TLR9 agonists. It can be reasonable assumed that intracellular localization of R848 and polyU be different, although it is not formally clarified.

5. dsRNA recognition system

TLR9-deficient mice lack all effects induced by CpG DNA, indicating that TLR9 is an essential receptor for CpG DNA. Meanwhile, TLR3-deficient mice retain some effects of dsRNA [12]. This means that TLR3 is not the only receptor for dsRNA, but other molecules such as RIG-I are also involved in recognizing dsRNA [13]. This makes it obscure to evaluate how TLR3 signaling contributes to the effects of dsRNA.

Murine bone marrow (BM)-derived DC can be obtained in the presence of either GM-CSF or Flt3 ligand (Flt3L). Wild-type GM-CSF-induced BM DC cannot produce IFN-α in response to CpG DNA, but can produce IFN-α in response to a synthesized dsRNA, polyinosinic–polycytidylic acid (poly(I:C)) (Fig. 6). This IFN-α production was not impaired in TLR3-deficient DCs. TLR3 can associate with an intracytoplasmic adapter, TRIF, but TRIF-deficient DC still can produce IFN-α in response to poly(I:C). Wild-type GM-CSF-induced BM DC can secrete IL-12p40 in response to LPS, but fail to produce IL-12p40 in response to poly(I:C). Thus, GM-CSF-induced BM DC can respond to dsRNA in a TLR3-independent manner by producing IFN-α, but not IL-12p40.

Wild-type Flt3L-induced BM DC can produce IFN-α in response to CpG DNA, but cannot in response to poly(I:C). However, the DC can produce IL-12p40 after stimulation with poly(I:C). This poly(I:C)-induced IL-12p40 production was abolished in TLR3-deficient DC. The results suggest that Flt3L-induced BM DC can respond to dsRNA in a

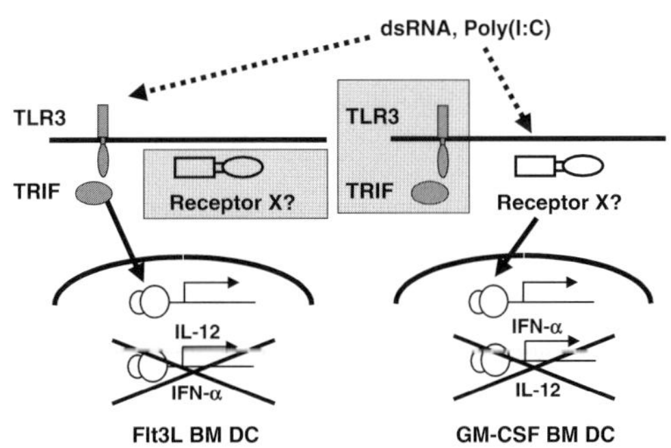

Fig. 6. Distinct types of DCs show differential responses against poly(I:C).

TLR3-dependent manner by producing IL-12p40. Taken together with these results on poly(I:C)-induced effects, DCs process dsRNA-induced signals in a cell-type specific manner (Fig. 6).

In addition to poly(I:C), polyadenylic–polyuridylic acids (polyA:U) can also activate DC. Poly(A:U) can induce IFN-α and IL-12p40 from wild-type Flt3L-induced BM DC. The effects were dependent on TLR7, but not on TLR3, indicating that TLR7 is critical for poly(A:U)-induced effects. It can be speculated that poly(A:U)-induced adjuvant activity can be ascribed to polyU-induced effects and that dsRNA formation should stabilize polyU or facilitate incorporation of polyU into DC. Thus, two types of ds RNAs are processed by distinct recognition systems.

6. Conclusion

Nucleic acid TLR ligands are different from lipid or protein TLR ligands. The characteristics are featured by endosomal recognition, restricted expression pattern, type I IFN-inducing ability and similarity to host components. Notably the last one contributes to pathogenesis of autoimmune disorders. TLR ligands, especially CpG DNAs, are now promisingly applied for treating various diseases including cancers or allergy. Therefore, it is very important to clarify how these nucleic acids are recognized and processed in a variety of innate immune cells including DCs.

Acknowledgements

This work was supported by the Advanced and Innovative Research Program in Life Sciences, the Special Coordination Fund for Promoting Science and Technology, the Ministry of Education, Culture, Sports, Science, and Technology (MEXT), the Japan Science and Technology Corporation (JST), the Uehara Memorial Foundation, the Naito Foundation, and the Novartis Foundation for the Promotion of Science.

References

[1] C.A. Janeway Jr., R. Medzhitov, Innate immune recognition, Annu. Rev. Immunol. 20 (2002) 197–216.
[2] K. Takeda, T. Kaisho, S. Akira, Toll-like receptors, Annu. Rev. Immunol. 21 (2003) 335–376.
[3] T. Kaisho, S. Akira, Regulation of dendritic cell function through Toll-like receptors, Curr. Mol. Med. 3 (2003) 373–385.
[4] T. Taniguchi, A. Takaoka, The interferon-alpha/beta system in antiviral responses: a multimodal machinery of gene regulation by the IRF family of transcription factors, Curr. Opin. Immunol. 14 (2002) 111–116.
[5] M. Colonna, G. Trinchieri, J. Liu, Plasmacytoid dendritic cells in immunity, Nat. Immunol. 5 (2004) 1219–1226.
[6] I. Gursel, et al., Repetitive elements in mammalian telomeres suppress bacterial DNA-induced immune activation, J. Immunol. 171 (2003) 1393–1400.
[7] I.R. Rifkin, et al., Toll-like receptors, endogenous ligands, and systemic autoimmune disease, Immunol. Rev. 204 (2005) 27–42.
[8] D.M. Klinman, Immunotherapeutic uses of CpG oligodeoxynucleotides, Nat. Rev. Immunol. 4 (2004) 249–258.
[9] H. Hemmi, et al., The roles of Toll-like receptor 9, MyD88, and DNA-dependent protein kinase catalytic subunit in the effects of two distinct CpG DNAs on dendritic cell subsets, J. Immunol. 170 (2003) 3059–3064.

[10] M. Kerkmann, et al., Spontaneous formation of nucleic acid-based nanoparticles is responsible for high interferon-alpha induction by CpG-A in plasmacytoid dendritic cells, J. Biol. Chem. 280 (2005) 8086–8093.
[11] H. Hemmi, et al., Small anti-viral compounds activate immune cells via the TLR7 MyD88-dependent signaling pathway, Nat. Immunol. 3 (2002) 196–200.
[12] L. Alexopoulou, Recognition of double-stranded RNA and activation of NF-kappaB by Toll-like receptor 3, Nature 413 (2001) 732–738.
[13] M. Yoneyama, et al., The RNA helicase RIG-I has an essential function in double-stranded RNA-induced innate antiviral responses, Nat. Immunol. 5 (2004) 730–737.

ELSEVIER

International Congress Series 1285 (2005) 42–49

www.ics-elsevier.com

The role of toll-like receptors in systemic autoimmune disease

A. Marshak-Rothstein [a,*], L. Busconi [a], C.M. Lau [a], M. Uccellini [a], G.A. Viglianti [a], I.R. Rifkin [b]

[a] *Department of Microbiology, Boston University School of Medicine, Boston, MA 02118, USA*
[b] *Department of Medicine, Boston University School of Medicine, Boston, MA 02118, USA*

Abstract. The AM14 B cell receptor, derived from an autoimmune Fas-deficient mouse, is a rheumatoid factor specific for IgG2a. B cells expressing the AM14 receptor have been effectively activated by immune complexes (ICs) consisting of IgG2a associated with endogenous TLR ligands that essentially serve as autoadjuvants. One source of endogenous ligand is DNAse-sensitive material, presumably chromatin, released from dead/dying mammalian cells. The chromatin response was blocked by endosome acidification inhibitors, eliminated in MyD88-deficient cells and markedly reduced, in TLR9-deficient cells; residual activity appeared to depend on a TLR(s) other than TLR9. Sources of TLR9-reactive mammalian DNA have been explored. AM14 B cells also responded to ICs consisting of IgG2a bound to RNA-associated autoantigens. These responses were eliminated in MyD88-deficient cells but unaffected by TLR9 deficiency. Thus, activation depends on BCR-directed delivery of the ICs to vesicular compartments that contain an appropriate TLR. Intriguingly, such BCR/TLR co-engagement leads to the expression of gene products not elicited by independent activation of the BCR (anti-IgM $F(ab')_2$) or TLR9 (CpG s-ODN) alone. The effects of nucleic acid-associated ICs on both B cells and antigen presenting cells indicate that the TLR9 subfamily may be a key target for therapeutic intervention in patients with systemic autoimmune diseases. © 2005 Published by Elsevier B.V.

Keywords: Toll-like receptor; Autoantibody; Immune complex; Cytokine; Chromatin

1. Introduction

Systemic autoimmune diseases such as SLE are frequently associated with the production of high titers of autoantibodies specific for nuclear and/or cytoplasmic cellular

* Corresponding author. Tel.: +1 617 638 4299; fax: +1 617 638 4286.
E-mail address: amrothst@bu.edu (A. Marshak-Rothstein).

0531-5131/ © 2005 Published by Elsevier B.V.
doi:10.1016/j.ics.2005.07.101

components. Such antibodies subsequently form immune complexes (ICs), deposit in the blood vessel walls, joints, and glomeruli, and thereby contribute to the vasculitis, arthritis, and glomerulonephritis characteristic of systemic disease. Remarkably, in both animal models and human disease, the autoantibody repertoire consistently targets a relatively limited set of DNA and RNA associated autoantigens [1,2]. A better understanding of the mechanisms by which these particular molecules activate autoreactive B cells is critical to the design of more effective therapeutics.

A number of recent studies have linked the antigenicity of particular autoantigens to the process of apoptotic cell death and subsequent conformational changes of many of the prominent autoantigens. Apoptosis can be induced by environmental insults or by cytotoxic effector cells; in either case, many potential autoantigens are cleaved by caspases or granzymes, or undergo post-translational modifications such as oxidation, citrullination, or phosphorylation [3,4]. It has been proposed that such alterations may lead to the creation of neo-epitopes that are then recognized as foreign by the adaptive immune system. The process of epitope spreading can then effectively break tolerance to the actual self-determinants. However, it has recently been shown that autoantibodies specific for granzyme B target proteins are just as prevalent in granzyme B-deficient autoimmune mice as in granzyme B-sufficient autoimmune prone mice [5]. It follows that autoantigen cleavage may be a fingerprint of apoptosis but not necessarily a trigger for autoantibody production.

Alternatively, some aspect of the apoptotic process may directly prime the innate immune system to initiate an adaptive response, perhaps by converting autoantigens into "autoadjuvants", or by promoting the redistribution or aberrant accumulation of pre-existing autoadjuvants. In this context, normally benign self-determinants may appear foreign. The potential adjuvanticity of mammalian nucleic acids was originally revealed by the pivotal studies of Ronnblom et al. who first demonstrated the potent effects of DNA- and RNA-containing ICs on IFNα-producing dendritic cells [6,7]. Our laboratory has extended this analysis by taking advantage of a B cell receptor transgenic line designated AM14 [8].

AM14 B cells recognize IgG2a with relatively low affinity and can be activated in vitro only by IgG2a presented as a multivalent IC. Importantly, the type of antigen contained in the IC plays a critical role in the cell activation process. IgG2a mAbs specific for histones, nucleosomes, or DNA bind to DNAse sensitive material released from dead or dying cells that is present in the supernatant of primary B cell cultures [9,10]. These "chromatin" ICs are potent ligands for AM14 B cells under conditions in which IgG2a bound to protein antigens, or protein ICs, have little effect. The stimulatory capacity of the chromatin ICs can be explained by their ability to effectively engage both the AM14 B cell receptor and one or more chloroquine/bafilomycin sensitive receptors. Ongoing studies from our laboratory have focused on the identification or the relevant receptor(s) and the nature of the mammalian DNA ligand.

2. The role of TLR9 in the activation of AM14 B cells

The first indication that TLRs might be involved in B cell autoantibody production came from the observation that MyD88-deficient AM14 B cells completely failed to proliferate in

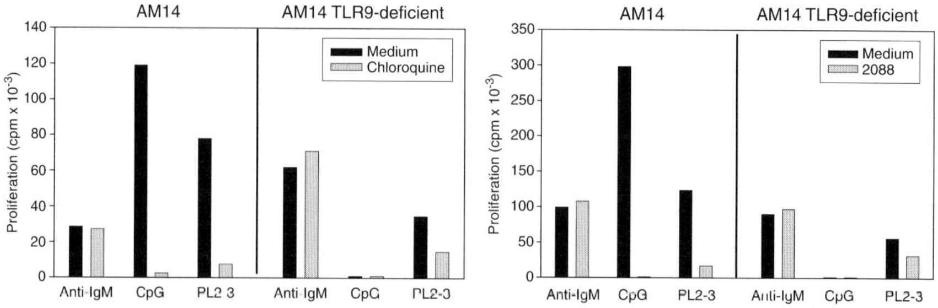

Fig. 1. The residual response of AM14 TLR9-deficient B cells can be partially blocked by chloroquine or s-ODN 2088.

response to anti-nucleosome/histone monoclonal antibodies such as PL2-3. In addition, the PL2-3 response of wild-type AM14 B cells could be very effectively blocked by the phosphorothioate oligodeoxynucleotide (s-ODN) 2088 [10]. Even though 2088 incorporates a CpG dinucleotide, the upstream CCT and 5′GGGG render this s-ODN a TLR9 inhibitor [11]. As DNA, albeit bacterial DNA, was known to be a potent ligand for TLR9, TLR9 seemed to be a reasonable candidate for the BCR co-receptor in the response of AM14 B cells to chromatin complexes. We were subsequently able to confirm a role for TLR9 when the AM14 receptor was bred onto a TLR9-deficient background. However, although the response of TLR9-deficient AM14 cells was markedly reduced relative to wild-type B cells, it was consistently higher than the response of AM14 MyD88-deficient cells [12]. Importantly, the residual activity of the AM14 TLR9-deficient cells could be further reduced by chloroquine and s-ODN 2088 (Fig. 1). Overall the data implicated TLR9, and at least one additional member of the TLR9 subfamily, in autoreactive B cell activation.

3. TLRs and mammalian DNA

TLR9 was first identified as a pattern recognition receptor capable of distinguishing bacterial DNA from mammalian DNA. These initial studies were carried out with non-transgenic B cells via a mechanism that did not depend on the B cell receptor for DNA uptake [13]. However, even in experimental systems involving the BCR-mediated delivery of bacterial and mammalian genomic DNA to the relevant endosomal/lysosomal compartments, we have found a dramatic difference in the stimulatory capacity of bacterial and mammalian DNA [14].

There are a number of reasons for the relative inability of mammalian DNA to activate TLR9. The first is the relative paucity of stimulatory hypomethylated CpG motifs. The overall CG content of mammalian DNA is low, only about 41% of total DNA. Moreover, while the predicted frequency of the dinucleotide CpG is 4%, the actual frequency in mammalian genomes is less than 1% [15]. Although only 3% of the cytosines in the human genome are methylated, 80% of these CpGs are thought to incorporate methylated C. Not only does mammalian DNA contain a remarkably low frequency of hypomethylated CpG motifs, it also contains a relatively high frequency of inhibitory DNA motifs. These include CG dinucleotides flanked on the 3′ end with a poly-G region (similar to s-ODN 2088), which are capable of neutralizing the effects of both bacterial DNA and stimulatory s-ODN [16], as well as telomeric repeats that can suppress B cell activation by TLR9 and non-TLR9 ligands [17,18]. Finally, there is the issue of availability. TLR9 is sequestered in internal vesicular compartments that presumably fuse with bacterial phagosomes, thereby allowing TLR9 access to bacterial DNA. By contrast, host DNA, released from apoptotic or dying cells, remains extracellular where it can be degraded by circulating DNAse. In addition, a very effective scavenger system normally clears apoptotic debris before it can accumulate to a dangerous level.

Nevertheless, data from a variety of experimental systems point to a pivotal role for abnormally elevated levels of chromatin and/or apoptotic debris in etiology of SLE and SLE-associated diseases. Significantly, both apoptotic low molecular weight DNA and DNA isolated from ICs obtained from the sera of SLE patients have a higher than normal CG-content [19,20]. Therefore it is possible that preferential release of CpG-enriched DNA may account for at least part of the stimulatory chromatin apparent in our AM14/chromatin IC studies. Potential sources of CG-rich DNA include CpG islands—regions of DNA frequently located near transcriptional start sites that are CG rich (an average of 60–70% C+G), contain the expected frequency of CpG dinucleotides, and are hypomethylated. In this context, it is intriguing that chromosomal regions associated with actively transcribed genes may be preferentially cleaved early in apoptosis [21].

B cells that express the transgene-encoded 3H9 heavy chain in combination with a variety of light chains can recognize DNA and charged phospholipids [22]. We have found that a reasonably high frequency of 3H9 B cells directly bind DNA and proliferate robustly in response to DNA fragments constructed to incorporate multiple repetitive copies of the stimulatory CpG 1826 motif [14]. By contrast, the response to calf thymus DNA was found to be minimal at best. However, a significantly higher response was observed when the 3H9 cells were cultured with DNA fragments amplified from a CpG island library and therefore enriched for sequences representative of mammalian CpG islands (MBU and GAV, unpublished results), even though these sequences did not incorporate high levels of previously identified strong stimulatory CpG motifs. These data indicate that a fraction of mammalian DNA can effectively engage TLR9.

4. TLR activation as a result of DNA modification

There is also evidence that certain modifications in mammalian DNA structure may enhance TLR reactivity. Loxoribine, and other guanosine analogs, have been found to activate TLR7 [23]. Loxoribine is structurally related to 8-hydroxy-2′-deoxyguanosine (8OHdG), and its presence correlates with ROS-mediated DNA damage. Intriguingly, 8OHdG has been detected in the circulating ICs of SLE patient sera [24]. ROS-modified DNA has been shown to be more immunogenic than unmodified DNA [25,26] and to be preferentially recognized by the anti-DNA antibodies present in certain SLE sera [26,27].

Potential sources of ROS-modified DNA include sites of infection or inflammation where cells have been targeted by activated macrophages or neutrophils [28]. 8OHdG is also a marker for cells damaged by UV irradiation [29]. Coincidentally, exposure to UV irradiation is often associated with exacerbated disease in patients with SLE. Due to the absence of protective histones and direct exposure to respiratory chain metabolism, mitochondrial DNA is subject to more extensive oxidative damage than nuclear DNA

[30,31]. It has been recently shown that mitochondrial DNA and oxidatively damaged (8-OHdG) DNA can be detected in the synovial fluids of patients with rheumatoid arthritis [32]. To further establish the connection between oxidative damage and autoimmunity, mice were injected intra-articularly with mitochondrial DNA or 8OHdG modified-DNA. Both the mitochondrial and 8OHdG DNA were found to induce arthritis via a mechanism dependent on direct activation of monocytes and/or macrophages [33]. Moreover, mice lacking NFR2, a transcription factor linked to the activation of numerous anti-oxidant and detoxification genes, develop SLE-like autoimmune diseases [34].

To determine whether oxidized DNA could serve as a "non-CpG-motif" ligand for one of the Toll-like receptors, we stimulated wild-type B cells with 8OHdG-modified and unmodified oligodeoxynucleotides. The 8OHdG-modified DNA induced a significantly stronger proliferative response than unmodified DNA. The 8OHdG-modified DNA did not stimulate either MyD88-deficient or TLR9-deficient cells, further implicating modified DNA as an efficient trigger of the innate immune system (LB, unpublished results).

5. RNA-associated autoantigens and TLR activity

Just as TLR9 plays a critical role in the recognition of bacterial and viral DNA, TLR3 and TLR7 have been shown to respond to double stranded and single-stranded RNA, respectively [35–37]. At the moment, the sequence specificity of the RNA-reactive receptors is somewhat unresolved. Particularly strong RNA stimulatory motifs have not yet been identified although it is known that TLR7-expressing cells appear to preferentially recognize GU-rich stretches of RNA. Although it might be assumed that TLR7 is particularly attuned to the presence of viral RNA, TLR7 has been shown to recognize mammalian RNA [35]. To what extent viral RNA sequence and/or the dearth of inhibitory motifs might account for TLR7 discrimination of viral and mammalian DNA remains to be determined. However, it is known that TLR7 is sequestered in vesicular compartments, just as in the case of TLR9, and thus inaccessible to circulating RNA or RNA/protein macromolecules that might be released from dead or dying host cells. Nevertheless, again as initially demonstrated by Ronnblom et al., receptor mediated uptake of RNA-containing ICs can be a potent stimulus for the innate immune system [38].

We have used AM14 B cells to further explore the contribution of Toll-like receptors to the B cell autoantibody response. Just as chromatin and DNA containing IgG2a ICs provide a potent stimulus, we have found that ICs containing common RNA autoantigens can also effectively stimulate AM14 cells. AM14 MyD88-deficient B cells fail to respond

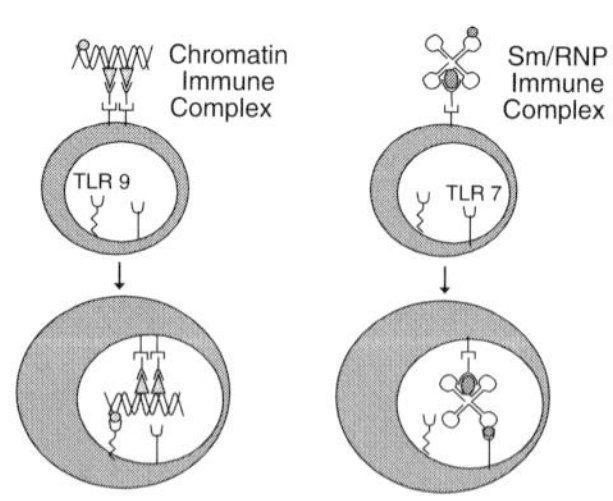

Fig. 2. Activation of AM14 autoreactive B cells by DNA- and RNA-containing immune complexes.

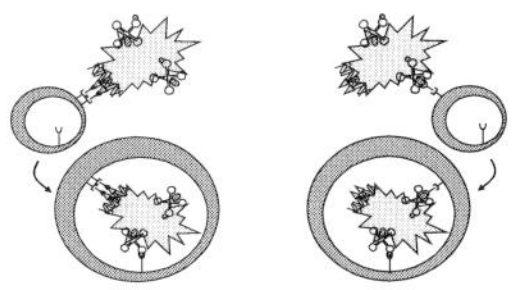

Fig. 3. Activation of AM14 B cells by IgG2a bound to apoptotic cells or debris.

to the RNA ICs although the response is intact in AM14 TLR9-deficient cells. The data clearly point to a role for TLR7 in the RNA IC response, but the definitive studies with TLR7-deficient AM14 B cells are still in progress.

6. Summary and speculation

Extrapolating from the AM14 chromatin IC data and what is currently known about the cell biology of TLR7 and TLR9 expression, it is reasonable to propose that the AM14 receptor (specific for IgG2a) can bind IgG2a specific for either a chromatin-associated protein (such as histone) (Fig. 2, left), or an RNA-associated protein, (such as the Sm antigen) (Fig. 2, right). Uptake by the AM14 BCR then directs the complex to a vesicular compartment where the nucleic acid in the complex can engage either TLR9 or TLR7. This scheme can be termed the "solution model" as the autoantigens are depicted as independent complexes available in the lymphoid circulation. Based on this model, one would predict a clear dependence of the chromatin response on TLR9 and a clear dependence of the Sm response on TLR7. However, as shown previously, PL2-3 stimulation of AM14 B cells is reduced on a TLR9-deficient background, but not entirely eliminated (Fig. 1).

A second possibility, referred to as the "apoptotic body model", assumes that the physiologically relevant form of the autoantigen stimulus is an apoptotic body that might incorporate more than one autoantigen. In this case, it is possible that recognition of either the chromatin or Sm could lead to the uptake of the apoptotic body and thus the combination of autoantigens. In a TLR9-deficient cell, uptake mediated by chromatin (Fig. 3, left) or by Sm (Fig. 3, right) could synergize with a second signal delivered to TLR7.

It will be important to gain a better understanding of exactly how autoantigen engages both the BCR and the relevant TLR and how the combination of signals emanating from the two receptors can modify the function, differentiation, and death of the B cell. Moreover, the parameters that enhance autoantigen TLR engagement need to be further elucidated. However, it is clear that TLRs play a key role in the activation of autoreactive B cells and represent an important future target for therapeutic intervention in systemic diseases such as SLE.

References

[1] E. Tan, Antinuclear antibodies: diagnostic markers for autoimmune diseases and probes for cell biology, Adv. Immunol. 44 (1989) 93–151.

[2] P.H. Plotz, The autoantibody repertoire: searching for order, Nat. Rev., Immunol. 3 (2003) 73–78.

[3] L.A. Casciola-Rosen, et al., Cleavage by granzyme B is strongly predictive of autoantigen status: implication for initiation of autoimmunity, J. Exp. Med. 190 (1999) 815–825.

[4] P.J. Utz, T.J. Gensler, P. Anderson, Death, autoantigen modifications, and tolerance, Arthritis Res. 2 (2000) 101–114.

[5] K.L. Graham, et al., Granzyme B is dispensable for immunologic tolerance to self in a murine model of systemic lupus erythematosus, Arthritis Rheum. 52 (2005) 1684–1693.
[6] H. Vallin, et al., Patients with systemic lupus erythematosus (SLE) have a circulating inducer of interferon-alpha (IFN-a) production acting on leucocytes resembling immature dendritic cells, Clin. Exp. Immunol. 115 (1999) 196–202.
[7] U. Bave, et al., Fc gamma RIIa is expressed on natural IFN-alpha-producing cells (plasmacytoid dendritic cells) and is required for the IFN-alpha production induced by apoptotic cells combined with lupus IgG, J. Immunol. 171 (2003) 3296–3302.
[8] L.G. Hannum, et al., A disease-related rheumatoid factor autoantibody is not tolerized in a normal mouse: implications for the origins of autoantibodies in autoimmune disease, J. Exp. Med. 184 (1996) 1269–1278.
[9] I.R. Rifkin, et al., Immune complexes present in the sera of autoimmune mice activate rheumatoid factor B cells, J. Immunol. 165 (2000) 1626–1633.
[10] E.A. Leadbetter, et al., Immune complexes activate autoreactive B cells by co-engagement of sIgM and Toll-like receptors, Nature 419 (2002) 603–607.
[11] P. Lenert, et al., CpG stimulation of primary mouse B cells is blocked by inhibitory oligodeoxyribonucleotides at a site proximal to NF-kB activation, Antisense Nucleic Acid Drug Dev. 4 (2001) 247–256.
[12] A. Marshak-Rothstein, et al., Comparison of CpG s-ODNs, chromatin immune complexes, and dsDNA fragment immune complexes in the TLR9-dependent activation of rheumatoid factor B cells, J. Endotoxin Res. 10 (2004) 247–251.
[13] S. Bauer, et al., Human TLR9 confers responsiveness to bacterial DNA via species-specific CpG motif recognition, Proc. Natl. Acad. Sci. U. S. A. 98 (2001) 9237–9242.
[14] G.A. Viglianti, et al., Activation of autoreactive B Cells by CpG dsDNA, Immunity 19 (2003) 837–847.
[15] IHGSC, Initial sequencing and analysis of the human genome, Nature 409 (2001) 860–922.
[16] A.M. Krieg, et al., Sequence motifs in adenoviral DNA block immune activation by stimulatory CpG motifs, Proc. Natl. Acad. Sci. U. S. A. 95 (1998) 12631–12636.
[17] I. Gursel, et al., Repetitive elements in mammalian telomeres suppress bacterial DNA-induced immune activation, J. Immunol. 171 (2003) 1393–1400.
[18] H. Shirota, et al., Suppressive oligodeoxynucleotides protect mice from lethal endotoxic shock, J. Immunol. 174 (2005) 4579–4583.
[19] H. Sano, C. Morimoto, DNA isolated from DNA/anti-DNA antibody immune complexes in systemic lupus erythematosus is rich in guanine-cytosine content, J. Immunol. 128 (1982) 1341–1345.
[20] H. Sano, et al., Accumulation of guanine-cytosine-enriched low M.W. DNA fragments in lymphocytes of patients with systemic lupus erythematosus, J. Immunol. 130 (1983) 187–190.
[21] A. Krystosek, Preferential sites of early DNA cleavage in apoptosis and the pathway of nuclear damage, Histochem. Cell Biol. 111 (1999) 265–276.
[22] M.Z. Radic, et al., Ig H and L chain contributions to autoimmune specificities, J. Immunol. 146 (1991) 176–182.
[23] H. Hemmi, et al., Small anti-viral compounds activate immune cells via the TLR7 MyD88-dependent signaling pathway, Nat. Immunol. 3 (2002) 196–200.
[24] J. Lunec, et al., 8-Hydroxydeoxyguanosine: a marker of oxidative DNA damage in systemic lupus erythematosus, FEBS Lett. 348 (1994) 131–138.
[25] M.S. Cooke, et al., Immunogenicity of DNA damaged by reactive oxygen species—implications for anti-DNA antibodies in lupus, Free Radic. Biol. Med. 22 (1997) 151–159.
[26] D.K. Garg, R. Ali, Reactive oxygen species modified polyguanylic acid: Immunogenicity and implications for systemic autoimmunity, J. Autoimmun. 11 (1998) 371–378.
[27] S. Blount, et al., Reactive oxygen species modify human DNA, eliciting a more discriminating antigen for the diagnosis of systemic lupus erythematosus, Clin. Exp. Immunol. 81 (1990) 384–389.
[28] H. Wiseman, B. Halliwell, Damage to DNA by reactive oxygen and nitrogen species: role in inflammatory disease and progression to cancer, Biochem. J. 313 (1996) 17–29.
[29] T.D. Golan, et al., Solar ultraviolet radiation induces enhanced accumulation of oxygen radicals in murine SLE-derived splenocytes in vitro, Lupus 3 (1994) 103–106.
[30] C. Richter, J.-W. Park, B.N. Ames, Normal oxidative damage to mitochondrial and nuclear DNA is extensive, Proc. Natl. Acad. Sci. U. S. A. 85 (1988) 6465–6467.

[31] F.M. Yakes, B. Van Houten, Mitochondrial DNA damage is more extensive and persists longer than nuclear DNA damage in human cells following oxidative stress, Proc. Natl. Acad. Sci. U. S. A. 94 (1997) 514–519.
[32] S. Hajizadeh, et al., Extracellular mitochondrial DNA and oxidatively damaged DNA in synovial fluid of patients with rheumatoid arthritis, Arthritis Res. Ther. 5 (2003) R234–R240.
[33] L.V. Collins, et al., Endogenously oxidized mitochondrial DNA induces in vivo and in vitro inflammatory responses, J. Leukoc. Biol. 75 (2004) 995–1000.
[34] J. Li, T.D. Stein, J.A. Johnson, Genetic dissection of systemic autoimmune disease in Nrf2 deficient mice, Physiol. Genomics 18 (2004) 261–272.
[35] S.S. Diebold, et al., Innate antiviral responses by means of TLR7-mediated recognition of single-stranded RNA, Science 303 (2004) 1529–1531.
[36] F. Heil, et al., Species-specific recognition of single-stranded RNA via Toll-like receptor 7 and 8, Science 303 (2004) 1526–1529.
[37] J.M. Lund, et al., Recognition of single-stranded RNA viruses by Toll-like receptor 7, Proc. Natl. Acad. Sci. U. S. A. 101 (2004) 6835–6856.
[38] T. Lovgren, et al., Induction of interferon-alpha production in plasmacytoid dendritic cells by immune complexes containing nucleic acid released by necrotic or late apoptotic cells and lupus IgG, Arthritis Rheum. 50 (2004) 1861–1872.

International Congress Series 1285 (2005) 50–54

ELSEVIER

www.ics-elsevier.com

Role of innate immunity cytokines in systemic lupus and systemic onset arthritis

Virginia Pascual *, Karolina Palucka, Jacques Banchereau

Baylor Institute for Immunology research, Dallas, TX, USA

Abstract. Cytokines of the innate immune system, like TNF and type I interferon (IFN-alpha/beta), have been described to be key players in autoimmunity. IFN-alpha/beta may drive many of the immune alterations described in systemic lupus erythematosus (SLE), a prototype autoimmune disease characterized by a break of tolerance to nuclear components. The recognition of the fundamental role of immature dendritic cells (DCs) in the control of peripheral tolerance led to the hypothesis that SLE may be driven through unabated DC activation. Indeed, CD14+ monocytes isolated from SLE blood, but not those from healthy individuals, act as DCs. Their activation is driven by IFN-α secreted by plasmacytoid DCs that have been shown to infiltrate SLE skin lesions. The importance of IFN-α in SLE is further shown by the presence of an IFN-α signature in the blood of all SLE patients, and by its extinction upon therapy with high-dose steroids. The excess of IFN-α may also contribute to the hypergammaglobulinemia that characterizes SLE patients, as pDCs triggered with virus induce activated B cells to differentiate into plasma cells. We have also explored the role of an innate immunity cytokine, interleukin-1 (IL-1), in the pathogenesis of systemic onset juvenile idiopathic arthritis (SOJIA), one of the major forms of chronic inflammatory arthritis in childhood. Our results indicate that this cytokine is at the center of SOJIA pathogenesis, as these patients produce an excess of IL-1 and treatment with IL-1 receptor antagonist (IL-1Ra) results in disease resolution. © 2005 Published by Elsevier B.V.

Keywords: Interferon-α; TNF-α; Interleukin-1; Systemic lupus erythematosus; Systemic onset juvenile idiopathic arthritis

1. Systemic lupus erythematosus (SLE), a disease of innate and adaptive immunity

SLE is a systemic autoimmune disease clinically characterized by a waxing and waning course and by involvement of multiple organs including skin, kidneys and central nervous

* Corresponding author.
E-mail address: Virginip@baylorhealth.edu (V. Pascual).

0531-5131/ © 2005 Published by Elsevier B.V.
doi:10.1016/j.ics.2005.08.018

system [1,2]. The etiopathogenesis of SLE is poorly understood and current therapies are based on non-specific immunosuppression prompting the search for pathogenic factors as well as novel therapeutic targets.

Among the immunological features of SLE are high titers of autoantibodies predominantly specific for DNA and nucleosomes. Paradoxically, polyclonal hypergammaglobulinemia and high number of plasma cells coexist with considerable B lymphopenia and an increased frequency of pre-germinal center B cells [3]. Likewise, autoreactive T cells are found in spite of a profound reduction of circulating T cells [4,5]. The systemic autoimmune reaction in SLE together with the presence of autoreactive T and B cells made us consider that SLE patients could display alterations of dendritic cells (DCs), the controllers of immune reaction at both non-antigen specific and antigen-specific stages [6]. Accordingly, monocytes from SLE blood act as DCs. Furthermore, SLE sera induce normal monocytes to differentiate into DCs. These DCs capture and present antigens from dying cells leading to proliferation of autologous CD4 T cells. The capacity of SLE sera to induce DC differentiation correlates with disease activity and depends on IFN-α [7]. Using microarray analysis of blood leukocytes we confirmed that the majority of pediatric SLE patients display evidence of in vivo exposure to this cytokine [8]. Thus, unabated DCs induction may drive the autoimmune response in SLE and may be controlled by targeting IFN-α.

Plasmacytoid DCs (pDCs) represent a unique DC subset able to promptly release large amounts of type I interferon (IFN-αβ) upon viral encounter [9]. We have described that depletion of pDCs from human blood mononuclear cells abrogates the secretion of specific and polyclonal IgGs in response to influenza virus. Furthermore, purified DCs (pDCs) triggered with virus induce CD40-activated B cells to differentiate into plasma cells. Two pDC cytokines act sequentially, with IFN-αβ generating non-Ig-secreting plasma blasts and IL-6 inducing their differentiation into Ig-secreting plasma cells. These plasma cells

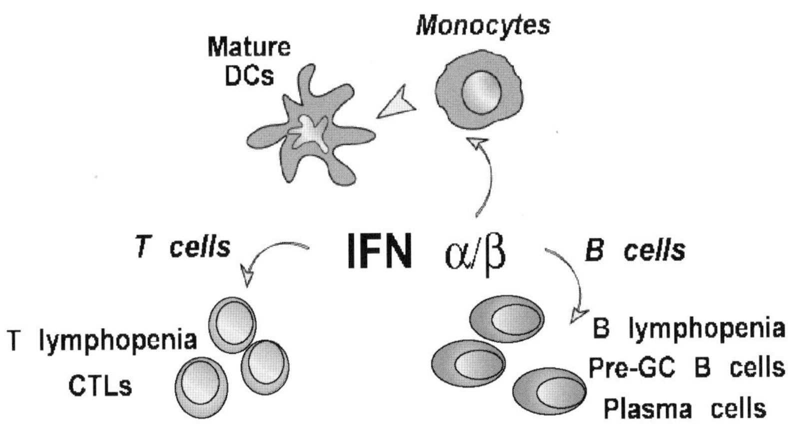

Fig. 1. Interferon alpha is at the center of many of the immune alterations in SLE: (i) it drives monocytes to mature into DCs, (ii) it induces the expression of germinal center markers like CD38 on mature B cells and the differentiation of mature B cells into plasma cell precursors, (iii) it induces lymphopenia, (iv) it enhances cytotoxic T cell differentiation.

display the high levels of CD38 found on tissue plasma cells. Thus, pDCs are critical for the generation of plasma cells and antibody responses, two key features of SLE [10]. The central role of IFN-α in driving immune alterations that characterize SLE is summarized in Fig. 1.

2. Interplay between IFN-α and TNF-α in autoimmune diseases

The identification of TNF as a major factor in the pathogenesis of rheumatoid arthritis and the development of anti-TNF therapy represent a success of immunology. Yet, a fraction of RA patients treated with anti-TNF develop anti-dsDNA antibodies and some of them present clinical symptoms of SLE [11], suggesting a potential interplay between TNF and IFN-α. TNF regulates IFN-α production in vitro at two levels. First, it inhibits IFN-α release by immature pDCs exposed to Influenza virus, and secondly, it inhibits the generation of pDCs from $CD34^+$ hematopoietic progenitors. These findings are clinically relevant, as we have reported that five out of five patients with systemic juvenile arthritis treated with TNF antagonists display overexpression of IFN-α-regulated genes in their blood leukocytes (Fig. 2) [12]. These results may provide a mechanistic explanation for the development of anti-dsDNA antibodies and lupus-like syndrome in patients undergoing anti-TNF therapy.

These findings led us to propose that an excess of either IFN-alpha or TNF may result in the activation of immature DCs into cells with different pathogenic capacities. Therefore, understanding DC heterogeneity is critical to a better understanding of the immune responses, most particularly as it applies to immunopathology and immunotherapy.

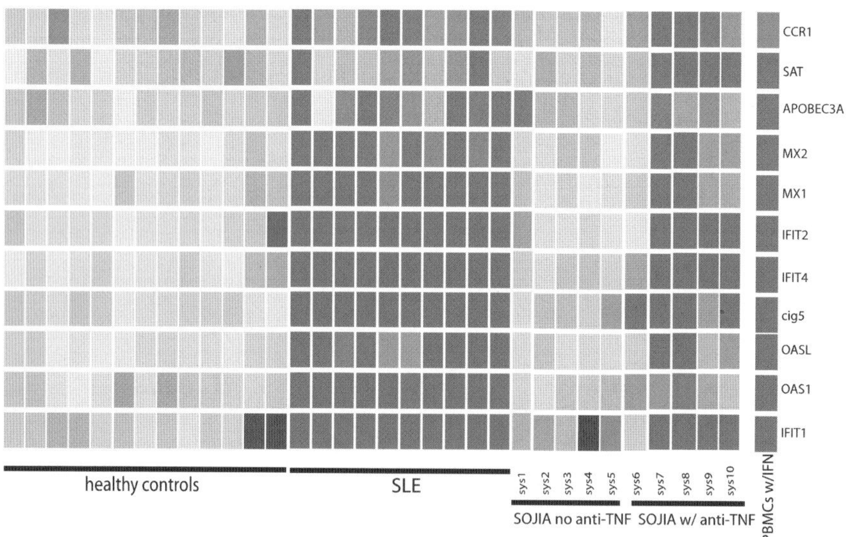

Fig. 2. Cross-regulation of IFN-α and TNF-α in autoimmune diseases. PBMCs from SOJIA patients treated with anti-TNF therapy display increased transcription of IFN-α-regulated genes. Gene expression was analyzed using U95Av2 and U133 Affymetrix chips and was normalized to the median of healthy controls. A set of IFN-α-regulated genes, identified by the analysis of SLE patients as described in Ref. [8] was compared in patients with and without anti-TNA therapy.

3. Systemic onset juvenile idiopathic arthritis is an interleukin-1 mediated disease

Systemic onset juvenile idiopathic arthritis (SOJIA) remains one of the most enigmatic pediatric rheumatic diseases [13]. Although the disease can be self-limited, about half of the patients develop a chronic, polyarticular type of arthritis that may be very difficult to control with available therapies, including methotrexate and anti-TNF agents. Blocking IL-1 is only partially effective in the treatment of patients with inflammatory chronic arthritis as assessed in clinical trials performed in adults with rheumatoid arthritis and children with diverse forms of juvenile arthritis [14,15]. SOJIA patients experiencing systemic symptoms have been excluded from these studies, as the disease symptoms can mimic drug reactions.

In order to gain insight into the pathogenesis of this disease, we analyzed the gene expression changes induced by SOJIA serum on healthy blood cells. Healthy PBMCs were incubated with the serum of 4 active SOJIA patients in vitro, and the serum-induced changes in gene transcription were assessed using gene expression profiling. The most significantly altered genes were analyzed in vivo in 38 SOJIA patients and in 12 healthy controls using microarray analysis and/or real-time PCR. Healthy and SOJIA patient's PBMCs were exposed in vitro to LPS and PMA and the cytokine levels in the corresponding supernatants were assessed by Luminex technology. Based on the results of these experiments, 8 SOJIA patients were treated with a commercially available IL-1 antagonist (Anakinra®) for 3–12 months.

SOJIA serum induced the upregulation of transcription of a series of innate immunity genes that included IL-1 a and IL-1 b. IL-1 b protein was also released into the supernatant of SOJIA serum incubated healthy PBMCs. Incubation of SOJIA patient's PBMCs with LPS and PMA induced a significantly increased release of IL-1 b compared with healthy controls. Most importantly, treatment of 9 SOJIA patients with active systemic and arthritic symptoms with Anakinra for a period of 3–12 months induced a complete disease remission in 7/9 patients and a partial response in the remaining two patients [16].

We therefore conclude that SOJIA patients produce excessive IL-1, and blocking the bioavailability of this cytokine is an effective treatment for this disease.

References

[1] G.M. Kammer, G.C. Tsokos, Lupus: Molecular and Cellular Pathogenesis, Humana Press, 1999.

[2] R.G. Lahita, Systemic Lupus Erythematosus, 3rd edition, Academic Press, 1999.

[3] E. Arce, et al., Increased frequency of pre-germinal center b cells and plasma cell precursors in the blood of children with systemic lupus erythematosus, J. Immunol. 167 (2001) 2361–2369.

[4] G.M. Kammer, et al., Abnormal T cell signal transduction in systemic lupus erythematosus, Arthritis Rheum. 46 (2002) 1139–1154.

[5] S.K. Datta, A. Kaliyaperumal, A. Desai-Mehta, T cells of lupus and molecular targets for immunotherapy, J. Clin. Immunol. 17 (1997) 11–20.

[6] J. Banchereau, R.M. Steinman, Dendritic cells and the control of immunity, Nature 392 (1998) 245–252.

[7] P. Blanco, et al., Induction of dendritic cell differentiation by IFN-alpha in systemic lupus erythematosus, Science 294 (2001) 1540–1543.

[8] L. Bennett, et al., Interferon and granulopoiesis signatures in systemic lupus erythematosus blood, J. Exp. Med. 197 (2003) 711–723.

[9] F.P. Siegal, et al., The nature of the principal type 1 interferon-producing cells in human blood, Science 284 (1999) 1835–1837.

[10] G. Jego, et al., Plasmacytoid dendritic cells induce plasma cell differentiation through type I interferon and interleukin 6, Immunity 19 (2003) 225–234.
[11] D.S. Pisetsky, Tumor necrosis factor alpha blockers and the induction of anti-DNA autoantibodies, Arthritis Rheum. 43 (2000) 2381–2382.
[12] A.K. Palucka, et al., Cross-regulation of TNF and IFN-{alpha} in autoimmune diseases, Proc. Natl. Acad. Sci. U. S. A. 102 (2005) 3372–3377.
[13] J.T. Cassidy, R.E. Petty, Textbook of Pediatric Rheumatology, W.B. Saunders, Philadelphia, 2001.
[14] M.C. Genovese, et al., Combination therapy with etanercept and Anakinra in the treatment of patients with rheumatoid arthritis who have been treated unsuccessfully with methotrexate, Arthritis Rheum. 50 (2004) 1412–1419.
[15] M.H. Buch, et al., Lack of response to Anakinra in rheumatoid arthritis following failure of tumor necrosis factor alpha blockade, Arthritis Rheum. 50 (2004) 725–728.
[16] V. Pascual, et al., Role of interleukin-1 (IL-1) in the pathogenesis of systemic onset juvenile idiopathic arthritis and clinical response to IL-1 blockade, J. Exp. Med. 201 (2005) 1479–1486.

International Congress Series 1285 (2005) 55–59

www.ics-elsevier.com

Apoptotic cell clearance by phagocytes

Masato Tanaka *

Laboratory for Innate Cellular Immunity, RIKEN Research Center for Allergy and Immunology, 1-7-22, Suehiro, Tsurumi-ku, Yokohama, Kanagawa 230-0045, Japan

Abstract. Macrophages and dendritic cells recognize not only microorganisms foreign to the body but also dying self-cells, which they eliminate by engulfment. This phenomenon prevents dying cells from releasing potentially harmful or immunogenic intracellular materials. We found that milk fat globule-EGF-factor 8 (MFG-E8) linked apoptotic cells and phagocytes, and promoted the phagocytosis of cell corpses. MFG-E8 is expressed in tingible body macrophages (TBM) in the germinal centers of the spleen and lymph nodes. In MFG-E8-deficient mice, a large number of apoptotic lymphocytes were associated with TBM but were not engulfed, indicating that MFG-E8 was involved in the clearance of apoptotic B cells by TBM. The MFG-E8-deficient mice developed splenomegaly and produced autoantibodies such as antinuclear antibodies as well as anti-DNA antibodies in an age-dependent manner. To further examine the consequences of failure in apoptotic cell clearance, we produced a recombinant MFG-E8 mutant protein (D89E), which had inhibitory effects on the phagocytosis of apoptotic cells by a wide variety of phagocytes. When intravenously injected into mice, the D89E protein induced the production of autoantibodies. The autoantibodies production was enhanced by the coinjection of syngeneic apoptotic thymocytes. These results indicated that the impairment of apoptotic cell phagocytosis led to autoantibody production.

Keywords: Apoptosis; Phagocytosis; MFG-E8; Autoimmune disease

1. Introduction

Programmed cell death, or apoptosis, is essential for the elimination of unwanted or potentially harmful cells from multicellular organisms [1]. Apoptosis is a cell-suicide mechanism, and its process is thought to be cell-autonomous. When apoptotic signals are

* Tel.: +81 45 503 9686; fax: +81 45 503 9685.
E-mail address: mtanaka@rcai.riken.jp.

0531-5131/
doi:10.1016/j.ics.2005.07.080

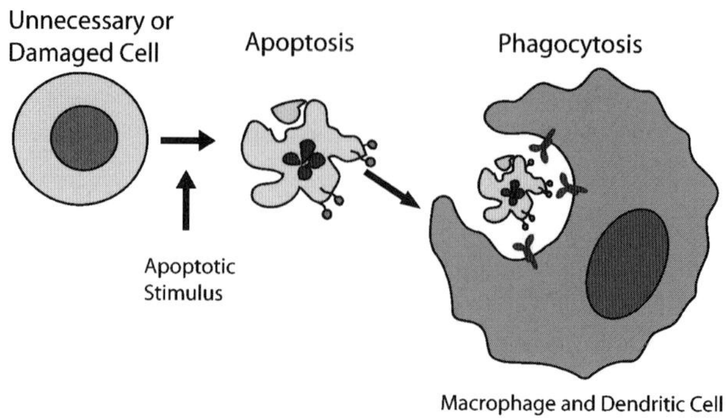

Fig. 1. The elimination of unwanted or potentially harmful cells.

transduced into cells, caspases, members of a family of cysteine proteases, are sequentially activated, and active caspases cleave their target molecules to induce cell death [2]. Apoptotic cells are rapidly engulfed by professional phagocytes, such as macrophages and dendritic cells, or by neighboring cells [3,4] (Fig. 1). The clearance of dead cells by phagocytes occurs so rapidly that it is very difficult to find apoptotic cells that are not associated with phagocytes even in the thymus. This phagocytosis prevents the release of potentially toxic or immunogenic intracellular materials from dead cell corpses. In addition, the phagocytosis of apoptotic cells renders the phagocytes immunosuppressive by producing anti-inflammatory cytokines, such as IL-10 [5–7]. Therefore, even tissues with high cell turnover rates are free from inflammation.

2. Molecular mechanisms for apoptotic cell engulfment

Based on the evidence that phagocytes engulf dead cell corpses but not living cells, the mechanisms by which phagocytes recognize apoptotic cell corpses have been extensively studied. It is most likely that phagocytes express specific receptors that recognize cell surface molecules exposed on apoptotic cells as "eat me" signals. To identify the molecules involved in the phagocytosis of apoptotic cells by macrophages, we raised monoclonal antibodies against molecules expressed on thioglycollate-elicited mouse peritoneal macrophages by immunizing the cells in Armenian hamsters and screened them with a quantitative phagocytosis assay. One antibody, designated 2422, was found to accelerate the phagocytosis of apoptotic thymocytes by macrophages when it was added to the assay. A molecule recognized by 2422 Ab was purified by affinity chromatography, and a mass spectrometry analysis of the protein identified it as mouse milk fat globule-EGF-factor 8 (MFG-E8), a secreted protein [8].

MFG-E8, also called lactadherin or BA46, was originally identified as a component of milk fat globules [9–11], and it is also produced and secreted by activated macrophages and immature dendritic cells [8,12]. MFG-E8 has two factor VIII-homologous domains in the C-terminus (Fig. 2A). These domains have high affinity to anionic phospholipids, such as phosphatidylserine (PS). PS is located in the inner leaflet of living cells. When cells undergo apoptosis, PS is translocated to the outer leaflet by unknown mechanisms and

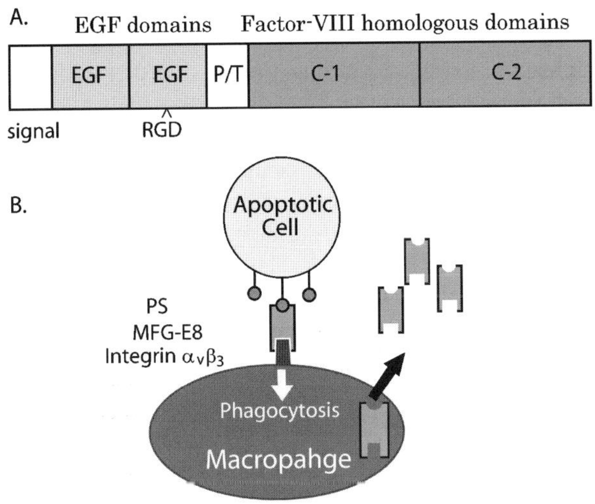

Fig. 2. (A) Structure of MFG-E8. (B) Model for the molecular mechanisms of apoptotic cell engulfment with MFG-E8.

thus become exposed on the surface of apoptotic cells. MFG-E8 specifically binds to PS exposed on apoptotic cells. When MFG-E8 is engaged by apoptotic cells, it binds to $\alpha_v\beta_3$ integrin expressed on phagocytes via N-terminal EGF-like domains containing an RGD motif and promotes the phagocytosis of apoptotic cells (Fig. 2B). Consistent with this model, MFG-E8 carrying a point mutation in the RGD motif (see below) behaved as a dominant negative form, and it inhibited the phagocytosis of apoptotic cells by activated peritoneal macrophages in vitro and in vivo.

3. Injection of the MFG-E8 mutant protein

To reveal the function of MFG-E8, the mutant MFG-E8, designated D89E, carrying a point mutation in an RGD motif, was produced in 293T cells. D89E inhibited the phagocytosis of apoptotic cells by various kinds of macrophages in a dose-dependent manner [7]. Since another mutant, E1E2PT, lacking the C1 and C2 domains, had no effect on the phagocytosis of these macrophages, D89E's inhibitory effects were dependent on its binding activity to PS. These results indicated that a wide variety of macrophages recognize PS on apoptotic cells as “eat me” signals for phagocytosis, and that the D89E protein can inhibit apoptotic cell engulfment by phagocytes by masking the PS on dead cells.

When the rapid removal of apoptotic cells by phagocytes is impaired, intracellular materials from secondary necrotic cells might be released to induce autoantibody production. In fact, D89E induced the production of autoantibodies, including antiphospholipid and antinuclear antibodies, when intravenously injected into mice [7]. The production of autoantibodies was enhanced by the coinjection of syngeneic apoptotic thymocytes, indicating that the impairment of apoptotic cell phagocytosis led to autoantibody production.

4. The function of MFG-E8 in vivo

MFG-E8 is expressed in tingible body macrophages (TBM) in the germinal centers of the spleen and lymph nodes in mice [13]. TBM is CD68-positive and F4/80-negative and contains apoptotic corpses (tingible bodies). The cell is thought to be responsible for removing apoptotic B cells in the germinal centers. In MFG-E8-deficient mice, a large number of apoptotic lymphocytes were associated with TBM in the germinal centers, but they were not engulfed by the macrophages, indicating that MFG-E8 was involved in the clearance of apoptotic B cells by TBM. The MFG-E8-deficient mice developed splenomegaly and spontaneously produced autoantibodies, such as antinuclear antibodies and anti-DNA antibodies in an age-dependent manner. These results indicate that the clearance of apoptotic cells plays an important role in the maintenance of self-tolerance.

5. Tethering molecules for apoptotic cell engulfment

By screening monoclonal antibodies, we found that SHPS-1 is involved in the phagocytosis of apoptotic cells by BAM3 cells, a macrophage cell line [14]. SHPS-1 belongs to the immunoglobulin superfamily, and it binds to CD47 [15]. The inhibition of interaction between CD47 and SHPS-1 prevents the macrophages from engulfing apoptotic cells, indicating that the interaction between CD47 on preys and SHPS-1 expressed on phagocytes is required for efficient engulfment of apoptotic cells. However, the expression level of CD47 is not different between living cells and apoptotic cells. Furthermore, CD47 not only on apoptotic thymocytes but also on those living cells can bind to SHPS-1, suggesting that phagocytes cannot distinguish dying cells from healthy cells by SHPS-1. The masking of PS on apoptotic cells with D89E, the MFG-E8 mutant protein, completely inhibits phagocytosis by BAM3 cells, indicating that recognition of PS is also required for the phagocytosis of dead cells by macrophages. The reconstitution assay with 3T3 cells revealed that interaction between CD47 and SHPS-1 was required for apoptotic cells to bind to phagocytes, while PS recognition played a critical role in the engulfment of dead cells. These results indicate that phagocytes require two different steps for the phagocytosis of apoptotic cells; first, target cells are tethered to phagocytes by the interaction between CD47 and SHPS-1. Then, phagocytes exclusively engulf dead cells by recognition of PS. These results are consistent with the two-step model proposed by Hoffmann et al. [16].

Acknowledgments

I would like to thank all of my colleagues who contributed to the work in this review. This study is supported in part by grants from the Ministry of Education, Science, Sports, and Culture of Japan, and by the Uehara Foundation.

References

[1] M.D. Jacobson, M. Weil, M.C. Raff, Programmed cell death in animal development, Cell 88 (3) (1997) 347–354.

[2] S. Nagata, Apoptosis by death factor, Cell 88 (3) (1997) 355–365.

[3] MO. Hengartner, Apoptosis: corralling the corpses, Cell 104 (3) (2001) 325–328.

[4] K. Lauber, et al., Clearance of apoptotic cells: getting rid of the corpses, Mol. Cell 14 (3) (2004) 277–287.
[5] R.E. Voll, et al., Immunosuppressive effects of apoptotic cells, Nature 390 (6658) (1997) 350–351.
[6] A. Byrne, D.J. Reen, Lipopolysaccharide induces rapid production of IL-10 by monocytes in the presence of apoptotic neutrophils, J. Immunol. 168 (4) (2002) 1968–1977.
[7] K. Asano, et al., Masking of phosphatidylserine inhibits apoptotic cell engulfment and induces autoantibody production in mice, J. Exp. Med. 200 (4) (2004) 459–467.
[8] R. Hanayama, et al., Identification of a factor that links apoptotic cells to phagocytes, Nature 417 (6885) (2002) 182–187.
[9] N. Aoki, et al., Immunologically cross-reactive 57 kDa and 53 kDa glycoprotein antigens of bovine milk fat globule membrane: isoforms with different N-linked sugar chains and differential glycosylation at early stages of lactation, Biochim. Biophys. Acta 1200 (2) (1994) 227–234.
[10] N. Aoki, et al., Molecular cloning of glycoprotein antigens MGP57/53 recognized by monoclonal antibodies raised against bovine milk fat globule membrane, Biochim. Biophys. Acta 1245 (3) (1995) 385–391.
[11] J.D. Stubbs, et al., cDNA cloning of a mouse mammary epithelial cell surface protein reveals the existence of epidermal growth factor-like domains linked to factor VIII-like sequences, Proc. Natl. Acad. Sci. U. S. A. 87 (21) (1990) 8417–8421.
[12] K. Miyasaka, et al., Expression of milk fat globule epidermal growth factor 8 in immature dendritic cells for engulfment of apoptotic cells, Eur. J. Immunol. 34 (5) (2004) 1414–1422.
[13] R. Hanayama, et al., Autoimmune disease and impaired uptake of apoptotic cells in MFG-E8-deficient mice, Science 304 (5674) (2004) 1147–1150.
[14] K. Tada, et al., Tethering of apoptotic cells to phagocytes through binding of CD47 to Src homology 2 domain-bearing protein tyrosine phosphatase substrate-1, J. Immunol. 171 (11) (2003) 5718–5726.
[15] P. Jiang, C.F. Lagenaur, V. Narayanan, Integrin-associated protein is a ligand for the P84 neural adhesion molecule, J. Biol. Chem. 274 (2) (1999) 559–562.
[16] P.R. Hoffmann, et al., Phosphatidylserine (PS) induces PS receptor-mediated macropinocytosis and promotes clearance of apoptotic cells, J. Cell Biol. 155 (4) (2001) 649–659.

International Congress Series 1285 (2005) 60–67

www.ics-elsevier.com

Regulation of innate immunity by paired receptors

Hisashi Arase

Department of Immunochemistry, Research Institute for Microbial Diseases, Osaka University, Japan
PRESTO, Japan Science and Technology Corporation, Japan

Abstract. NK cells show cytotoxicity and cytokine production upon recognition of virus-infected cells. When NK cells are removed from cytomegalovirus-resistant mice, the virus titer after infection is markedly increased and the mice are likely to die due to infection. However, the exact mechanism of how NK cells recognize virus-infected cells has remained unclear for a long time. Recent findings of the presence of virus-specific NK cell receptors and their ligands on virus-infected cells have provided a new vision of a protective role of NK cells in virus infection. Furthermore, the recognition of virus-infected cells by paired receptors consisting of activating and inhibitory receptors was found to correlate with the degree of host susceptibility to virus infection. Here, we would like to discuss the role of NK cells in anti-virus immunity. © 2005 Published by Elsevier B.V.

Keywords: NK cells; Virus infection; Cytomegalovirus; Herpesvirus

1. Introduction

Immune-compromised patients who lack normal NK cells are susceptible to severe infectious diseases caused by several viruses even if they have functional T cells and B cells [1]. Similarly, certain mouse strains become susceptible to infection by some viruses, such as cytomegalovirus, when NK cells are deleted although NK cell-deficient mice are not always susceptible to virus infections [2]. From these observations, NK cells are thought to be a critical lymphocyte population for protection against certain virus infections [1]. Indeed, NK cells specifically recognize virus-infected cells and directly kill them. In addition, NK cells produce such cytokines as IFN-γ and regulate the immune response of T cells or B cells. Because NK cells show such effector functions against virus infection without prior sensitization, they play a role in immune response early in infection before the immune responses of T cells and B cells are established. Recent studies have

E-mail address: arase@biken.osaka-u.ac.jp.

0531-5131/ © 2005 Published by Elsevier B.V.
doi:10.1016/j.ics.2005.08.005

revealed that virus-induced activation of NK cells may involve direct recognition of virus-infected cells via activating receptors such as Ly49H or NKG2D, or stimulation of NK cells by interferon-α/β and the cytokines, IL-12 and IL-18 and which are produced by myeloid or other cells at the site of infection.

2. NK cells in anti-virus immunity

The role of NK cells in anti-virus immunity has been well characterized using the MCMV system [1,3,4]. Newborn mice or NK cell-deficient mice are highly susceptible to MCMV infection. The adoptive transfer of mature NK cells into these mice protects the mice against MCMV infection. C57BL/6 mice are relatively resistant to MCMV infection; however, the virus titer after infection is increased by approximately one-thousand folds when NK cells are depleted. On the other hand, mice of inbred mouse strains such as BALB/c, DBA/2 and 129/J mice are quite susceptible to cytomegalovirus infection. They show a peak virus titer approximately one thousand times higher than that in resistant C57BL/6 mice. The genetic locus responsible for resistance to MCMV infection segregated as a single locus and was detected on mouse chromosome 6 and named *cmv-1* [5].

Recently, *cmv-1* has been reported to encode Ly49H, one of the activating NK receptors (see below). The *Ly49* gene family encodes receptors belonging to the C-type lectin superfamily and is polygenic and polymorphic [6]. Although Ly49 receptors are highly homologous to each other in amino acid sequence, different *Ly49* genes encode either inhibitory or activating receptors that are expressed on subsets of NK cells and T cells. Activating Ly49 receptors possess positively charged amino acids, lysine or arginine, in its transmembrane region and associate with the DAP12 adaptor molecule that has negatively charged amino acids in the transmembrane region [7]. DAP12 has an ITAM possessing a consensus sequence, Y-x-x-(L/I)-x(6-8)-Y-x-x-(L/I) in the cytoplasmic region and delivers activation signals by the recruitment of the Syk and ZAP70 tyrosine kinases. Activating Ly49 receptors require DAP12 for their cell surface expression as well as for activating signal transduction. On the other hand, inhibitory Ly49 receptors contain an ITIM with a consensus sequence, (I/V/L/S)-x-Y-x-x-(L/V), in the cytoplasmic region and delivers inhibitory signals via the SHP-1 or SHP-2 tyrosine phosphatase [8]. Inhibitory Ly49 receptors do not have positively charged amino acids in the transmembrane region and hence do not associate with DAP12. Daniels et al. showed that NK cells expressing the activating Ly49H receptors produce IFN-γ upon MCMV infection [9]. Furthermore, they showed that resistance to MCMV infection is lost when Ly49H-positive cells are removed. These results indicated that *cmv-1* gene encodes Ly49H. Other groups also identified Ly49H as a *cmv-1* gene by genomic mapping of the MCMV-resistance gene using BXD-8 recombinant inbred mouse [10,11]. BXD-8, a recombinant inbred strain generated by a cross between MCMV-resistant C57BL/6 mice and MCMV-sensitive DBA/2 mice, had a defect in the C57BL/6-derived Ly49H gene that rendered the mice susceptible to MCMV. Namely, MCMV-resistant mice expressed Ly49H whereas MCMV-susceptible mice did not. These results are also supported by the observation that DAP12-deficient mice are susceptible to MCMV infection [12].

To address the question of how Ly49H-expressing NK cells recognize MCMV-infected cells, we generated NFAT-GFP reporter cells transfected with Ly49H and DAP12 and used as Ly49H reporter cells [13]. The Ly49H reporter cells expressed the reporter GFP when co-cultured with MCMV-infected cells, indicating the presence of a ligand on the infected cells that binds to Ly49H. Using those Ly49H reporter cells, we further found that Ly49H recognizes m157, one of the uncharacterized MCMV gene products. The soluble recombinant form of m157 binds to Ly49H-expressing cells, thereby indicating that the recognition of m157 by Ly49H involves direct binding [13]. Smith et al. also identified m157 as a ligand for Ly49H using a similar NFAT reporter system [14].

Within the Ly49 family, the activating and inhibitory receptors are highly homologous, usually exhibiting more than 90% amino acid identity in the extracellular domains. Especially, sequence similarity between inhibitory Ly49I and activating Ly49H is very high among Ly49 receptors. Therefore, we considered the possibility that the viral m157 protein may be similar to MHC class I because Ly49I recognizes MHC class I. However, the primary structure of m157 does not show any appreciable homology to known mammalian molecules. Interestingly, when analyzed by the 3D-PSSM program that detects structurally homologous proteins based on their secondary structures, m157 was found to be similar to non-classical MHC class I molecules, such as CD1 or H-2M3. The relationship of m157 to some MHC class I proteins suggests that CMV may have originally acquired the *m157* gene from a mammalian host and adapted it for use in the host.

3. Virus evasion from NK cells by mimicking normal cells

The activation of NK cell responses is regulated by inhibitory receptors. Therefore, virus-infected cells that have lost MHC class I expression in order to escape from CTL may be more susceptible to attack by NK cells. In order to avoid this, it appears that viruses may have acquired MHC-like molecules to serve as ligands for these inhibitory receptors.

As described above, NK cells expressing the activating Ly49H receptor recognize m157, an MHC-like molecule of MCMV, and this plays a critical role in protection against MCMV. This, however, leads to the following question: why does cytomegalovirus possess m157, a target molecule of NK cells? m157 is conserved between at least two independently derived MCMV strains. In addition, m157 is not involved in viral replication in vitro because a large deletion mutant virus that lacks sixteen genes between m150 and m165 efficiently infects cells in vivo. Therefore, m157 should play some beneficial role in MCMV infection in vivo. When NK cells from various MCMV-susceptible mouse strains were stained with a soluble m157-Ig fusion protein, NK cells from 129/J and NZB mouse strains were stained by soluble m157-Ig, although they did not express Ly49H and did not kill m157-expressing cells. Binding analysis of soluble m157 to several Ly49 receptors from 129/J mice revealed that the inhibitory Ly49I receptor from 129/J mice recognizes m157. From those findings, m157 appears to be a molecule that MCMV has acquired as a ligand for inhibitory NK receptors in order to escape from attack by NK cells [13]. In other words, m157 may make MCMV-infected cells appear like normal to NK cells.

Although m157 was newly identified as an MHC-like molecule, MCMV is known to express another viral glycoprotein, m144, that is highly homologous to the MHC class I molecule. Unlike m157, m144 exhibits homology to MHC at the primary structure level and like conventional MHC class I associates with β2-microblobulin. Interestingly, the m144 deletion virus is less virulent than the wild-type cytomegalovirus [15]. This suggests that m144 is also recognized by certain inhibitory receptors expressed on the immune system, although the receptors for m144 have not been identified to date. Similarly, a human cytomegalovirus glycoprotein, UL18, is also homologous to MHC class I [16]. An inhibitory receptor, LIR-1 (ILT-2/CD85I), that is expressed by all monocytes and macrophages binds to UL18 with high affinity [17]. In this way, cytomegalovirus escapes from the immune system by expressing MHC-like proteins that serve as ligands for inhibitory receptors.

4. Virus-driven evolution of NK receptors

As described above, MCMV seems to have originally acquired m157 from a host MHC class I gene to serve as a ligand for inhibitory NK receptors. The observations that m157 is recognized by an inhibitory Ly49 receptor in MCMV-susceptible mice and by an activating Ly49 receptor in MCMV-resistant mice prompted us to hypothesize that the activating Ly49 receptors may have evolved from an ancestral inhibitory receptors. This may have been caused by selective pressure imposed by MCMV infection and resulted in host protection against this pathogen. The process of evolving from an inhibitory receptor to an activating receptor is a relatively easy one. This would involve a point mutation in the transmembrane segment of the inhibitory receptor to acquire a charged amino acid, permitting association with the pre-existing activating adaptor protein, DAP12. A point mutation, introducing a stop codon, or missense mutation would result in deletion of the ITIM sequences in the cytoplasmic domain of the inhibitory receptor to abolish this function. By this mechanism, it would be possible to convert inhibitory into activation NK receptors.

Although it is difficult to formally show direct evidence to support this hypothesis, our genome contains clues that are consistent with this idea. For example, the human *KIR* genes are the functional orthologs of the rodent *Ly49* genes (which no longer exist in our genome). When the sequence of the 3′ untranslated (UT) region of an activating KIR gene, is translated, ITIM sequences are found at the same position as that in a highly related inhibitory KIR, but are rendered non-functional by an upstream stop codon in the activating *KIR* gene that prevents incorporation of the ITIM in the protein. Because there is no reason to explain why the activating KIR has an ITIM sequence in the 3′UT region, it is likely that the activating KIR evolved from the inhibitory KIR. Therefore, inhibitory receptors seem to have evolved into activating receptors, in some cases possibly for protection against virus infection.

These NK receptors, both in humans and mice, are composed of exons that separate the extracellular domains, the transmembrane domains, and the cytoplasmic domains. Therefore, by gene duplication and recombination, it is possible to generate novel receptors comprised of the exons encoding the extracellular domain of an inhibitory receptor and the transmembrane and cytoplasmic domain of a DAP12-associated activating receptor. Such conversion has been proposed for a Ly49 receptor in C57/L mice that has an extracellular domain similar to Ly49D, but an inhibitory cytoplasmic domain similar to Ly49A [18]. The danger inherent to this strategy is the generation of activating receptors that will recognize self-MHC class I and trigger autoimmunity. However, it appears that subtle alternations have also occurred in the extracellular domains of the activating receptors to ensure that they do not bind self-MHC class I with high affinity, thereby avoiding this problem.

If the original function of m157 is to engage inhibitory Ly49 receptors to give the virus a growth advantage, the passage of MCMV in C57BL/6 mice expressing an activating Ly49H receptor should result in the loss of this gene or mutation such that it cannot bind to Ly49H. Alternatively, an m157-deficient MCMV strain should be less virulent than the wild-type virus in a mouse strain that expresses an inhibitory Ly49 receptor on a large fraction of the NK cell population. It would be relevant to determine whether the m157 gene exists in 'clinical isolates' of MCMV established from field mice and whether there is a correlation between CMV susceptibility and Ly49 receptor expression in the natural environment of mice. Finally, it will be of interest to determine whether HCMV has influenced the evolution of the human KIR genes in a similar fashion.

5. Regulation of virus infection by 'paired receptors'

In addition to Ly49, there are several other examples of highly related receptors with inhibiting and activating counterparts in NK cells [8,19]. Similar to the case of Ly49, the inhibitory KIR binds to polymorphic HLA-A, -B, and -C ligands, whereas the activating KIR either do not bind to HLA class I or do so with weak affinity [20]. The extracellular domains of the activating KIR are very similar to those of the inhibitory KIR, again suggesting a common origin. A majority of the activating KIRs are present in the genome of only a subset of the human population [20]. The possibility that the extensive and rapid diversification of KIR genes is driven by human pathogens has been suggested by Khakoo et al. based on a comparison of KIR between human and chimpanzee [21].

Another related pair of NK receptors is the inhibitory CD94/NKG2A and the activating CD94/NKG2C/DAP12 complex [22]. Unlike the case of Ly49 and KIR, both CD94/NKG2A and CD94/NKG2C bind to a common ligand, HLA-E [23]. The rationale for activating and inhibitory receptors having the same ligand specificity is unclear; however, it has been suggested that those related receptors may have different affinities for HLA-E [24] and may be influenced by different peptides [25] bound in the HLA-E groove. If pathogen-encoded peptides bound by HLA-E preferentially engage the activating CD94/NKG2C but not the inhibitory CD94/NKG2A receptor, this may provide a rationale for this phenomenon. Rodents also possess receptors encoded by the *NKR-P1* gene family that can potentially activate [26] or inhibit [27] NK cell function. Although this potential has been clearly demonstrated by the ligation of the NKR-P1 receptors with mAbs, the natural ligands for these receptors are only beginning to be appreciated.

Related inhibitory and activating 'paired receptors' are present in many cell types other than NK cells. For example, the SIRP, PIR, and the CD85 (ILT, LIR) receptor families have activating and inhibitory receptors [28,29]. SIRPα expressed on macrophages recognizes CD47 and prevents phagocytosis of CD47-bearing red blood cells [30–32]. By contrast, DAP12 is associated with the related SIRPβ receptor and can activate macrophages when ligated with anti-SIRP mAb [33,34]. The activating SIRPβ receptor does not bind to CD47, and its ligand has not been identified so far. It is intriguing to note that human smallpox virus has a gene related to CD47. Similarly, some inhibitory CD85 (ILT/LIR) receptors are known to recognize MHC class I [35,36], but as yet the ligands for the activating CD85 isoforms are unknown [37]. Those receptors are expressed predominantly on macrophages or dendritic cells, suggesting a role in the innate immune response against pathogens. The demonstration that other activating and inhibitory 'paired receptors' recognize pathogens would provide support for the hypothesis that pathogens have driven the evolution of immune genes.

6. Future direction

'Paired receptor' families consisting of activating and inhibitory receptors are widely distributed in various immune cells. According to our hypothesis, we propose that pathogens have specifically acquired ligands that function to engage the inhibitory receptors and suppress an immune response. In turn, the host has responded by converting an inhibitory receptor into an activating receptor to foil this process. Currently, only the interaction between mouse Ly49H and MCMV m157 serves to support this idea; the function of other 'paired receptors' remains unclear. Thus, the discovery of additional paired receptors that recognize virus-infected cells will be needed to validate this general concept. If proven correct, the elucidation of virus-specific receptors and their virus ligands will be useful in designing vaccines for viruses and developing therapies for virus infection. Further study on virus-specific 'paired receptors' promises to provide a new vision for anti-virus immunity.

Acknowledgements

This work was supported in part by Uehara Memorial Foundation, Japan to H. Arase.

References

[1] C.A. Biron, et al., Natural killer cells in antiviral defense: function and regulation by innate cytokines, Annu. Rev. Immunol. 17 (1999) 189–220.
[2] A.R. French, W.M. Yokoyama, Natural killer cells and viral infections, Curr. Opin. Immunol. 15 (2003) 45–51.
[3] J.F. Bukowski, et al., Adoptive transfer studies demonstrating the antiviral effect of natural killer cells in vivo, J. Exp. Med. 161 (1985) 40–52.
[4] R.M. Welsh, et al., Natural killer (NK) cell response to virus infections in mice with severe combined immunodeficiency. The stimulation of NK cells and the NK cell-dependent control of virus infections occur independently of T and B cell functions, J. Exp. Med. 173 (1991) 1053–1063.
[5] A.A. Scalzo, et al., The effect of the Cmv-1 resistance gene, which is linked to the natural killer cell gene complex, is mediated by natural killer cells, J. Immunol. 149 (1992) 581–589.
[6] W.M. Yokoyama, B.F. Plougastel, Immune functions encoded by the natural killer gene complex, Nat. Rev., Immunol. 3 (2003) 304–316.

[7] K.M. Smith, et al., Ly49D and Ly49H associate with mouse DAP12 and form activating receptors, J. Immunol. 161 (1998) 7–10.
[8] J.V. Ravetch, L.L. Lanier, Immune inhibitory receptors, Science 290 (2000) 84–89.
[9] K.A. Daniels, et al., Murine cytomegalovirus is regulated by a discrete subset of natural killer cells reactive with monoclonal antibody to Ly49H, J. Exp. Med. 194 (2001) 29–44.
[10] H.-S. Lee, et al., Susceptibility to mouse cytomegalovirus is associated with depletion of an activating natural killer cell receptor of the C-type lectin superfamily, Nat. Genet. 28 (2001) 42–45.
[11] M.G. Brown, et al., Vital involvement of a natural killer cell activation receptor in resistance to viral infection, Science 292 (2001) 934–937.
[12] H. Sjolin, et al., Pivotal role of KARAP/DAP12 adaptor molecule in the natural killer cell-mediated resistance to murine cytomegalovirus infection, J. Exp. Med. 195 (2002) 825–834.
[13] H. Arase, et al., Direct recognition of cytomegalovirus by activating and inhibitory NK cell receptors, Science 296 (2002) 1323–1326.
[14] H.R. Smith, et al., Recognition of a virus-encoded ligand by a natural killer cell activation receptor, Proc. Natl. Acad. Sci. U. S. A. 99 (2002) 8826–8831.
[15] H.E. Farrell, et al., Inhibition of natural killer cells by a cytomegalovirus MHC class I homologue in vivo, Nature 386 (1997) 510–514.
[16] S. Beck, B.G. Barrell, Human cytomegalovirus encodes a glycoprotein homologous to MHC class-I antigens, Nature 331 (1988) 269–272.
[17] D. Cosman, et al., A novel immunoglobulin superfamily receptor for cellular and viral MHC class I molecules, Immunity 7 (1997) 273–282.
[18] I.K. Mehta, et al., A "chimeric" c57l-derived ly49 inhibitory receptor resembling the ly49d activation receptor, Cell. Immunol. 209 (2001) 29–41.
[19] L.L. Lanier, Face off—the interplay between activating and inhibitory immune receptors, Curr. Opin. Immunol. 13 (2001) 326–331.
[20] C. Vilches, P. Parham, KIR: diverse, rapidly evolving receptors of innate and adaptive immunity, Annu. Rev. Immunol. 20 (2002) 217–251.
[21] S.I. Khakoo, et al., Rapid evolution of NK cell receptor systems demonstrated by comparison of chimpanzees and humans, Immunity 12 (2000) 687–698.
[22] L.L. Lanier, et al., Association of DAP12 with activating CD94/NKG2C NK cell receptors, Immunity 8 (1998) 693–701.
[23] V.M. Braud, et al., HLA-E binds to natural killer cell receptors CD94/NKG2A, B, and C, Nature 391 (1998) 795–798.
[24] M. Valés-Gómez, et al., Kinetics and peptide dependency of the binding of the inhibitory NK receptor CD94/NKG2-A and the activating receptor CD94/NKG2-C to HLA-E, EMBO J. 18 (1999) 4250–4260.
[25] M. Llano, et al., HLA-E-bound peptides influence recognition by inhibitory and triggering CD94/NKG2 receptors: preferential response to an HLA-G-derived nanomer, Eur. J. Immunol. 28 (1998) 2854–2863.
[26] N. Arase, et al., Association with FcRg is essential for activation signal through NKR-P1 (CD161) in natural killer (NK) cells and NK1.1$^+$ T cells, J. Exp. Med. 186 (1997) 1957–1963.
[27] J.R. Carlyle, et al., Mouse NKR-P1B, a novel NK1.1 antigen with inhibitory function, J. Immunol. 162 (1999) 5917–5923.
[28] H. Kubagawa, P.D. Burrows, M.D. Cooper, A novel pair of immunoglobulin-like receptors expressed by B cells and myeloid cells, Proc. Natl. Acad. Sci. U. S. A. 94 (1997) 5261–5266.
[29] A. Maeda, M. Kuorsaki, T. Kurosaki, Paired immunoglobulin-like receptor (PIR)-A is involved in activating mast cells through its association with Fc receptor g chain, J. Exp. Med. 188 (1998) 991–995.
[30] X. Han, et al., CD47, a ligand for the macrophage fusion receptor, participates in macrophage multinucleation, J. Biol. Chem. 275 (2000) 37984–37992.
[31] E.F. Vernon-Wilson, et al., CD47 is a ligand for rat macrophage membrane signal regulatory protein SIRP (OX41) and human SIRPalpha 1, Eur. J. Immunol. 30 (2000) 2130–2137.
[32] P.A. Oldenborg, et al., Role of CD47 as a marker of self on red blood cells, Science 288 (2000) 2051–2054.
[33] E. Tomasello, et al., Association of signal-regulatory proteins beta with KARAP/DAP-12, Eur. J. Immunol. 30 (2000) 2147–2156.

[34] J. Dietrich, et al., Cutting edge: signal-regulatory protein beta1 is a DAP12-associated activating receptor expressed in myeloid cells, J. Immunol. 164 (2000) 9–12.
[35] L. Borges, et al., A family of human lymphoid and myeloid Ig-like receptors, some of which bind to MHC class I molecules, J. Immunol. 159 (1997) 5192–5196.
[36] M. Colonna, et al., A common inhibitory receptor for major histocompatibility complex class I molecules on human lymphoid and myelomonocytic cells, J. Exp. Med. 186 (1997) 1809–1818.
[37] H. Nakajima, et al., Human myeloid cells express an activating ILT receptor (ILT1) that associates with Fc receptor g-chain, J. Immunol. 162 (1999) 5–8.

International Congress Series 1285 (2005) 68–77

www.ics-elsevier.com

Nod1 signaling to extracellular mucosal bacteria in epithelial cells

R.L. Ferrero [a,*], D.J. Philpott [b]

[a] *Department of Microbiology, Monash University, Building 53, Wellington Road, Clayton 3800, VIC, Australia*
[b] *Group d'Immunité Innée et Signalisation, Institut Pasteur, Paris, France*

Abstract. The mechanisms by which epithelial cells discriminate between pathogenic and commensal micro-organisms are still poorly understood. Nod1 (CARD4), a cytosolic molecule with homology to plant resistance proteins, was shown to initiate innate immune signaling in epithelial cells to invasive bacterial pathogens. We recently identified Nod1 as also playing a key role in epithelial cell responses to a non-invasive bacterium, *Helicobacter pylori*. The Nod1 signaling cascade was triggered by *H. pylori* delivery of peptidoglycan, a component of its cell wall, to host cells. It appeared that Nod1 recognition of *H. pylori* might represent a novel paradigm of host innate immune "sensing" of non-invasive bacteria that cause mucosal inflammation. We have tested this hypothesis by investigating epithelial cell responses to intestinal *Helicobacter* spp., several of which are known to induce colitis in animal hosts. Of the various isolates tested, only one (*Helicobacter muridarum*) induced Nod1-dependent signaling in intestinal epithelial cells. *H. muridarum* is a member of the intestinal flora of conventional rodents, yet has previously been associated with the development of colitis in mice. Taken together, the findings suggest that Nod1 may play a key role in the etiology of a variety of inflammatory conditions triggered by the host microflora.

Keywords: Nod1/CARD4; *Helicobacter pylori*; *Helicobacter* spp.; Innate immunity; Peptidoglycan

1. Introduction

Epithelial cells have long been considered to act as a physical barrier that protects the integrity of epidermal or mucosal surfaces. It is now clear that these cells also play an

* Corresponding author. Tel.: +61 3 9905 4842; fax: +61 3 9905 4811.
E-mail address: Richard.Ferrero@med.monash.edu.au (R.L. Ferrero).

doi:10.1016/j.ics.2005.07.097

active role in host defense. Indeed, epithelial cells express a variety of signaling molecules [1] that are essential components of the mammalian innate immune system [2]. The recognition by these molecules of conserved structures on micro-organisms represents a key event in the initiation of innate immune responses against microbial aggression. Such responses are thought to play a dual role in host defense by mediating effector mechanisms that directly limit pathogen dissemination, and by regulating the development of adaptive immunity. These responses are triggered by molecules, often referred to as pathogen recognition molecules (PRMs), which sense invariant microbial structures via leucine-rich repeat motifs (LRR) situated at their C-terminus. Microbial stimulation of PRMs initiates intracellular signaling cascades in host cells leading to the activation of eukaryotic transcription factors, such as nuclear factor-κB (NF-κB). These factors in turn regulate changes in gene expression that culminate in the activation of various pro-inflammatory and host defense molecules, including cytokines/chemokines, co-stimulatory molecules, and adhesion factors.

The best characterized PRMs, Toll-like receptor 2 (TLR2) and TLR4, are transmembrane molecules that recognize bacterial lipoproteins (or lipoteichoic acid) and lipopolysaccharide (LPS), respectively. More recently, a family of cytoplasmic PRMs, termed Nod proteins, has been discovered [3]. Nod proteins share homology with the plant resistance R proteins and Apaf-1/Ced-4 apoptosis regulators, and play a major role in the detection of bacteria [4,5]. Two of the members of this family, Nod1 (CARD4) and Nod2 (CARD15), have been shown to detect bacteria through different peptidoglycan motifs; the former senses the disaccharide-tripeptide motif of Gram-negative bacterial peptidoglycan [6,7], whereas the latter is a general sensor of peptidoglycan through its detection of muramyl dipeptide (MDP), the minimal bioactive motif of peptidoglycan [8]).

Pathogen recognition molecules are widely expressed within the gastrointestinal tract [1,9]. Moreover, intestinal epithelial cells have been shown to utilize a diverse array of TLRs to respond to microbial products. Nevertheless, it has yet to be elucidated how such cells, which are in constant contact with a large and diverse microflora, are able to distinguish between the products of pathogenic micro-organisms and those of commensal organisms in vivo. Recently, it was shown that TLR recognition of the commensal microflora could actually serve a beneficial role, by regulating intestinal epithelial homeostasis and protection from injury, suggesting broader functions for these molecules beyond simply host defense [10]. Conversely, micro-organisms that are able to overcome the epithelial barrier through cell invasion are recognized as pathogens, and thus trigger strong pro-inflammatory responses in host cells. Significantly, the invasive intestinal pathogens *Shigella flexneri* and enteroinvasive *Escherichia coli* were shown to not signal through transmembrane TLRs in epithelial cells, but instead to be recognized by the cytosolic host molecule, Nod1 [11,12]. Nod1 responds to peptidoglycan which was presented within the cytoplasmic compartment of epithelial cells by these invasive bacteria. Until recently, it was unclear how pathogenic bacteria that are non-invasive might induce innate immune responses in epithelial cells. This review will focus on the role of Nod1 as an important signaling molecule in epithelial cell recognition of mucosal pathogens that cause inflammation in the gastrointestinal tracts of animal hosts.

2. *Helicobacter pylori* infection of gastric epithelial cells: a paradigm for extracellular mucosal pathogens

H. pylori infects the stomach of more than half of the world's population and is a major etiological factor in the development of gastritis, peptic ulcer disease and gastric cancer in humans. Gastritis is characterized by the presence of mixed populations of polymorphonuclear and mononuclear cells in the gastric mucosa. The initial trigger for this inflammatory condition is likely to be mediated by epithelial cells, which provide a first line of defense against bacterial aggression. Although *H. pylori* has been reported to invade epithelial cell lines in vitro [13], this bacterium is most commonly found adhering to epithelial cells in gastric biopsies.

2.1. Surface TLRs are not involved in epithelial cell responses to H. pylori

Given the extracellular location of *H. pylori* bacteria, logic would dictate that a transmembrane TLR would most likely be responsible for epithelial cell recognition of this pathogen. Indeed, TLR4 molecules expressed by epithelial cells were shown to respond to *E. coli* LPS [9,14] and early reports indicated that gastric pit cells isolated from guinea pigs were responsive to *H. pylori* LPS [15]. Gastric epithelial cell lines that normally develop strong pro-inflammatory responses to stimulation by *H. pylori* bacteria were, however, non-responsive to *H. pylori* LPS, even when relatively high concentrations (1 μg/ml) of this endotoxin were added to the cells [16]. Consistent with this, a TLR4-neutralising antibody did not block *H. pylori*-induced secretion of an NF-κB-dependent chemokine, CXC chemokine ligand 8 (CXCL-8; also known as interleukin-8), in the AGS gastric epithelial cell line [17]. Although *tlr4* mRNA was detected in human gastric epithelial cell lines, including AGS cells [16,17], these cells lacked cell membrane-bound CD14 [16,18]. The latter is critical for LPS loading onto complexes comprising TLR4 and its co-receptor, MD-2. The absence of TLR4 expression in primary human gastric epithelial cells [16] further reinforces the notion that this PRM is unlikely to play a significant role in epithelial cell responses to *H. pylori.*

H. pylori LPS was shown to have a 500- to 1000-fold lower endotoxic activity than that of a classical Gram-negative bacterium, *Salmonella typhimurium* [19]. The very low activity of *H. pylori* LPS in biological assays was attributed to its unusual phosphorylation pattern and lipid A acylation [19]. In common with other atypical LPS molecules, *H. pylori* LPS appears to be recognized by TLR2, and not by TLR4 [20,21]. TLR2 signaling to *H. pylori* was assessed by measuring NF-κB-luciferase reporter activity in HEK293 cells transfected to express exogenous TLR2 [20,21]. In contrast to intestinal cells [14,22,23], HEK293 cells do not produce this PRM [7,18,24] and therefore do not normally respond to stimulation with TLR2 agonists [7,24]. Nevertheless, HEK293 cells are as responsive to stimulation by *H. pylori* bacteria as AGS gastric epithelial cells [18,25]. Thus, further work is warranted to determine the contribution of TLR2 to epithelial cell responses to *H. pylori*.

Another important surface-associated PRM in epithelial cell responses to Gram-negative pathogens is the flagellin-sensing TLR5 molecule. Several lines of experimental evidence, however, suggest that this molecule is not involved in host cell recognition of *H. pylori*. Firstly, isogenic *H. pylori* mutants devoid of flagellar proteins were still able to induce pro-inflammatory responses in various gastric epithelial cell lines shown to express *tlr5* mRNA [26,27]. Secondly, purified native and recombinant *H. pylori* flagellar preparations were very poor inducers of CXCL-8 synthesis in gastric or intestinal epithelial cell lines, when compared with *Salmonella typhimurium* flagellin, a known TLR5 agonist [26,27]. Thirdly, *H. pylori* flagellin was shown to harbor a polypeptide domain that facilitates its evasion from TLR5 recognition [28]. Taken together, it is possible to exclude a significant role for the major Gram-negative sensing molecules (TLR2, TLR4 or TLR5) in epithelial cell recognition of *H. pylori* bacteria. Nevertheless, the possibility that other TLRs may be involved in signaling to this pathogen still needs to be formally excluded.

2.2. *H. pylori initiates pro-inflammatory responses in epithelial cells from the inside*

H. pylori strains harboring a pathogenicity island ("*cag*PAI") are particularly effective at inducing NF-κB activation and CXCL-8 synthesis in gastric epithelial cells in vitro [29,30]. These strains are also more frequently associated with the severe forms of *H. pylori*-related disease [31]. The *cag*PAI was shown to encode a type IV secretion (TFSS) apparatus, capable of translocating at least one effector molecule into gastric epithelial cells [32]. While it appeared that the translocation or delivery of an effector molecule by the *H. pylori* TFSS was required for the induction of pro-inflammatory responses in gastric epithelial cells, the precise mechanism was unknown.

It was recently reported that Nod1/CARD4, a cytosolic PRM with homology to plant resistance proteins, mediated epithelial cell responses to the invasive bacteria, *S. flexneri* and enteroinvasive *E. coli* [11,12]. Given that a functional TFSS was required for *H. pylori*-mediated induction of pro-inflammatory responses in epithelial cells, and that surface-associated PRMs did not appear to play a significant role in *H. pylori* recognition, we speculated that intracellular Nod1 might be involved in epithelial cell responses to this gastric pathogen. This hypothesis was tested in HEK293 cells, which express endogenous levels of Nod1 [7,12,25], but which do not express TLR2 nor TLR4 [7,18,24]. Consistent with previous work in gastric epithelial cells, we showed that the induction of NF-κB activation in HEK293 cells by *H. pylori* was mediated by a *cag*PAI-dependent mechanism [25]. Moreover, *H. pylori*-induced NF-κB activation in HEK293 cells was significantly diminished following co-transfection of cells with a Nod1 dominant negative construct. Thus, Nod1 appeared to be the PRM involved in epithelial cell signaling to this bacterium. This finding was confirmed using small interfering RNA (siRNA) specific to human Nod1 [25].

2.3. *H. pylori peptidoglycan is recognized by Nod1 in epithelial cells*

Nod1 specifically recognizes a disaccharide-tripeptide motif of bacterial peptidoglycan which is found almost exclusively in Gram-negative bacteria [6,7]. In agreement with this, *H. pylori* peptidoglycan, which was delivered into HEK293 cells using a liposome-based transfection procedure, induced NF-κB reporter activity in the cells [25]. Significantly, *H. pylori* LPS that was delivered within cells had no effect on NF-κB reporter activity. Moreover, an *H. pylori* mutant that released lower amounts of the disaccharide-tripeptide motif into the surrounding medium was significantly affected in its ability to induce pro-inflammatory responses in epithelial cells. Bacterial invasion of the cells was not required for these host responses, suggesting that the *cag*PAI secretion apparatus might serve to deliver *H. pylori* peptidoglycan into the cytosol of host cells. This was confirmed by performing β-imager analyzes on AGS cells that were co-cultured with *H. pylori* bacteria in which the disaccharide-tripeptide motif of peptidoglycan had been tritiated. As compared with *H. pylori* bacteria with a functional TFSS, bacteria in which the system had been rendered non-functional by genetic disruption or heat-inactivation delivered significantly reduced (50–93%) levels of ^{3}H labeled material to the cells [25]. These data confirm the importance of a functional *cag*PAI for peptidoglycan delivery to host epithelial cells and are consistent with the findings above regarding the role of internalized *H. pylori* peptidoglycan in NF-κB responses of host cells. These are the first experimental data suggestive of bacterium-mediated translocation of peptidoglycan in epithelial cells.

2.4. Nod1 signaling in epithelial cells and host defense

Pathogen recognition molecules are thought to play a key role in host defense to microbial pathogens. The role of Nod1 in host defense against *H. pylori* was investigated in Nod1-deficient and wild-type counterpart mice. Mice deficient in Nod1 were found to be significantly more susceptible to infection by *cag*PAI-positive *H. pylori* bacteria, when compared with wild-type animals [25]. In contrast, no differences were observed in colonization levels between Nod1-deficient and wild-type animals for *H. pylori* lacking a functional TFSS. These data indicated a function for Nod1 in host defense against *H. pylori* bacteria with a functional TFSS. It also provided indirect evidence to suggest that murine Nod1 is capable of recognizing *H. pylori* peptidoglycan. This was confirmed by measuring in primary gastric epithelial cells from Nod1-deficient and wild-type mice the production of MIP-2, an NF-κB-dependent CXC chemokine with analogous biological activities to human CXCL-8 [25]. The cells from Nod1-deficient mice produced lower levels of MIP-2 in response to stimulation with *H. pylori* bacteria [25].

Despite recent advances in knowledge concerning the role of PRMs in innate immune signaling to microbial pathogens, it is still unclear how these signaling processes contribute to host defense mechanisms. Amongst the most important effectors of the innate immune system are microbicidal compounds. An example of this are a family of anti-microbial peptides, the defensins, which are widely distributed amongst the phagocytic and epithelial cells of mammalian hosts [33,34]. Studies on Nod2 have shown that this PRM is required for the expression of intestinal anti-microbial peptides (α-defensins and cryptdins) [35,36]. Preliminary studies suggest that members of the family of anti-microbial peptides, the β-defensins [33,34], which are known to contribute significantly to innate host defenses in epithelial cells, may be regulated by Nod1 signaling to *H. pylori* (unpublished data). This finding would provide a mechanistic basis for the increased susceptibility of Nod1-deficient mice to *H. pylori* infection.

We propose that Nod1 recognition of *H. pylori* in epithelial cells represents a paradigm for other infectious causes of mucosal inflammation due to non-invasive pathogens.

3. The role of the host microflora in the induction of chronic intestinal inflammation

Idiopathic inflammatory disorders of the lower gastrointestinal tract, generally referred to as inflammatory bowel disease (IBD), represent a substantial cause of human morbidity, affecting up to 0.2% of the population in developed countries [37]. These disorders have a multi-factorial etiology involving environmental, genetic and immunological factors.

Deregulated mucosal immune responses to the host's microflora represent a major initiator in the formation of the chronic intestinal inflammation observed in human IBD [38]. Altered host recognition of microbial components has been reported to occur as a result of structural modifications in the innate immune signaling molecule Nod2. Specifically, it was shown that mutations in the LRR-coding region of *NOD2* render the molecule insensitive to bacteria or their products, predisposing the host to the development of a form of IBD known as Crohn's disease (CD) [39,40]. Several mouse models can reproduce the intestinal lesions (colitis) observed in human IBD. While the majority of these models utilize animals with genetic defects in specific immunological functions, all were dependent on an intestinal microflora for the development of colitis [38]. These data reinforce the role of the host microflora in the development of chronic intestinal inflammation.

Bacterial species forming part of the indigenous microflora of mice have been shown to induce colitis in this animal host. These include *Helicobacter bilis* and *Helicobacter hepaticus*, two species that are phylogenetically related to *H. pylori* [41]. *H. bilis* and *H. hepaticus* were shown to induce particularly severe forms of colitis and typhlocolitis (inflammation of the cecum) in IL-10-deficient mice [42,43]. These bacterial species have also been associated with hepatitis, and even hepatocarcinoma, in certain mouse strains [1]. For the majority of intestinal *Helicobacter* spp., however, the role of these bacteria in pathogenesis has yet to be clearly defined. One such isolate is *Helicobacter muridarum*, which was initially described as a member of the normal flora of conventional rodents [44,45]. More recent evidence suggests that this bacterium can cause colitis in mice [46].

3.1. Nod1 signaling to intestinal Helicobacter spp. associated with colitis

Animal hosts infected with intestinal *Helicobacter* spp. develop colitis, yet the mechanism by which these bacteria induce inflammatory lesions is currently unknown. For this reason, we investigated epithelial cell responses to mouse and human intestinal *Helicobacter* spp. The *Helicobacter* mouse pathogens, *H. bilis* and *H. hepaticus*, up-regulated CXC chemokine (KC, MIP-2) production in a murine intestinal epithelial cell line (m-IC_{cl2}; unpublished data). These chemokines are key promoters of leukocyte recruitment in mice [47,48] and are likely to represent important mediators of the inflammatory responses observed in *Helicobacter* colitis models. Most strikingly, it was *H. muridarum*, and not the two pathogenic species, that consistently induced the highest levels of CXC chemokine production in these cells. These responses were dependent on direct contact between the bacteria and the epithelial cells. The ability of *H. muridarum* to induce pro-inflammatory responses in epithelial cell lines is consistent with the findings from animal model studies [46,49,50]. It is particularly noteworthy that mice monoassociated with *H. muridarum*, but not those colonized with other members of the intestinal microflora of mice, exhibited an accelerated development of IBD-like lesions in a $CD45RB^{high}$ $CD4^{+}$ T cell transfer model of experimental colitis [46]. It was suggested that *H. muridarum* could serve as a "provocateur" of IBD in this model.

Consistent with the data of Hornef and co-workers [14], the m-IC_{cl2} cells were responsive to *H. muridarum* LPS. The kinetics and magnitude of the cellular responses to this molecule were, however, different to those induced by live *H. muridarum* bacteria, suggesting the presence of an LPS-independent mechanism in epithelial cell responses to *H. muridarum* (unpublished data). This mechanism was investigated in HEK293 cells using intestinal *Helicobacter* spp. of murine (*H. bilis*, *H. hepaticus*, *H. muridarum*) and human (*Helicobacter cinaedi*, *Helicobacter fennelliae*) origins. Strikingly, *H. muridarum* was the only one of these isolates to induce significant levels of NF-κB reporter activity and CXCL-8 production in HEK293 cells. Such responses were inhibited in a dose-dependent manner by co-transfection of the cells with dominant-negative Nod1-encoding DNA, thus implicating Nod1 in epithelial cell signaling to *H. muridarum*.

The mechanism by which *H. muridarum* induces Nod1 signaling in HEK293 cells is, at present, unknown. In contrast to *H. pylori*, it is unlikely that *H. muridarum* utilizes a TFSS to deliver peptidoglycan to host cells as genomic studies have failed to reveal the presence of a homolog of the *H. pylori* TFSS in this bacterium (unpublished data). Furthermore, *H. muridarum* bacteria do not appear to invade epithelial cell lines to any significant degree in vitro (unpublished data). The fact that this bacterium seems to be less efficient at inducing NF-κB reporter activity in HEK293 cells, when compared with TFSS-positive *H. pylori* bacteria, suggests that the former may use an alternative strategy to stimulate Nod1 signaling in epithelial cells. Further studies are needed to identify the strategies by which non-invasive bacteria trigger epithelial cell responses via the signaling molecule Nod1.

3.2. Is there cross-talk between Nod1 and TLR signaling pathways?

Primary intestinal epithelial cells from Nod1-deficient mice produced significantly augmented levels of CXC chemokines in response to stimulation with *H. muridarum*, when compared with cells from congenic wild-type animals. This differs to the findings reported previously for *H. pylori* [25]. The difference between the studies may be attributed to the differing roles of Nod1 in pathogen recognition in these two infection models. For example, it is possible that besides playing a direct role in *H. muridarum* recognition, Nod1 may play an additional role in the down-regulation of TLR-mediated responses to this bacterium. In contrast, TLRs are unlikely to play a major role in epithelial cell responses to *H. pylori*. The proposed regulation of TLR signaling by Nod1 is consistent with recent studies in which exaggerated responses were reported in Nod2-defective host cells stimulated with bacterial components [51,52]. Defects in Nod and/or TLR signaling pathways may affect the ability of host cells to recognize and respond to the intestinal microflora, thus favoring the development of inflammatory conditions such as IBD. Indeed, it was reported that *tlr4* gene polymorphisms increased the relative risk of IBD development in individuals with CD-associated *NOD2* variants [53].

4. Conclusions and future perspectives

The identification of Nod1 in host recognition of *H. pylori* infection has important implications for an understanding of the mechanisms by which epithelial cells distinguish between pathogenic and commensal micro-organisms [25]. Indeed, this work has demonstrated for the first time how the internalization of a non-protein microbial product (peptidoglycan) per se might act as an alarm signal for the induction of host immune responses against microbial aggression. The implication of Nod1 in epithelial cell responses to *H. muridarum* is significant because it provides a second example in which Nod1 has been shown to be involved in host recognition of a non-invasive micro-organism capable of causing mucosal inflammation in animal hosts [46,49,50]. This work has also demonstrated how, under certain circumstances, Nod1 recognition of a member of the intestinal microflora of conventional animals may lead to the induction of pro-inflammatory responses in the host. A recent study provided evidence for the involvement of Nod1 in the genesis of inflammatory lesions of the intestine. It was observed that certain polymorphisms in the LRR-encoding exons of *NOD1* could be linked to the development of IBD, suggesting that structural changes in the microbe-sensing LRR regions of this PRM may alter the reactivity of the protein to bacterial components [54]. This would be expected to result in the induction of inappropriate responses by host cells to the microflora.

A major challenge for the future will be to better understand how Nod1, indeed PRMs in general, recognize and respond to microbial products. Moreover, it will be important to determine how modifications in these products contribute to altered pathogen recognition by signaling molecules such as Nod1. Another important challenge for the future will be to clarify the roles of these molecules in the regulation of host immune response functions, in particular, those associated with host defense against microbial infections. Given the findings of a recent study in mice with defective TLR signaling [10], it is likely that PRMs have evolved to participate in a diverse array of normal host cell functions.

References

[1] F. Backhed, M. Hornef, Toll-like receptor 4-mediated signaling by epithelial surfaces: necessity or threat?, Microbes Infect. 5 (11) (2003) 951–959.

[2] S. Akira, K. Hoshino, T. Kaisho, The role of Toll-like receptors and MyD88 in innate immune responses, J. Endotoxin Res. 6 (5) (2000) 383–387.

[3] N. Inohara, et al., Human Nod1 confers responsiveness to bacterial lipopolysaccharides, J. Biol. Chem. 276 (4) (2001) 2551–2554.

[4] S.E. Girardin, P.J. Sansonetti, D.J. Philpott, Intracellular vs. extracellular recognition of pathogens—common concepts in mammals and flies, Trends Microbiol. 10 (4) (2002) 193–199.

[5] N. Inohara, G. Nunez, NODs: intracellular proteins involved in inflammation and apoptosis, Nat. Rev., Immunol. 3 (5) (2003) 371–382.

[6] M. Chamaillard, et al., An essential role for NOD1 in host recognition of bacterial peptidoglycan containing diaminopimelic acid, Nat. Immunol. 4 (7) (2003) 702–707.

[7] S.E. Girardin, et al., Nod1 detects a unique muropeptide from gram-negative bacterial peptidoglycan, Science 300 (5625) (2003) 1584–1587.

[8] S.E. Girardin, et al., Peptidoglycan molecular requirements allowing detection by Nod1 and Nod2, J. Biol. Chem. 278 (43) (2003) 41702–41708.

[9] E. Cario, et al., Commensal-associated molecular patterns induce selective Toll-like receptor-trafficking from apical membrane to cytoplasmic compartments in polarized intestinal epithelium, Am. J. Pathol. 160 (1) (2002) 165–173.

[10] S. Rakoff-Nahoum, et al., Recognition of commensal microflora by Toll-like receptors is required for intestinal homeostasis, Cell 118 (2) (2004) 229–241.

[11] S.E. Girardin, et al., CARD4/Nod1 mediates NF-kappaB and JNK activation by invasive *Shigella flexneri*, EMBO Rep. 2 (8) (2001) 736–742.

[12] J.G. Kim, S.J. Lee, M.F. Kagnoff, Nod1 is an essential signal transducer in intestinal epithelial cells infected with bacteria that avoid recognition by Toll-like receptors, Infect. Immun. 72 (3) (2004) 1487–1495.

[13] M.R. Amieva, et al., *Helicobacter pylori* enter and survive within multivesicular vacuoles of epithelial cells, Cell. Microbiol. 4 (10) (2002) 677–690.
[14] M.W. Hornef, et al., Toll-like receptor 4 resides in the Golgi apparatus and colocalizes with internalized lipopolysaccharide in intestinal epithelial cells, J. Exp. Med. 195 (5) (2002) 559–570.
[15] T. Kawahara, et al., Type I *Helicobacter pylori* lipopolysaccharide stimulates Toll-like receptor 4 and activates mitogen oxidase 1 in gastric pit cells, Infect. Immun. 69 (7) (2001) 4382–4389.
[16] F. Bäckhed, et al., Gastric mucosal recognition of *Helicobacter pylori* is independent of Toll-like receptor 4, J. Infect. Dis. 187 (2003) 829–836.
[17] B. Su, et al., *Helicobacter pylori* activates Toll-like receptor 4 expression in gastrointestinal epithelial cells, Infect. Immun. 71 (6) (2003) 3496–3502.
[18] S. Maeda, et al., Distinct mechanism of *Helicobacter pylori*-mediated NF-kB activation between gastric cancer cells and monocytic cells, J. Biol. Chem. 276 (48) (2001) 44856–44864.
[19] A. Muotiala, et al., Low biological activity of *Helicobacter pylori* lipopolysaccharide, Infect. Immun. 60 (4) (1992) 1714–1716.
[20] L. Mandell, et al., Intact Gram-negative *Helicobacter pylori*, *Helicobacter felis*, and *Helicobacter hepaticus* bacteria activate innate immunity via Toll-like receptor 2 but not Toll-like receptor 4, Infect. Immun. 72 (11) (2004) 6446–6454.
[21] M.F. Smith Jr., et al., Toll-like receptor (TLR) 2 and TLR5, but not TLR4, are required for *Helicobacter pylori*-induced NF-kappa B activation and chemokine expression by epithelial cells, J. Biol. Chem. 278 (35) (2003) 32552–32560.
[22] E. Cario, et al., Lipopolysaccharide activates distinct signaling pathways in intestinal epithelial cell lines expressing Toll-like receptors, J. Immunol. 164 (2) (2000) 966–972.
[23] M. Hershberg, The epithelial cell cytoskeleton and intracellular trafficking: V. Polarized compartmentalization of antigen processing and Toll-like receptor signaling in intestinal epithelial cells, Am. J. Physiol.: Gasterointest. Liver Physiol. 283 (4) (2002) 833–839.
[24] M. Fujita, et al., Involvement of leucine residues at positions 107, 112, and 115 in a leucine-rich repeat motif of human Toll-like receptor 2 in the recognition of diacylated lipoproteins and lipopeptides and *Staphylococcus aureus* peptidoglycans, J. Immunol. 171 (7) (2003) 3675–3683.
[25] J. Viala, et al., Nod1 responds to peptidoglycan delivered by the *Helicobacter pylori* cag pathogenicity island, Nat. Immunol. 5 (2004) 1166–1174.
[26] A.T. Gewirtz, et al., *Helicobacter pylori* flagellin evades Toll-like receptor 5-mediated innate immunity, J. Infect. Dis. 189 (10) (2004) 1914–1920.
[27] S.K. Lee, et al., *Helicobacter pylori* flagellins have very low intrinsic activity to stimulate human gastric epithelial cells via TLR5, Microbes Infect. 5 (15) (2003) 1345–1356.
[28] E. Andersen-Nissen, et al., Evasion of Toll-like receptor 5 by flagellated bacteria, Proc. Natl. Acad. Sci. U. S. A. 102 (26) (2005) 9247–9252.
[29] C. Audibert, et al., Correlation between IL-8 induction, cagA status and vacA genotypes in 153 French *Helicobacter pylori* isolates, Res. Microbiol. 151 (3) (2000) 191–200.
[30] S. Backert, et al., Functional analysis of the cag pathogenicity island in *Helicobacter pylori* isolates from patients with gastritis, peptic ulcer, and gastric cancer, Infect. Immun. 72 (2) (2004) 1043–1056.
[31] R.M. Peek Jr., M.J. Blaser, *Helicobacter pylori* and gastrointestinal tract adenocarcinomas, Nat. Rev., Cancer 2 (1) (2002) 28–37.
[32] S. Odenbreit, et al., Translocation of *Helicobacter pylori* CagA into gastric epithelial cells by type IV secretion, Science 287 (2000) 1497–1500.
[33] R.N. Cunliffe, Y.R. Mahida, Expression and regulation of antimicrobial peptides in the gastrointestinal tract, J. Leukoc. Biol. 75 (1) (2004) 49–58.
[34] T. Ganz, Defensins: antimicrobial peptides of innate immunity, Nat. Rev., Immunol. 3 (9) (2003) 710–720.
[35] K.S. Kobayashi, et al., Nod2-dependent regulation of innate and adaptive immunity in the intestinal tract, Science 307 (2005) 731–734.
[36] J. Wehkamp, et al., NOD2 (CARD15) mutations in Crohn's disease are associated with diminished mucosal a-defensin expression, Gut 53 (2004) 1658–1664.
[37] D.K. Podolsky, Inflammatory bowel disease (1), N. Engl. J. Med. 325 (13) (1991) 928–937.
[38] R.S. Blumberg, L.J. Saubermann, W. Strober, Animal models of mucosal inflammation and their relation to human inflammatory bowel disease, Curr. Opin. Immunol. 11 (6) (1999) 648–656.

[39] J.P. Hugot, et al., Association of NOD2 leucine-rich repeat variants with susceptibility to Crohn's disease, Nature 411 (2001) 599–603.

[40] Y. Ogura, et al., A frameshift mutation in NOD2 associated with susceptibility to Crohn's disease, Nature 411 (6837) (2001) 603–606.

[41] R.L. Ferrero, J.G. Fox, In vivo modeling of *Helicobacter*-associated gastrointestinal diseases, in: H.L.T. Mobley, G.L. Mendz, S.L. Hazell (Eds.), *Helicobacter pylori*: Physiology and Genetics, ASM Press, Washington, DC, 2001, pp. 565–582.

[42] A. Burich, et al., *Helicobacter*-induced inflammatory bowel disease in IL-10- and T cell-deficient mice, Am. J. Physiol.: Gasterointest. Liver Physiol. 281 (2001) G764–G778.

[43] M.C. Kullberg, et al., *Helicobacter hepaticus*-induced colitis in interleukin-10 (IL-10)-deficient mice: cytokine requirements for the induction and maintenance of intestinal inflammation, Infect. Immun. 69 (7) (2001) 4232–4241.

[44] M. Phillips, A. Lee, W.D. Leach, The mucosa-associated microflora of the rat intestine: a study of normal distribution and magnesium sulphate induced diarrhoea, Aust. J. Exp. Biol. Med. Sci. 56 (6) (1978) 649–662.

[45] M.W. Phillips, A. Lee, Isolation and characterization of a spiral bacterium from the crypts of rodent gastrointestinal tracts, Appl. Environ. Microbiol. 45 (2) (1983) 675–683.

[46] H.Q. Jiang, et al., Monoassociation of SCID mice with *Helicobacter muridarum*, but not four other enterics, provokes IBD upon receipt of T cells, Gastroenterology 122 (5) (2002) 1346–1354.

[47] Y. Ohtsuka, et al., MIP-2 secreted by epithelial cells increases neutrophil and lymphocyte recruitment in the mouse intestine, Gut 49 (4) (2001) 526–533.

[48] D.G. Remick, et al., CXC chemokine redundancy ensures local neutrophil recruitment during acute inflammation, Am. J. Pathol. 159 (3) (2001) 1149–1157.

[49] A. Lee, et al., Long term infection of the gastric mucosa with *Helicobacter* species does induce atrophic gastritis in an animal model of *Helicobacter pylori* infection, Zentralbl. Bakteriol. 280 (1–2) (1993) 38–50.

[50] D.M. Queiroz, et al., Spiral bacterium associated with gastric, ileal and caecal mucosa of mice, Lab Anim. 26 (4) (1992) 288–294.

[51] M.G. Netea, et al., NOD2 mediates anti-inflammatory signals induced by TLR2 ligands: implications for Crohn's disease, Eur. J. Immunol. 34 (7) (2004) 2052–2059.

[52] T. Watanabe, et al., NOD2 is a negative regulator of Toll-like receptor 2-mediated T helper type 1 responses, Nat. Immunol. 5 (2004) 800–808.

[53] D. Franchimont, et al., Deficient host-bacteria interactions in inflammatory bowel disease? The Toll-like receptor (TLR)-4 Asp299gly polymorphism is associated with Crohn's disease and ulcerative colitis, Gut 53 (7) (2004) 987–992.

[54] D.P. McGovern, et al., Association between a complex insertion/deletion polymorphism in NOD1 (CARD4) and susceptibility to inflammatory bowel disease, Hum. Mol. Genet. 14 (10) (2005) 1245–1250.

International Congress Series 1285 (2005) 78–83

www.ics-elsevier.com

Fcα/μR, a novel Fc receptor for innate antibodies IgM and IgA

Shin-ichiro Honda [a], Akitomo Miyamoto [a,b], Akira Shibuya [a,*]

[a] *Department of Immunology, Institute of Basic Medical Sciences, Graduate School of Comprehensive Human Sciences and Center for TARA, University of Tsukuba, Japan*

[b] *Subteam for Manipulation of Cell Fate, BioResource Center, RIKEN Tsukuba Institute, Japan*

Abstract. Natural antibody that mainly belongs to IgM class is involved in the prevention of pathogen dissemination to vital organs. However, it has been a mystery how it protects us against infection. We previously identified a novel Fc receptor for IgM and IgA, designated Fcα/μ receptor (Fcα/μR), which might be involved in IgM-mediated immune defenses against infection. Fcα/μR is a new member of Fc receptors family on the chromosome 1. The Fcα/μR is constitutively expressed on the majority of B-lymphocytes and macrophages. The Fcα/μR mediates endocytosis *Staphylococcus aureus*/anti-*S. aureus* IgM antibody immune complexes by B-lymphocytes. These results reveal a new mechanism in the primary stage of immune defense against microbes.

Keywords: IgM; IgA; Fc receptor; Fcα/μ receptor; B cell

1. Introduction

IgM is the first antibody to be produced in a humoral immune response and plays an important role in the primary stage of immunity. In addition, IgM is a major isotype of natural antibodies, which already exist in innate animal and are involved in the prevention of pathogen dissemination to vital organs [1,2]. On the other hand, IgA is a secreted antibody at mucosal membrane and a protection from initial invasion of microbes. However, how these "innate type" of antibodies are involved in immunity has not necessarily been elucidated.

* Corresponding author. 1-1-1 Tennodai, Tsukuba Science-City, Ibaraki 305-8575, Japan. Tel.: +81 29 853 3474; fax: +81 29 853 3410.

E-mail address: ashibuya@md.tsukuba.ac.jp (A. Shibuya).

0531-5131/ © 2005 Published by Elsevier B.V.
doi:10.1016/j.ics.2005.08.038

The antibodies or immune complexes bind to cell surface Fc receptors on hematopoietic cells and play important roles in a wide array of immune responses, including antibody-dependent cellular cytotoxicity, mast cell degranulation, phagocytosis, cell proliferation, antibody secretion and enhancement of antigen presentation [3]. Functional Fc receptors for IgM have been reported on subpopulations of human and rodent T, B and NK cells [4–9]. In contrast to the well-defined Fcγ and Fcε receptors, a gene encoding an Fcμ receptor has not previously been identified, although a polymeric Ig receptor able to bind IgM and IgA has been described [10]. Similarly, although a human Fcα receptor (*CD89*) gene has been reported [11], a homologous rodent Fcα receptor has not yet been found. We have recently cloned a novel Fc receptor for IgM and IgA, designated Fcα/μR [12]. Here, we describe a molecular and functional characteristics of Fcα/μR (Fig. 1).

2. Identification of Fcα/μR gene

To identify an Fc receptor for IgM, we screened COS-7 cells transfected with a cDNA library prepared from the mouse T cell leukemia BW5147 by using a mouse IgM monoclonal antibody (mAb) as a probe. We isolated a cDNA clone of 2361 bp that contains an open reading frame encoding a type I transmembrane protein [12]. A pair of

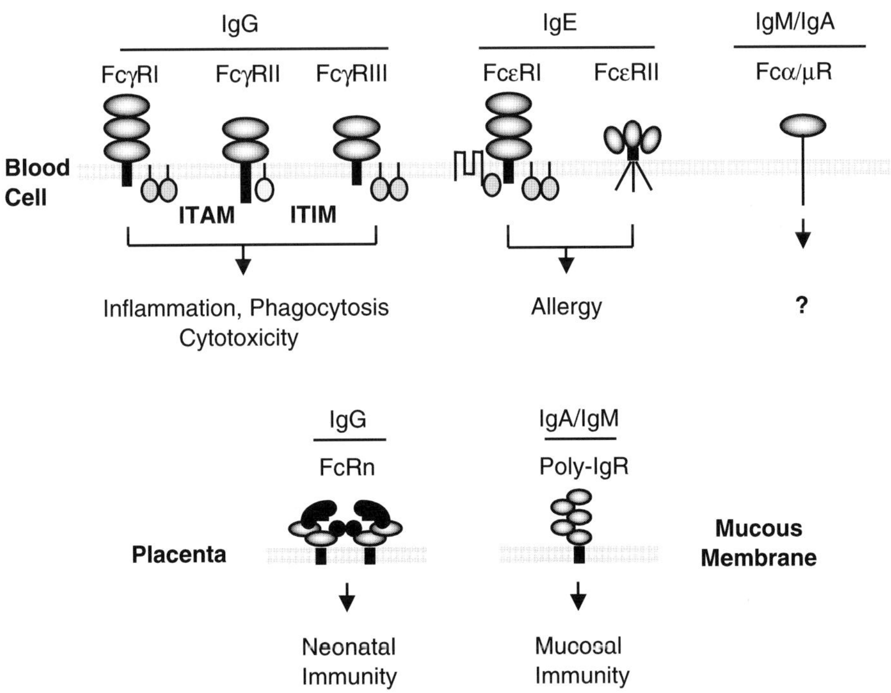

Fig. 1. Structure and function of Fc receptors on hematopoietic cells (FcγRs, FcεR and Fcα/μR) and nonhematopoietic cells (FcRn and poly-IgR).

cysteine residues in the extracellular domain was flanked by the consensus sequence for Ig-like domains, indicating that this molecule, designated mFcα/μR, is a member of the Ig supergene family. A human cDNA with homology to the mFcα/μR (hFcα/μR) was identified in a database [12] and was found to encode a protein with 49% amino acid identity to the mFcα/μR. These genes were mapped by FISH to syntenic regions of mouse chromosome 1 (1F) and human chromosome 1 (1q32.1), near several other Fc receptors, including Fcγ receptors I, II, and III, Fcε receptor, and the polymeric Ig receptor (Fig. 2).

The Fcα/μR is unique, demonstrating no significant homology to other proteins or nucleotide sequences in databases. However, we observed a motif in the Ig-like domain conserved in the first Ig-like domain of the human, bovine, and rodent polymeric Ig receptor, which binds to the Fc of IgA and IgM. Overall, the Fcα/μR has less than 10% amino acid homology with the mouse and human polymeric Ig receptor.

Because *FcγR* has rich diversity of structures encoded by corresponding genes on chromosome 1, a question has been raised whether the *Fcα/μR* is a single or multiple gene-family member [13]. To address this issue, we searched the *Fcα/μR* gene in the database of human genome project. The *Fcα/μR* gene containing the entire coding regions was found in the locus from the 194,644 kbp to 194,653 on chromosome 1 (GenBank and DDBJ accession number; NT004787). However, we could not detect any gene fragments with significant homology with *Fcα/μR* in other chromosomal regions, suggesting that the *Fcα/μR* is a single gene-family member [14]. Comparison of human *Fcα/μR* cDNA with the genome sequence on chromosome 1 in the database revealed that the human *Fcα/μR* gene composed of 6 exons. It is of interest that the human *Fcα/μR* gene is located just 12 kb apart from the locus of the *Poly-IgR* gene [14]. Although Fcα/μR and pIgR have less than 10% amino acid homology each other, both Fc receptors have a conserved motif in the Ig-like domain which binds to the Fc of IgA and IgM [12]. These results suggest the phylogenetic and functional relationship between *Fcα/μR* and *Poly-IgR*.

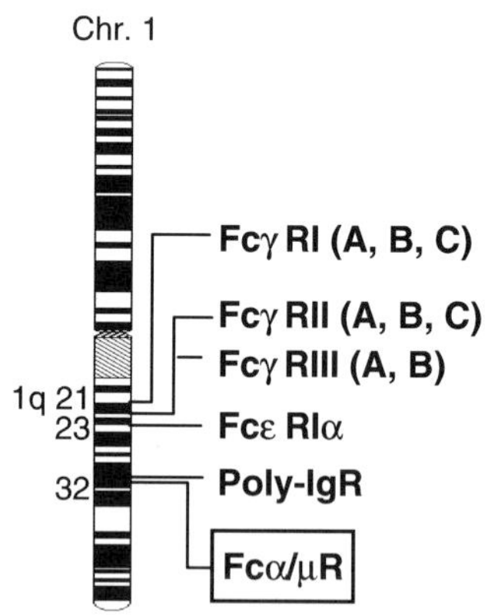

Fig. 2. The human Fcα/μR gene was mapped by FISH to chromosome 1 (1q32.3), near several other Fc receptors, including Fcγ receptors I, II, and III, Fcα receptor, and the polymeric Ig receptor. The mouse Fcα/μR gene was mapped to syntenic region of mouse chromosome 1 (1F).

3. Expression of Fcα/μR

RT-PCR analysis demonstrated that the Fcα/μR transcripts is expressed in several hematopoietic and nonhematopoietic tissues, including thymus, spleen, liver, kidney, small and large intestines, testis, and placenta [12,14]. Northern blot analysis further demonstrated that the Fcα/μR transcripts is abundantly expressed in kidney, small intestine and lymph node [15].

To confirm the cell surface expression of the Fcα/μR protein, we generated a monoclonal antibody against the Fcα/μR. Analysis of spleen cells by flow cytometry showed that the Fcα/μR is expressed on the majority of B cells and macrophages, but not on granulocytes, T cells or NK cells [12]. We compared the Fcα/μR expression between IgD^-, IgM^+ immature and IgD^+, IgM^+ mature B lymphocytes. While IgD^+ mature B lymphocytes expressed a significant amount of the mFcα/μR, it was not expressed on the majority of IgD^- immature B lymphocytes [15]. Further analyses on spleen cells showed that marginal zone B (MZB) cells, defined as $CD21/35^{high}$, $CD23^-$, also expressed the Fcα/μR [24]. Interestingly, Fcα/μR protein was detected not only on hematopoietic cells but also on nonhematopoietic cells, such as follicular dendritic cells [24], and oligodendrocytes and myelin [16], suggesting that Fcα/μR plays an important role for a variety of immune responses.

4. Endocytosis of IgM-immune complex by the mFcα/μR

The cytoplasmic domain of the Fcα/μR contains a di-leucine motif at residues 519 and 520, which has been implicated in endosome and lysosome targeting of diverse proteins and is involved in agonist-induced internalization [17–20]. A di-leucine motif is involved in FcγRIIB-mediated endocytosis [21]. In fact, Fcα/μR mediated endocytosis of IgM-coated fluorescent beads. However, the fluorescent beads were not detected in any of the Ba/F3 transfectants expressing Fcα/μR mutated (L–A) at residues 519, 520 or both [12]. These results indicate that both leucines at residues 519 and 520 are required for endocytosis by the mFcα/μR.

To examine the biological significance of the mFcα/μR expressed on primary B-lymphocytes, mouse spleen cells were incubated with immune complexes composed of FITC-labeled *Staphylococcus aureus* bacteria coated with IgM or IgG anti-*S. aureus* mAbs. $B220^+$ spleen cells cultured with the immune complex of IgM anti-*S. aureus* and FITC-labeled *S. aureus* bacteria contained one or more FITC-labeled *S. aureus* bacteria in the cytoplasm, as determined by immunofluorescent microscopy. By contrast, IgG immune complex of *S. aureus* was not detected in $B220^+$ spleen cells [12]. These results indicate that the mFcα/μR mediates endocytosis of IgM-coated microbial pathogens.

5. Concluding remarks

Previous reports demonstrated that mice deficient in the secretory form of IgM exhibit delayed development of specific IgG antibodies to T cell-dependent foreign antigens [22] and dissemination of micropathogens in peripheral organs but not in secondary lymphoid organs [23], suggesting that the Fcα/μR may play an essential role in the priming of helper T lymphocytes in secondary lymphoid organs and in the immune defense against bacteria in peripheral organs. To explore in vivo role of Fcα/μR in immune responses, we have recently established Fcα/μR-deficient and -transgenic mice. These mice suggested that Fcα/μR plays an important role in immune responses against T-independent antigens and is involved in development of autoimmune diseases [24]. Further studies are required to clarify a molecular basis of Fcα/μR function in immune responses in these mice.

References

[1] M.R. Ehrenstein, H.T. Cook, M.S. Neuberger, Deficiency in serum immunoglobulin (Ig)M predisposes to development of IgG autoantibodies, J. Exp. Med. 191 (7) (2000) 1253–1258.
[2] M. Boes, et al., Accelerated development of IgG autoantibodies and autoimmune disease in the absence of secreted IgM, Proc. Natl. Acad. Sci. U. S. A. 97 (3) (2000) 1184–1189.
[3] J.V. Ravetch, R.A. Clynes, Divergent roles for Fc receptors and complement in vivo, Annu. Rev. Immunol. 16 (1998) 421–432.
[4] C.A. Whelan, A functional role for Fc mu receptors on human lymphocytes, Immunol. Lett. 3 (4) (1981) 249–254.
[5] L. Ercolani, et al., Expression of Fc mu receptors by human T lymphocytes: effects of enzymes, metabolic inhibitors, and X-irradiation, J. Immunol. 127 (5) (1981) 2044–2051.
[6] A. Mathur, R.G. Lynch, G. Kohler, Expression, distribution and specificity of Fc receptors for IgM on murine B cells, J. Immunol. 141 (6) (1988) 1855–1862.
[7] T. Ohno, et al., Biochemical nature of an Fc mu receptor on human B-lineage cells, J. Exp. Med. 172 (4) (1990) 1165–1175.
[8] L. Pricop, et al., Characterization of the Fc mu receptor on human natural killer cells. Interaction with its physiologic ligand, human normal IgM, specificity of binding, and functional effects, J. Immunol. 151 (6) (1993) 3018–3029.
[9] T. Nakamura, et al., Characterization of an IgM Fc-binding receptor on human T cells, J. Immunol. 151 (12) (1993) 6933–6941.
[10] K.E. Mostov, Transepithelial transport of immunoglobulins, Annu. Rev. Immunol. 12 (1994) 63–84.
[11] C.R. Maliszewski, et al., Expression cloning of a human Fc receptor for IgA, J. Exp. Med. 172 (6) (1990) 1665–1672.
[12] A. Shibuya, et al., Fc alpha/mu receptor mediates endocytosis of IgM-coated microbes, Nat. Immunol. 1 (5) (2000) 441–446.
[13] J.P. Kinet, P. Launay, Fc alpha/microR: single member or first born in the family?, Nat. Immunol. 1 (5) (2000) 371–372.
[14] Y. Shimizu, et al., Fc(alpha)/mu receptor is a single gene-family member closely related to polymeric immunoglobulin receptor encoded on chromosome 1, Immunogenetics 53 (8) (2001) 709–711.
[15] N. Sakamoto, et al., A novel Fc receptor for IgA and IgM is expressed on both hematopoietic and non-hematopoietic tissues, Eur. J. Immunol. 31 (5) (2001) 1310–1316.
[16] J. Nakahara, et al., Expression of Fc receptor for immunoglobulin M in oligodendrocytes and myelin of mouse central nervous system, Neurosci. Lett. 337 (2) (2003) 73–76.
[17] C. Aiken, et al., Nef induces CD4 endocytosis: requirement for a critical dileucine motif in the membrane-proximal CD4 cytoplasmic domain, Cell 76 (5) (1994) 853–864.
[18] I. Hamer, et al., Dual role of a dileucine motif in insulin receptor endocytosis, J. Biol. Chem. 272 (35) (1997) 21685–21691.
[19] A.M. Gabilondo, et al., A dileucine motif in the C terminus of the beta2-adrenergic receptor is involved in receptor internalization, Proc. Natl. Acad. Sci. U. S. A. 94 (23) (1997) 12285–12290.
[20] H.M. Craig, M.W. Pandori, J.C. Guatelli, Interaction of HIV-1 Nef with the cellular dileucine-based sorting pathway is required for CD4 down-regulation and optimal viral infectivity, Proc. Natl. Acad. Sci. U. S. A. 95 (19) (1998) 11229–11234.
[21] W. Hunziker, C. Fumey, A di-leucine motif mediates endocytosis and basolateral sorting of macrophage IgG Fc receptors in MDCK cells, Embo J. 13 (13) (1994) 2963–2969.

[22] M.R. Ehrenstein, et al., Targeted gene disruption reveals a role for natural secretory IgM in the maturation of the primary immune response, Proc. Natl. Acad. Sci. U. S. A. 95 (17) (1998) 10089–10093.
[23] A.F. Ochsenbein, et al., Control of early viral and bacterial distribution and disease by natural antibodies, Science 286 (5447) (1999) 2156–2159.
[24] S. Honda, et al., Enhanced T-independent antibody responses and spontaneous autoantibody production in Fcα/μ receptor-deficient mice (submitted for publication).

ELSEVIER

International Congress Series 1285 (2005) 84–93

www.ics-elsevier.com

Linkage between innate and acquired immunities at the mucosa

Osamu Igarashi, Tomonori Nochi, Kazutaka Terahara, Hiroshi Kiyono*

Division of Mucosal Immunology, Institute of Medical Science, The University of Tokyo, 4-6-1 Shirokanedai, Minato-ku, 108-8639 Tokyo, Japan
Core Research for Evolutional Science and Technology Agency (CREST), Japan Science and Technology Corporation (JST), Saitama, Japan

Abstract. The epithelium covering mucosal tissues consists of epithelial cells (ECs) and intraepithelial lymphocytes (IELs), which constitutes the first line of defense against infection by microorganisms, through mucosal innate and acquired immunity. One of the principal roles of the mucosal epithelium is to form a strong physical barrier such as tight junction to prevent microbial penetration. While adhesion mechanisms between ECs have been extensively studied, there are few investigations on the mechanisms between ECs and IELs. Our findings indicate that a homophylic adhesion molecule termed epithelial cell adhesion molecule (Ep-CAM) is also expressed in IELs in addition to ECs, thus forming a physical interaction between ECs and IELs. In addition, we also characterized the expression and function of Toll-like receptors (TLRs) in mucosal epithelium using human corneal epithelial cells (HCEs). TLRs are mainly expressed by antigen presenting cells (APCs) and recognize pathogen-associated molecular patterns (PAMPs). However, responsiveness via TLR2 and TLR4 in HCEs was impaired, presumably due to restricted expression of the TLRs in the cytoplasm. These findings suggest that mucosal epithelium may create a state of tolerance in order to avoid unnecessary response to environmental and commensal antigens via TLRs. However, the mucosal surfaces that cover gut and respiratory lymphoid tissues such as Peyer's patch and nasopharynx-associated lymphoid tissue (NALT) are equipped with the gateway system which effectively uptake the outside antigens via M cells to initiate both the positive and negative immune responses. We recently identified M cell-like cells that are located within the villous epithelium and involved in antigen-transport into the lamina propria. Therefore, we designated them as villous M cells. These findings suggest that mucosal

* Corresponding author. 4-6-1 Shirokanedai, Minato-ku, Tokyo, 108-8639, Japan. Tel.: +81 3 5449 5271; fax: +81 3 5449 5411.

E-mail address: kiyono@ims.u-tokyo.ac.jp (H. Kiyono).

0531-5131/
doi:10.1016/j.ics.2005.08.017

immune system is equipped with multiple layers of induction/suppression mechanisms for the regulation of mucosal innate and acquired immunity.

Keywords: IEL; TLR; M cell; Epithelial cell adhesion molecule; (Ep-CAM)

1. Adhesion molecules between intestinal epithelial cells (IECs) and intraepithelial lymphocytes (IELs)

Intestinal epithelial cells (IECs) are originated from and are maintained by a small number of pluripotent stem cells residing in crypts and show a life span of 2 to 4 days [1]. IECs have long been known to absorb ingested nutrients and transport them into the circulation. More recently, IECs have also been found to act as an important immunological barrier against pathogens or non-self-antigens. To form the physically firm defensive barrier, mucosal epithelial cells are welded with each other by a number of adhesion mechanisms. For example, tight junctions consisting of occludin [2] and the family of claudin [3,4] have been shown to play a central role in sealing the intercellular space between epithelial cells [5–7]. E-cadherin, another adhesion molecule expressed by epithelial cells, contributes to a homophilic adhesion in a Ca^{2+}-dependent manner [8]. Epithelial cell adhesion molecules (Ep-CAM), which offer a Ca^{2+}-independent adhesion, also show a homophilic adhesive function among epithelial cells [9,10]. The adhesive structure mediated by Ep-CAM among epithelium is localized at the neighboring of E-cadherin, and these molecules form a junction called intermediate junction.

In addition to mucosal epithelial cells, high numbers of lymphocytes termed intraepithelial lymphocytes (IELs) are also integrated within the mucosal epithelium and believed to form the immunological barrier together with epithelial cells. The majority of the IELs are $CD3^+$ T cells that bear either αβ or γδ T cell receptor (TCR) and approximately 80% of the $CD3^+$ T cells belong to the CD8 subset [11]. In mice, IELs are found to be present every six epithelial cells [11]. The ratio of IEL expressing αβ TCR (αβIEL) and γδIEL is quite different from that observed in other systemic T cells. Because IELs are located adjacent to IECs, cell-to-cell communications between IECs and IELs would be important to maintain the epithelial barrier. For example, IECs are capable of producing IL-7 [12] and IL-15 [13], which are important for the stimulation and development of γδIELs, while γδIELs express keratinocyte growth factor (KGF), which stimulates the growth of IECs [14]. In addition, γδIELs have unique features to regulate mucosal immune system. For example, γδIELs are involved in the induction and regulation of antigen-specific IgA because $TCR\delta^{-/-}$ mice induce significantly lower levels of immune responses in both mucosal and systemic sites when immunized with antigens in combination with a mucosal adjuvant [15]. Furthermore, γδIELs are likely to regulate oral tolerance, a state where induction of systemic immune response is suppressed [16].

However, minimal information is currently available regarding the cellular and molecular mechanisms underlying the physical cell-to-cell interaction between epithelial cells and IELs. Recently, $\alpha_E\beta_7$ integrin was found to mediate T cell adhesion to epithelial

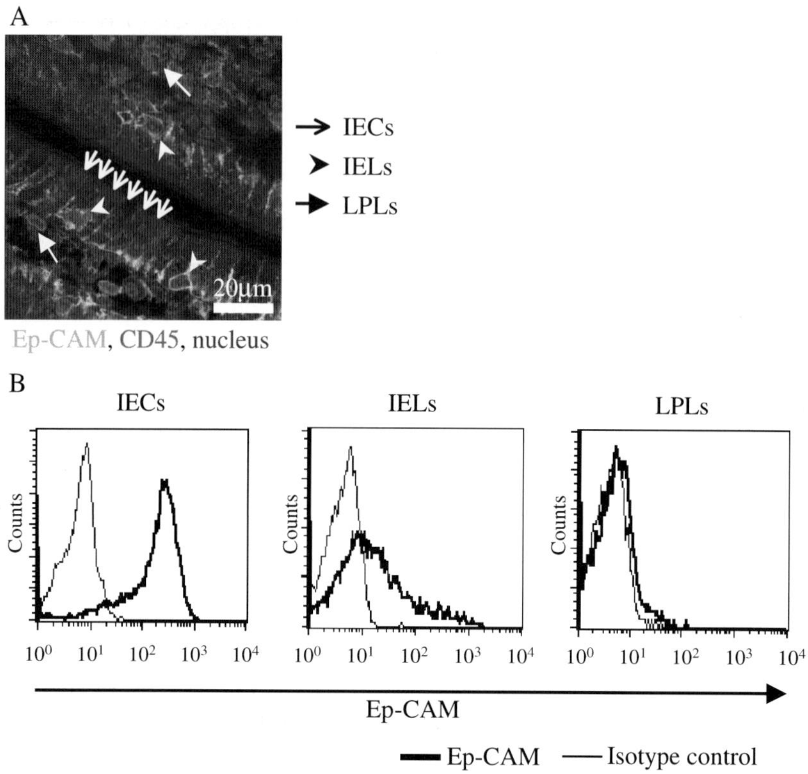

Fig. 1. Expression of epithelial cell adhesion molecule (Ep-CAM) in IECs, IELs and lamina propria lymphocytes (LPLs). Ep-CAM is expressed in $CD45^+$ IELs as well as IECs but not $CD45^+$ LPLs (A). Flow cytometric analysis also indicates that isolated IECs and IELs but not LPLs are reacted with anti-Ep-CAM monoclonal antibody (mAb).

cells through its binding to E-cadherin which was expressed selectively on epithelial cells [17–19]. In fact, the number of IELs was significantly decreased in α_E integrin-deficient mice [20]. These findings suggest that more complicated adhesive mechanisms are involved in the adhesion between IECs and IELs. Our novel findings indicate that Ep-CAM is also expressed by IELs as well as IECs and forms a homophilic adhesive structure between the two [21] (Fig. 1). Most recently, it was reported that IELs also expressed junctional adhesive molecules such as occludin and E-cadherin [22]. These suggest that adhesive mechanisms offered by IECs and IELs play an essential role in the constitution of a firm physical barrier at the mucosa.

2. Role of Toll-like receptors (TLRs) at the mucosa

The mucosal immune system has developed under the dual pressure for protecting the host from pathogenic infections and establishing symbiosis with otherwise harmless commensal microorganisms. Cells that constitute the first line of the protection through innate immunity are the epithelial cells that separate inner and outer body. In this regard, several molecules such as Toll-like receptors (TLRs) [23], defensins [24,25], and nucleotide oligomerization domains (NODs) [26,27] have been identified and shown to play a role in the host protection against microbial infections. For example, TLRs, the mammalian homologues of *Drosophila* Toll, recognize pathogen-associated molecular patterns (PAMPs) such as cell wall components and nucleic acids, and signal to trigger anti-microbial innate immunity [23]. Currently, the TLR family consists of at least 11 members (TLR1–11). Among them, most investigated are TLR2 and TLR4. Both of the TLRs are expressed in IECs and contribute to the recognition of peptideglycans (PGNs) and lipoproteins of Gram-positive bacteria [28], and recognition of LPS [29], a cell wall component of Gram-negative bacteria, respectively.

We have focused on the role of TLRs in ocular mucosal immunity and have shown that human corneal epithelial cells (HCEs) express TLR2 and TLR4 proteins intracellularly, but not at the surface level, and therefore unresponsive to the respective TLR ligands, PGN and LPS [30] (Table 1). Similar results have also been obtained with IECs; IECs are poorly responsive to PGN and LPS due to their expression of TLR2 and TLR4 at quite low levels [31,32]. Taken together, these findings suggest that there will be a negative regulatory mechanism(s) for mucosal TLRs by which host is protected from undesired induction of inflammation in response to commensal microorganisms.

The impaired surface expression of TLR2 and TLR4 in the HCEs and IECs also raises the possibility that epithelial cells have a defect in the transport of TLRs to the plasma membrane. In this point, a recent study clearly demonstrated that MD2, an accessory protein of TLR4, is essentially required for the transport of TLRs to the cell surface as well as responsiveness of the cells to LPS [33]. As expected, IECs were found defective in the expression of MD2 [34]. Moreover, expression of TLRs was also shown to be regulated by an endoplasmic reticulum chaperone gp96 [35]. Thus, our current interest is aimed at determining whether or not HCEs express these expression regulatory molecules.

In addition to the regulation at surface expression level, cellular responsiveness to TLR ligands seems to be regulated at the level of signal transduction. Hornef et al. have provided evidence that intestinal crypt epithelial m-IC$_{cl2}$ cells can internalize LPS in a clathrin-dependent pathway and respond to the LPS through cytoplasmic TLR4 [36]. This suggests a potential mechanism for intracellular recognition of TLR ligands by normal epithelial cells in an emergency such as pathogenic bacterial penetration. However, forced introduction of LPS into the HCEs resulted in no activation of NF-κB, the common TLR-signaling-associated transcription factor [30], suggesting that there may be a mechanism(s) by which signal transduction through TLRs is hampered. Accordingly, NF-κB-mediated inflammatory cytokine synthesis was not induced either. One explanation for the

Table 1
Expression of TLR2 and TLR4 proteins by human corneal epithelial cell line (HCE-T) and primary human corneal epithelial cells (HCEs)

Cells	TLR2		TLR4	
	Intracellular	Surface	Intracellular	Surface
HCE-T line	+	−	+	−
Primary HCEs	+	−	+	−

impaired responsiveness of the HCEs to LPS may be attributed to lack of gp96 in the HCEs since it is likely involved in the transport of TLR4 to the Golgi apparatus, the site where cytoplasmic TLR4 interact with internalized LPS [36]. Another explanation might be the presence of an inhibitor(s) for TLR-mediated signaling in the HCEs. Recently, Tollip, a Toll/IL-1R (TIR) domain-containing inhibitory protein [37], and TIR8/SIGIRR, single Ig IL-1R-related molecule [38], were identified as inhibitors for TLR signaling. Both of the inhibitors are highly expressed in IECs that poorly respond to LPS [34,38]. Moreover, mice deficient in TIR8/SIGIRR are more susceptible to dextran sodium sulfate (DSS)-induced colitis [39]. Thus, high expression of TLR-signaling inhibitors may limit TLR signaling and thereby control the TLR-mediated induction of inflammation at the mucosa.

In addition to TLR2 and TLR4, IECs were also shown to express TLR5, which recognizes bacterial flagellin at both apical and basolateral surfaces [40]. We are currently examining the expression as well as responsiveness in terms of the other TLRs in the HCEs. However, at least in the responsiveness, given that prolonged exposure of IEC lines to LPS or lipotechoic acid (LTA) leads not only to tolerance, but also to cross-tolerance to the other TLR ligands [41], the HCEs might be hyporesponsive to other PAMPs even if they express other members of TLRs.

Taken all together, these findings suggest that responsiveness of mucosal epithelial cells are negatively regulated by decreased surface expression of TLRs or increased intracellular expression of inhibitors or both in order to maintain the symbiosis with commensal microorganisms.

3. Antigen sampling sites at mucosal epithelium: Peyer's patch M cells and villous M cells

The uniqueness that distinguishes mucosal immunity from systemic immunity is characterized by the production of secretory IgA. Mucosa-associated lymphoid tissues (MALT) including Peyer's patches (PP) located in the small intestine have been considered to play a crucial role for the induction of antigen-specific mucosal immune responses and therefore called inductive site. With regard to the elicitation of specific mucosal immune responses, antigens must be transported across the epithelial layer of PP. Indeed, the follicle-associated epithelium (FAE) that lines mucosal lymphoid follicles contains M cells, specialized epithelial cells that are capable of uptaking foreign antigens. During more than 30 years from the discovery of M cells, some morphological, biochemical and biological features of M cells have been clarified. They have (I) a specific reactivity to the lectin *Ulex europaeus* agglutinin-1 (UEA-1), (II) short and irregular microvilli, (III) an endocytic activity to take up bacteria as well as macromolecules, (IV) a pocket structure, which allows a cluster of immunocompetent cells to be located in closer proximity to the lumen, and (V) low enzymatic activities of alkaline phosphatase and lysozyme [42]. Although it has been believed for a long time that M cells exist only in FAE, evidence have been provided that M cell-like cells are occasionally seen within villous epithelium adjacent to the lymphoid follicle [43] and UEA-1$^+$ cells are observed within the intestinal villous epithelium [44]. However, the functional properties of these cells remain unclear. Furthermore, our group recently demonstrated that antigen-specific IgA production was observed in PP null mice [45]. Taken together, these findings imply that M cells capable of sampling antigens also exist in villous epithelium.

Recently, we found epithelial cells that were located within the small intestinal villous epithelium and showed characteristics similar to those observed in conventional M cells (Fig. 2), and thus designated them as villous M cells [46]. Interestingly, villous M cells were located in the tip regions of intestinal villi of not only wild type mice but also various PP null mice such as in utero LTβR-Ig-treated, LTα$^{-/-}$, TNF/LTα$^{-/-}$ and Id2$^{-/-}$ mice. These findings provide evidence that villous M cells develop independently of organized mucosal lymphoid tissues, although development of M cells has been thought to be associated with that of these tissues. Furthermore, our results suggest that villous M cells can serve as an additional gateway for the entry of pathogenic bacteria such as *Salmonella typhimurium* and *Yersinia pseudotuberculosis*, both of which are known to invade through M cells. In addition, production of humoral antigen-specific antibodies was normally induced in TNF/LTα$^{-/-}$ mice, which lack PP and isolated lymphoid follicles (ILF), following oral administration of antigens such as recombinant *Salmonella* expressing the immunogenic C fragment of tetanus toxin. Similarly, M cells that are not associated with lymphoid follicles have been identified within respiratory epithelium in horse [47]. These findings also support the notion that M cells constantly exist in a variety of mucosal epithelium independently of association of the epithelium with lymphoid follicles, and play a role in the initiation of antigen-specific immune responses.

Another gateway for antigen sampling at the mucosa could be mucosal dendritic cells (DCs). Recent studies have clearly demonstrated that DCs residing within or adjacent to the intestinal villous epithelium take up luminal bacteria directly or by extending their arms across the epithelial layer, respectively [48,49].

Thus, various ways for antigen sampling may simultaneously occur at the entire mucosal surface and contribute to the induction of antigen-specific immune responses.

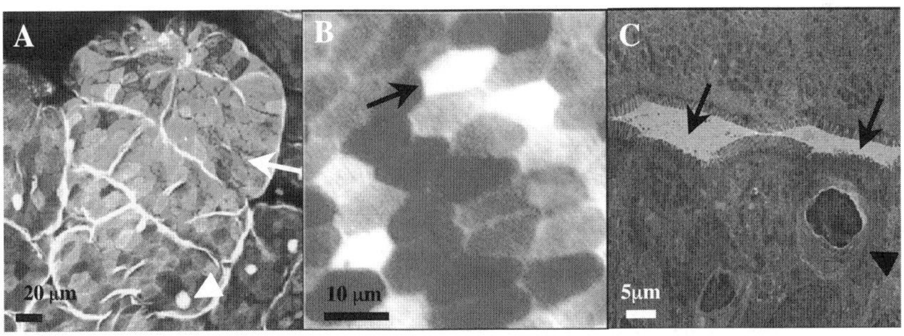

Fig. 2. Morphological characterization of small intestinal villous M cells in naïve BALB/c mice. (A) A confocal image of whole mount preparation of the small intestine stained with UEA-1-TRITC and WGA-FITC. Villous M cells are positive singly for UEA-1 (red, arrow), enterocytes singly for WGA (green), and goblet cells doubly for UEA-1 and WGA (yellow, arrowhead). (B) A light microscopic view of the whole mount preparation tested for alkaline phosphatase activity (red/pink) and alcian blue staining (blue). Villous M cells are doubly negative for alkaline phosphatase activity and alcian blue staining (white, arrow). (C) A transmission electron microscopic image of the villous epithelium. Villous M cells bear short stub-like microvilli at the luminal surface (arrows) and hold a mononuclear cell (arrowhead) in the pocket. (For interpretation of the references to colour in this figure legend, the reader is referred to the web version of this article.)

4. Concluding remarks

Mucosal surface is protected in multiple prudent ways from invasion by pathogens and antigens that induce undesired inflammation (Fig. 3). First, mucosal epithelium covering the associated tissues constitutes physical barriers that are tightly connected by a variety of intercellular adhesive mechanisms such as firm interactions between IELs and IECs and between IECs. Further, mucosal epithelium is covered by thick layers of mucus. Second, responsiveness of mucosal epithelial cells to PAMPs via TLRs are generally suppressed by decrease in the surface expression of TLRs and increase in the intracellular expression of inhibitors that are associated with TLR signaling, thus avoiding induction of unnecessary inflammation as a result of continuous signaling via TLRs. In general, the innate immunity at the mucosa may be negatively regulated and thus maintain the appropriate homeostasis between the host and outside environments.

In contrast, M cells that are located within the epithelium that covers lymphoid or non-lymphoid tissues can behave as a gateway for the transport of antigens and pathogenic microorganisms into the underlying lymphoid follicles or lamina propria, which leads to the initiation of mucosal acquired immunity. DCs located within or in close proximity to

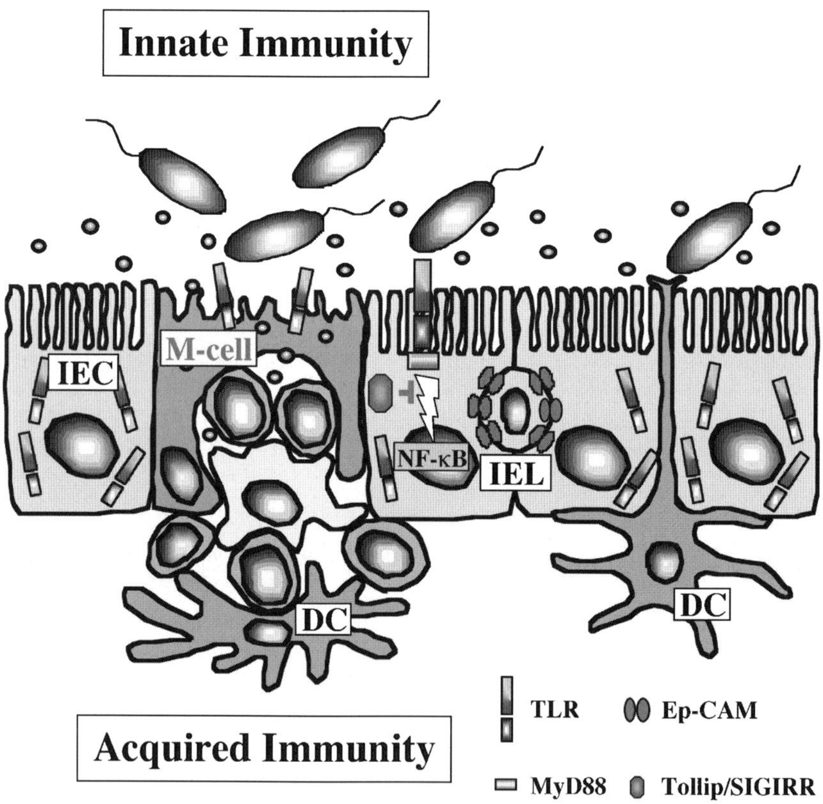

Fig. 3. Dynamic linkage between innate and acquired immunities at mucosal surface.

epithelium also sample antigens and contribute to the induction of acquired immunity. It is interesting to seek out the nature of acquired immunity against antigens taken up by PP-associated M cells, villous M cells, and mucosal DCs located in the different areas of intestinal tract.

It has been reported that DCs express tight junctional proteins to penetrate into epithelium [48] and a variety of TLRs to recognize a wide spectrum of PAMPs [23]. In addition, M cells located within the FAE of swine PP express TLR2 and TLR9 both at the apical and basolateral surfaces [50,51].

Taken all together, these findings suggest that M cells and DCs are key players that bridge innate and acquired immunities at the mucosa.

Acknowledgements

This work was supported by grants from Uehara Memorial Fundation, the Ministry of Education, Science, Sports and Cultures, the Ministry of Health and Welfare and CREST, JST, Japan.

References

[1] B. Creamer, The turnover of the epithelium of the small intestine, Br. Med. Bull. 23 (1967) 226–230.
[2] M. Furuse, et al., Occludin: a novel integral membrane protein localizing at tight junctions, J. Cell Biol. 123 (1993) 1777–1788.
[3] M. Furuse, et al., Claudin-1 and -2: novel integral membrane proteins localizing at tight junctions with no sequence similarity to occludin, J. Cell Biol. 141 (1998) 1539–1550.
[4] K. Morita, et al., Claudin multigene family encoding four-transmembrane domain protein components of tight junction strands, Proc. Natl. Acad. Sci. U. S. A. 96 (1999) 511–516.
[5] J.M. Anderson, C.M. Van Itallie, Tight junctions and the molecular basis for regulation of paracellular permeability, Am. J. Physiol. 269 (1995) G467–G475.
[6] E.E. Schneeberger, R.D. Lynch, Structure, function, and regulation of cellular tight junctions, Am. J. Physiol. 262 (1992) L647–L661.
[7] S. Tsukita, et al., Multifunctional strands in tight junctions, Nat. Rev., Mol. Cell Biol. 2 (2001) 285–293.
[8] M. Takeichi, Cadherin cell adhesion receptors as a morphogenetic regulator, Science 251 (1991) 1451–1455.
[9] S.V. Litvinov, et al., Ep-CAM: a human epithelial antigen is a homophilic cell–cell adhesion molecule, J. Cell Biol. 125 (1994) 437–446.
[10] S.V. Litvinov, et al., Evidence for a role of the epithelial glycoprotein 40 (Ep-CAM) in epithelial cell–cell adhesion, Cell Adhes. Commun. 2 (1994) 417–428.
[11] J. Mestecky, et al., The mucosal immune system, in: W.E. Paul (Ed.), Fundamental Immunology, 5th edn., Lipponcott Williams & Wilkins, Philadelphia, 2003, pp. 965–1020.
[12] K. Fujihashi, et al., Interleukin 2 (IL-2) and interleukin 7 (IL-7) reciprocally induce IL-7 and IL-2 receptors on γδ T-cell receptor-positive intraepithelial lymphocytes, Proc. Natl. Acad. Sci. U. S. A. 93 (1996) 3613–3618.
[13] K. Inagaki-Ohara, et al., Interleukin-15 preferentially promotes the growth of intestinal intraepithelial lymphocytes bearing γδ T cell receptor in mice, Eur. J. Immunol. 27 (1997) 2885–2891.
[14] H. Yang, et al., Intestinal intraepithelial lymphocyte γδ-T cell-derived keratinocyte growth factor modulates epithelial growth in the mouse, J. Immunol. 172 (2004) 4151–4158.
[15] K. Fujihashi, et al., γδ T cell-deficient mice have impaired mucosal immunoglobulin A responses, J. Exp. Med. 183 (1996) 1929–1935.
[16] K. Fujihashi, et al., γδ T cells regulate mucosally induced tolerance in a dose-dependent fashion, Int. Immunol. 11 (1999) 1907–1916.

[17] K.L. Cepek, et al., Adhesion between epithelial cells and T lymphocytes mediated by E-cadherin and the $\alpha_E\beta_7$ integrin, Nature 372 (1994) 190–193.
[18] P.I. Karecla, et al., Recognition of E-cadherin on epithelial cells by the mucosal T cell integrin alpha M290β7 ($\alpha_E\beta_7$), Eur. J. Immunol. 25 (1995) 852–856.
[19] J.M. Higgins, et al., Direct and regulated interaction of integrin $\alpha_E\beta_7$ with E-cadherin, J. Cell Biol. 140 (1998) 197–210.
[20] M.P. Schon, et al., Mucosal T lymphocyte numbers are selectively reduced in integrin α_E (CD103)-deficient mice, J. Immunol. 162 (1999) 6641–6649.
[21] T. Nochi, et al., Biological role of Ep-CAM in the physical interaction between epithelial cells and lymphocytes in intestinal epithelium, Clin. Immunol. 113 (2004) 326–339.
[22] K. Inagaki-Ohara, et al., Intraepithelial lymphocytes express junctional molecules in murine small intestine, Biochem. Biophys. Res. Commun. 331 (2005) 977–983.
[23] R. Medzhitov, C. Janeway Jr., Innate immune recognition: mechanisms and pathways, Immunol. Rev. 173 (2000) 89–97.
[24] D. Yang, et al., Beta-defensins: linking innate and adaptive immunity through dendritic and T cell CCR6, Science 286 (1999) 525–528.
[25] T. Ayabe, et al., Secretion of microbicidal α-defensins by intestinal Paneth cells in response to bacteria, Nat. Immunol. 1 (2000) 113–118.
[26] N. Inohara, et al., Human Nod1 confers responsiveness to bacterial lipopolysaccharides, J. Biol. Chem. 276 (2001) 2551–2554.
[27] S.E. Girardin, et al., Nod2 is a general sensor of peptidoglycan through muramyl dipeptide (MDP) detection, J. Biol. Chem. 278 (2003) 8869–8872.
[28] O. Takeuchi, et al., Differential roles of TLR2 and TLR4 in recognition of Gram-negative and Gram-positive bacterial cell wall components, Immunity 11 (1999) 443–451.
[29] A. Poltorak, et al., Defective LPS signaling in C3H/HeJ and C57BL/10ScCr mice: mutations in Tlr4 gene, Science 282 (1998) 2085–2088.
[30] M. Ueta, et al., Intracellularly expressed TLR2s and TLR4s contribution to an immunosilent environment at the ocular mucosal epithelium, J. Immunol. 173 (2004) 3337–3347.
[31] M.T. Abreu, et al., Decreased expression of Toll-like receptor-4 and MD-2 correlates with intestinal epithelial cell protection against dysregulated proinflammatory gene expression in response to bacterial lipopolysaccharide, J. Immunol. 167 (2001) 1609–1616.
[32] G. Melmed, et al., Human intestinal epithelial cells are broadly unresponsive to Toll-like receptor 2-dependent bacterial ligands: implications for host-microbial interactions in the gut, J. Immunol. 170 (2003) 1406–1415.
[33] Y. Nagai, et al., Essential role of MD-2 in LPS responsiveness and TLR4 distribution, Nat. Immunol. 3 (2002) 667–672.
[34] M.T. Abreu, et al., TLR4 and MD-2 expression is regulated by immune-mediated signals in human intestinal epithelial cells, J. Biol. Chem. 277 (2002) 20431–20437.
[35] F. Randow, B. Seed, Endoplasmic reticulum chaperone gp96 is required for innate immunity but not cell viability, Nat. Cell Biol. 3 (2001) 891–896.
[36] M.W. Hornef, et al., Intracellular recognition of lipopolysaccharide by Toll-like receptor 4 in intestinal epithelial cells, J. Exp. Med. 198 (2003) 1225–1235.
[37] K. Burns, et al., Tollip, a new component of the IL-1RI pathway, links IRAK to the IL-1 receptor, Nat. Cell Biol. 2 (2000) 346–351.
[38] D. Wald, et al., SIGIRR, a negative regulator of Toll-like receptor-interleukin 1 receptor signaling, Nat. Immunol. 4 (2003) 920–927.
[39] C. Garlanda, et al., Intestinal inflammation in mice deficient in Tir8, an inhibitory member of the IL-1 receptor family, Proc. Natl. Acad. Sci. U. S. A. 101 (2004) 3522–3526.
[40] A.T. Gewirtz, et al., Cutting edge: bacterial flagellin activates basolaterally expressed TLR5 to induce epithelial proinflammatory gene expression, J. Immunol. 167 (2001) 1882–1885.
[41] J.M. Otte, et al., Mechanisms of cross hyporesponsiveness to Toll-like receptor bacterial ligands in intestinal epithelial cells, Gastroenterology 126 (2004) 1054–1070.
[42] A. Gebert, et al., M cells in Peyer's patches of the intestine, Int. Rev. Cytol. 167 (1996) 91–159.
[43] C. Borghesi, et al., Rapid appearance of M cells after microbial challenge is restricted at the periphery of the follicle-associated epithelium of Peyer's patch, Lab. Invest. 79 (1999) 1393–1401.

[44] L. Bry, et al., A model of host-microbial interactions in an open mammalian ecosystem, Science 273 (1996) 1380–1383.
[45] M. Yamamoto, et al., Alternate mucosal immune system: organized Peyer's patches are not required for IgA responses in the gastrointestinal tract, J. Immunol. 164 (2000) 5184–5191.
[46] M.H. Jang, et al., Intestinal villous M cells: an antigen entry site in the mucosal epithelium, Proc. Natl. Acad. Sci. U. S. A. 101 (2004) 6110–6115.
[47] P. Kumar, J.F. Timoney, Histology, immunohistochemistry and ultrastructure of the equine tubal tonsil, Anat. Histol. Embryol. 34 (2005) 141–148.
[48] M. Rescigno, et al., Dendritic cells express tight junction proteins and penetrate gut epithelial monolayers to sample bacteria, Nat. Immunol. 2 (2001) 361–367.
[49] J.H. Niess, et al., CX3CR1-mediated dendritic cell access to the intestinal lumen and bacterial clearance, Science 307 (2005) 254–258.
[50] M. Tohno, et al., Toll-like receptor 2 is expressed on the intestinal M cells in swine, Biochem. Biophys. Res. Commun. 330 (2005) 547–554.
[51] T. Shimosato, et al., Toll-like receptor 9 is expressed on follicle-associated epithelia containing M cells in swine Peyer's patches, Immunol. Lett. 98 (2005) 83–89.

Interfaces between innate and acquired immunity

International Congress Series 1285 (2005) 97–103

www.ics-elsevier.com

The IκB kinase (IKK) complex as a critical regulator of immune responses

Michael Karin *

Laboratory of Signal Transduction and Gene Regulation, Department of Pharmacology, School of Medicine, University of California, San Diego, 9500 Gilman Drive MC 0723, La Jolla, CA 92093-0723, USA

Abstract. The IκB kinase (IKK) is a tripartite signaling complex composed of two catalytic (protein kinase) subunits, IKKα and IKKβ, and a regulatory subunit, IKKγ (a.k.a. NEMO). The major function of IKK is to connect pro-inflammatory stimuli and signals generated by pathogen-associated molecular patterns (PAMPs) to the activation of transcription factor NF-κB. This function is mainly dependent on the IKKβ catalytic subunit, whose activation requires the ubiquitination of IKKγ. IKKβ is the major kinase that leads to phosphorylation-induced degradation of IκBs, the inhibitors of NF-κB, and the consequent translocation of NF-κB dimers, containing RelA or c-Rel as activating subunits, to the nucleus. This results in induction of pro-inflammatory cytokines, chemokines, inhibitors of apoptosis, and other molecules required for a successful innate immune response. The function of IKKα in this pathway has been puzzling, but we recently found that IKKα serves an anti-inflammatory function by phosphorylating RelA and c-Rel at sites that accelerate their nuclear turnover. This seems to occur concomitantly with IκB phosphorylation by IKKβ. Thus, the IKK complex is responsible both for the onset of NF-κB activation and for the proper termination of this response. Another function unique for IKKα, which occurs independently of IKKβ and IKKγ, is the phosphorylation and processing of the NF-κB2/p100 protein, leading to specific activation of p52:RelB dimers. This response is critical for coupling innate immunity to certain adaptive responses involving B cells.

Keywords: NF-κB; IKK; Inflammation; Immunity

1. Introduction

Nuclear factor κB (NF-κB) was first identified as a B-lymphocyte-specific transcription factor but was soon recognized as an inducible activity present within all cell types [1].

* Tel.: +1 85 534 1361; fax: +1 858 534 8158.
E-mail address: karinoffice@ucsd.edu.

doi:10.1016/j.ics.2005.07.088

The most common and potent inducers of NF-κB activity are proinflammatory cytokines, such as tumor necrosis factor (TNF)α and interleukin (IL)-1 and a variety of molecules characteristic of bacteria, fungi and viruses collectively known as pathogen-associated molecular patterns (PAMPs). Whereas TNFα elicits NF-κB activation mostly through its type 1 receptor (TNFR1), a prototype of a large family of cytokine receptors [2,3], IL-1 and PAMPS signal via structurally related IL-1 receptor (IL-1R) and Toll-like receptors (TLRs) [4,5]. Engagement of all of these receptors results in activation of the IκB kinase (IKK) complex, a signaling machine responsible for the activation and modulation of NF-κB activity [6,7].

The IKK complex consists of two catalytic subunits IKKα and IKKβ and a regulatory/structural subunit called IKKγ or NEMO [7]. IKKα and IKKβ are structurally related but functionally distinct polypeptides that contain a serine/theonine kinase domain at their N-terminus and protein–protein interaction motifs including a leucine zipper (LZ) and a helix-loop-helix (HLH) at their C-terminal portion [7]. IKKγ by contrast lacks catalytic activity and instead contains several coiled-coil motifs that mediate its oligomerization. IKKα and IKKβ first form homo- or heterodimers (the heterodimer is the most common species in cells that express similar amounts of both kinases). These dimers then bind two molecules of IKKγ via decapeptide motifs at the extreme C-terminus of each kinase subunit. The IKKγ subunit then mediates further dimerization of the above complex such that the holoenzyme contains four catalytic subunits. Assembly of this complex based on the interaction between the catalytic subunits and IKKγ is essential for kinase activation [8,9]. Once activated, the IKK complex phosphorylates the inhibitor of kB (IκB) proteins, which associate with NF-κB dimers in the cytoplasm [7]. The ability of IKK to recognize the IκB:NF-κB ternary complex depends on its association with the substrate docking auxiliary protein ELKS [10]. The phosphorylated IκB proteins are then recognized by the βTrCP subunit of the $SCF^{\beta TrCP}$ E3 ligase complex which facilitates the polyubiquitination of the IκBs by an E2 ubiquitin-conjugating enzyme [11]. This process results in proteasomal degradation of IκBs and nuclear translocation of the spared and liberated NF-κB dimer. This pathway is known as the classical NF-κB signaling pathway and, in addition to IKKγ/NEMO, its activation by most stimuli in most cell types depends on the IKKβ rather than the IKKα subunit [6].

2. IKKβ and immunity

The IKKβ-dependent classical pathway is mostly responsible for the activation of NF-κB heterodimers consisting of the NF-κB1-p50, RelA(p65) and c-Rel subunits. These dimers are involved in induction of numerous target genes encoding enzymes involved in induction of inflammatory mediators, adhesion molecules, cell surface receptors, cytokines, chemokines, and anti-apoptotic proteins [1,12]. Collectively, these targets mediate a variety of innate and adaptive immune functions [13,14]. One of the most critical functions of the classical NF-κB signaling pathway is the inhibition of programmed cell death (PCD) [15]. Mice deficient in RelA, IKKβ, or IKKγ die at mid-gestation due to massive liver apoptosis mediated by TNFα signaling via TNFR1 [8,16–19]. Biochemical studies have revealed that engagement of TNFR1 results in activation of several effector pathways including the classical NF-κB signaling pathway and the Jun kinase (JNK) pathway [20]. While NF-κB activation inhibits PCD, JNK activation promotes PCD. Furthermore, one of the mechanisms through which NF-κB prevents PCD depends on the inhibition of reactive oxygen species (ROS) accumulation within the cell, thereby ensuring transient rather than prolonged JNK activation [21]. In the absence of NF-κB activity, TNFα stimulation results in massive ROS accumulation, and the consequent oxidation and inhibition of MAPK phosphatases (MKPs), thereby giving rise to prolonged JNK activation. The inhibition of PCD by NF-κB is important for maintaining the viability of various inflammatory and immune cells involved in both innate and adaptive immunity [14,15]. In fact, TNFR1 is not the only immune receptor that uses NF-κB to prevent PCD; both the T- and B-cell receptors, as well as TLR4, use a similar strategy to inhibit the death of cells in which they were activated and instead promote various inflammatory and immune functions [22–24]. Thus, NF-κB activation seems to serve as a checkpoint that controls both the activation of immune cells and the duration of the period through which they remain functional and viable. Interestingly, various highly pathogenic bacteria have evolved mechanisms that prevent NF-κB activation, thereby allowing them to avoid detection by the innate immune system. By contrast, bacteria and other microorganisms that exist as intracellular parasites induce persistent NF-κB activation as a way to prevent the apoptotic elimination of their hosts.

Given the important survival functions of NF-κB, it is surprising that mice that are deficient in either RelA or IKKβ, and are also deficient in TNFR1 (to ensure their survival to term), are highly susceptible to opportunistic infections and die within a short time after birth [25,26]. One prevalent defect in such animals is the reduced viability of macrophages as well as T and B lymphocytes, whereas another defect is the inability to produce sufficient amounts of cytokines and chemokines.

3. IKKα and the alternative pathway

Unlike IKKβ-deficient mice, which exhibit a phenotype that is directly related to the inability to mount an NF-κB activation response [18,26,27], IKKα-deficient mice exhibit a developmental phenotype that includes perinatal lethality but is not due to a defect in NF-κB activation [28,29]. In fact, this developmental phenotype is not even related to the protein kinase activity of IKKα [29,30]. To determine whether the protein kinase activity of IKKα is completely redundant, we have generated $Ikk\alpha^{AA/AA}$ mutant mice, which retain normal expression levels of a variant form of IKKα that cannot be activated in response to upstream stimuli because it lacks the phosphoacceptor sites for its activating protein kinase-NIK [31]. As expected, $Ikk\alpha^{AA/AA}$ mice do not exhibit the developmental defects that are characteristic of $Ikk\alpha^{-/-}$ mice. Instead $Ikk\alpha^{AA/AA}$ mice exhibit defective development of secondary lymphoid organs and reduced survival of immature B cells [32]. Biochemical studies have revealed that these defects are due to the inability to properly process the NF-κB2-p100 precursor protein to the mature p52 subunit [32]. Furthermore, as p100 is mostly associated with the RelB NF-κB subunit in the cytoplasm of non-stimulated cells, $Ikk\alpha^{AA/AA}$ or $Ikk\alpha^{-/-}$ cells are unable to activate p52:RelB dimers, while showing normal activation of p50:RelA or p50:c-Rel dimers [33]. As similar defects are exhibited by B lymphocytes from $Nik^{Aly/Aly}$ mice, which express an inactive form of the IKKα-activating kinase NIK [13], these results established the existence of a specialized NIK-IKKα cascade required for activation of the alternative pathway.

This pathway was found to be selectively activated in response to engagement of a limited subset of TNFR family members including the lymphotoxin (LT) β receptor (LTβR), BAFF receptor (BAFF-R), and CD40 [6,34]. In turn, activation of this pathway results in selective induction of p52:RelB target genes that contain a specialized NF-κB binding site that exhibits preference for p52:RelB over p50:RelA or p50:c-Rel dimers [33]. The genes that are selectively induced in response to the alternative pathway encode several organogenic chemokines that are essential for proper generation and organization of secondary lymphoid organs [13]. Thus, the alternative pathway plays an important role in adaptive immune responses although it is not directly involved in innate immunity.

4. IKKα as a negative modulator of the classical pathway

IKKβ and IKKγ are not involved in activation of the alternative pathway. In fact, in their absence the alternative pathway is activated more efficiently [34]. Yet, the more common form of IKK contains equimolar amounts of IKKα and IKKβ [7], thus suggesting that IKKα has a function in regulation of the classical pathway after all. This function became obvious recently. Infection studies, using group B *Streptococcus* (GBS) as a model pathogen revealed that $Ikk\alpha^{AA/AA}$ mice clear infections more efficiently than WT counterparts but at the same time mount a more vigorous inflammatory response [35]. An elevated inflammatory response in $Ikk\alpha^{AA/AA}$ mice was also seen upon administration of LPS or immunocomplexes. Molecular and biochemical analyses revealed that $Ikk\alpha^{AA/AA}$ macrophages express most NF-κB target genes for a longer duration than WT counterparts. This was found to correlate with longer residence time of RelA- or c-Rel-containing NF-κB dimers in the nucleus or on promoters of NF-κB target genes [35]. Further investigation revealed that the basis for the delayed promoter clearance of RelA- and c-Rel-containing dimers is the substantial increase in the stability of these proteins. Previous work has shown that one of the mechanisms that contribute to the termination of the NF-κB activation response involves accelerated proteasome-dependent degradation of nuclear RelA and c-Rel [36]. We found that macrophage stimulation with LPS accelerates the proteasomal degradation of RelA and c-Rel in a manner dependent on IKKα kinase activity. In the case of RelA, this accelerated degradation requires the phosphorylation of Ser536 near its C-terminus. Importantly, the phosphorylation of this site is largely dependent on IKKα rather than IKKβ activity [35]. Thus, Ser536 of RelA, and presumably a similar site on c-Rel, is a preferential IKKα phosphorylation site, in contrast to Ser32 and Ser36 of IκBα, which are preferential IKKβ phosphorylation sites.

These results suggest the following mechanism through which the classical IKK complex controls both the amplitude and duration of NF-κB activation. In response to activation of TLR4, and possibly other TLRs, the IKK complex is activated and interacts with the IκB:NF-κB ternary complex through the ELKS subunit. While IKKβ phosphorylates the IκB proteins and thereby targets them to ubiquitin-dependent degradation in the cytoplasm, the IKKα subunit phosphorylates the RelA and c-Rel subunits, prior to their translocation to the nucleus. The nuclear RelA- and c-Rel-containing dimers bind to NF-κB sites and contribute to the transcriptional activation of specific target genes. If phosphorylated at the IKKα-dependent C-terminal sites (Ser536 for RelA), the Rel proteins undergo ubiquitination by a yet-to-be identified nuclear ubiquitin ligase and are subsequently degraded via nuclear proteasomes. This results in promoter clearance and termination of the NF-κB activation response. Thus, while IKKβ is crucial for NF-κB activation, IKKα kinase activity contributes to the termination of this activation response.

5. Conclusions and implications

The IKK complex is evolutionary conserved—a similar complex composed of a single catalytic subunit. D-IKK, homologous to both IKKα and IKKβ, and a regulatory subunit, Kenny, a homolog of IKKγ/NEMO has been identified in the fruit fly *Drosophila melanogaster* [37]. The fly IKK is involved in activation of the NF-κB protein Relish in response to bacteria infection and is therefore critical for innate immune responses to bacteria, but not other pathogens [38]. Therefore, the activation of innate immunity is an ancient function that has also been conserved in mammals. Curiously, however, the *Drosophila* IKK complex achieves its biological function through activation of a process that is akin to the alternative pathway of mammals—phosphorylation-induced Relish processing [37], whereas the mammalian complex achieves its innate immune function through phosphorylation-induced IκB degradation [11]. Inducible NF-κB2/p100 proteolysis, by contrast, is mostly involved in development of the adaptive immune system and does not require the classical IKK complex, as it is dependent on NIK-mediated activation of IKKα homodimers [13]. Clearly, the mammalian IKK system is more evolved and more complex, and therefore in charge of multiple regulatory functions.

One of the more amazing aspects of the mammalian IKK system is the presence of two catalytic subunits instead of one. Despite their structural and biochemical similarity, IKKα and IKKβ have distinct biological functions. While IKKβ is required for the rapid activation of NF-κB in response to a myriad of innate immune challenges, IKKα is involved in terminating this response [35]. However, this function of IKKα is complementary, rather than antagonistic, to that of IKKβ. By controlling the stability and nuclear turnover of the RelA and c-Rel proteins, IKKα modulates both the magnitude and the duration of the NF-κB activation response. While a rapidly triggered activation system that is under feed-forward control is essential for an instant and proper response to infection and injury, many of the cytokines whose expression is controlled by NF-κB are quite toxic and thereby their prolonged and unnecessary production can lead to tissue damage and even death. Thus, a control over the duration of the NF-κB activation response, which depends on several mechanisms in addition to IKKα-mediated RelA or c-Rel phosphorylation, is essential for proper recovery and for limiting the collateral damage associated with activation of the innate immune system. It is quite likely that the secret to many chronic inflammatory diseases may lie within the termination, rather than the activation, of innate immunity.

References

[1] A.S. Baldwin, The NF-κB and IκB proteins: new discoveries and insights, Annu. Rev. Immunol. 14 (1996) 649–681.

[2] J.L. Bodmer, P. Schneider, J. Tschopp, The molecular architecture of the TNF superfamily, Trends Biochem. Sci. 27 (1) (2002) 19–26.

[3] J.R. Muppidi, J. Tschopp, R.M. Siegel, Life and death decisions: secondary complexes and lipid rafts in TNF receptor family signal transduction, Immunity 21 (4) (2004) 461–465.

[4] R. Medzhitov, Toll-like receptors and innate immunity, Nat. Rev., Immunol. 1 (2001) 135–145.

[5] L. O'Neill, The Toll/interleukin-1 receptor domain: a molecular switch for inflammation and host defence, Biochem. Soc. Trans. 28 (5) (2000) 557–563.

[6] S. Ghosh, M. Karin, Missing pieces in the NF-κB puzzle, Cell 109 (2002) S81–S96.

[7] D.M. Rothwarf, M. Karin. The NF-κB activation pathway: a paradigm in information transfer from membrane to nucleus. Science's STKE 1999; www.stke.org/cgi/content/fullOC_sigtrans;1999/5/re1.

[8] C. Makris, et al., Female mice heterozygote for IKKγ/NEMO deficiencies develop a genodermatosis similar to the human X-linked disorder Incontinentia Pigmenti, Mol. Cell 15 (2000) 969–979.

[9] C. Makris, J.L. Roberts, M. Karin, The carboxyl-terminal region of IκB kinase gamma (IKKγ) is required for full IKK activation, Mol. Cell. Biol. 22 (2002) 6573–6581.

[10] J.L. Ducut Sigala, et al., Activation of transcription factor NF-kappaB requires ELKS, an IkappaB kinase regulatory subunit, Science 304 (5679) (2004) 1963–1967.

[11] M. Karin, Y. Ben-Neriah, Phosphorylation meets ubiquitination: the control of NF-κB activity, Annu. Rev. Immunol. 18 (2000) 621–663.

[12] P.J. Barnes, M. Karin, NF-κB—a pivotal transcription factor in chronic inflammatory diseases, New Engl. J. Med. 336 (1997) 1066–1071.

[13] G. Bonizzi, M. Karin, The two NF-κB activation pathways and their role in innate and adaptive immunity, Trends Immunol. 25 (2004) 280–288.

[14] Q. Li, M. Verma, NF-κB regulation in the immune system, Nat. Rev., Immunol. 2 (2002) 725–734.

[15] M. Karin, A. Lin, NF-κB at the crossroads of life and death, Nat. Immunol. 3 (3) (2002) 221–227.

[16] A.A. Beg, et al., Embryonic lethality and liver degeneration in mice lacking the RelA component of NF-κB, Nature 376 (1995) 167–169.

[17] Q. Li, et al., Severe liver degeneration in mice lacking the IκB kinase 2 gene, Science 284 (1999) 321–325.

[18] Z.W. Li, et al., The IKKbeta subunit of IkappaB kinase (IKK) is essential for nuclear factor kappaB activation and prevention of apoptosis, J. Exp. Med. 189 (11) (1999) 1839–1845.

[19] D. Rudolph, et al., Severe liver degeneration and lack of NF-κB activation in NEMO/IKKγ-deficient mice, Genes Dev. 14 (7) (2000) 854–862.

[20] Z.-G. Liu, et al., Dissection of TNF receptor 1 effector functions: JNK activation is not linked to apoptosis, while NF-κB activation prevents cell death, Cell 87 (1996) 565–576.

[21] H. Kamata, et al., Reactive oxygen species promote TNFα-induced death and sustained JNK activation by inhibiting MAP kinase phosphatases, Cell 120 (2005) 649–661.

[22] J. Ruland, et al., Bcl10 is a positive regulator of antigen receptor-induced activation of NF-κB and neural tube closure, Cell 104 (2001) 33–42.

[23] L.C. Hsu, et al., The protein kinase PKR is required for macrophage apoptosis after activation of Toll-like receptor 4, Nature 428 (6980) (2004) 341–345.

[24] R.E. Voll, et al., NF-κB activation by the pre-T cell receptor serves as a selective survival signal in T lymphocyte development, Immunity 13 (2000) 677–689.

[25] E. Alcamo, et al., Targeted mutation of TNF receptor I rescues the RelA-deficient mouse and reveals a critical role for NF-κB in leukocyte recruitment, J. Immunol. 167 (2001) 1592–1600.

[26] U. Senftleben, et al., IKKβ is essential for protecting T cells from TNFα-induced apoptosis, Immunity 14 (2001) 217–230.

[27] Q. Li, et al., IKK1-deficient mice exhibit abnormal development of skin and skeleton, Genes Dev. 13 (1999) 1322–1328.

[28] Y. Hu, et al., Abnormal morphogenesis but intact IKK activation in mice lacking the IKKα subunit of the IκB kinase, Science 284 (5412) (1999) 316–320.

[29] Y. Hu, et al., IKKα controls formation of the epidermis independently of NF-κB via a differentiation inducing factor, Nature 410 (2001) 710–714.

[30] A.K. Sil, et al., IκB kinase-α acts in the epidermis to control skeletal and craniofacial morphogenesis, Nature 428 (2004) 660–664.

[31] Y. Cao, et al., IKKα provides an essential link between RANK signaling and cyclin D1 expression during mammary gland development, Cell 107 (2001) 763–775.
[32] U. Senftleben, et al., Activation by IKKα of a second, evolutionary conserved, NF-κB signaling pathway, Science 293 (2001) 1495–1499.
[33] G. Bonizzi, et al., Activation of IKKα target genes depends on recognition of specific κB binding sites by RelB:p52 dimers, EMBO J. 23 (21) (2004) 4202–4210.
[34] E. Dejardin, et al., The lymphotoxin-β receptor induces different patterns of gene expression via two NF-κB pathways, Immunity 17 (2002) 525–535.
[35] T. Lawrence, et al., IKKα limits macrophage NF-κB activation and contributes to the resolution of inflammation, Nature 434 (7037) (2005) 1138–1143.
[36] S. Saccani, et al., Degradation of promoter-bound p65/RelA is essential for the prompt termination of the nuclear factor kappaB response, J. Exp. Med. 200 (1) (2004) 107–113.
[37] N. Silverman, T. Maniatis, NF-κB signaling pathways in mammalian and insect innate immunity, Genes Dev. 15 (2001) 2321–2342.
[38] S. Rutschmann, et al., Role of Drosophila IKK gamma in a toll-independent antibacterial immune response, Nat. Immunol. 1 (4) (2000) 342–347.

International Congress Series 1285 (2005) 104–113

www.ics-elsevier.com

IRF family transcription factors in type I interferon induction

Hideyuki Yanai, Tatsuaki Mizutani, Takayuki Inuzuka, Kenya Honda, Akinori Takaoka, Tadatsugu Taniguchi *

Department of Immunology, Graduate School of Medicine and Faculty of Medicine, University of Tokyo, Hongo 7-3-1, Bunkyo-ku, Tokyo 113-0033, Japan

Abstract. The type I interferon (IFN-α/β) gene family was identified about a quarter of century ago as the prototype of many cytokine gene families, and the gene induction mechanism for IFN-α/β was extensively studied in the context of host defense against viral infections. More recently, much attention has been focused on the induction and function of the IFN-α/β system regulated by Toll-like receptors (TLRs), which are critical for linking the innate and adaptive immunities. The understanding of mechanisms underlying *IFN-α/β* gene induction by TLRs is therefore an emerging theme, for which new insights have been gained over the past few years. We summarise recent progress on the role of interferon regulatory factors (IRFs) in the induction of *IFN-α/β* genes in normal cells and plasmacytoid dendritic cells (pDCs) that are specialized to produce IFN-α/β at very high levels upon stimulation by TLR9 and its subfamily members.

Keywords: Interferon; IRF; Toll-like receptor 9

1. Introduction

Type I interferons (IFNs), namely, IFN-α and -β, were originally identified as humoral factors that confer an antiviral state on cells, and these cytokines constitute a family that encompasses a group of structurally related genes [1–7]. In humans and mice, multiple functional IFN-α gene subtypes exist, whereas a single gene exists for IFN-β [1–7]. Although originally discovered for their activity to confer an antiviral state on cells, more

* Corresponding author. Tel.: +81 3 5841 3375; fax: +81 3 5841 3450.
E-mail address: tada@m.u-tokyo.ac.jp (T. Taniguchi).

0531-5131/
doi:10.1016/j.ics.2005.09.010

evidence has recently been emerging regarding IFN-α/β actions on cell growth, differentiation and many immunoregulatory activities, which are of even greater fundamental biological significance [8–11]. The discovery of Toll-like receptors (TLRs) has opened a new avenue of research on the IFN-α/β system, focusing much attention on this system in the context of TLR signaling that modulates the development of innate and adaptive immune systems [12–14].

The induction of and signaling by IFN-α/β are reciprocally coupled. Both involve transcriptional events, wherein the IRF family of transcription factors play central roles [15,16] (Fig. 1). Our knowledge concerning the mechanism underlying the coupling of

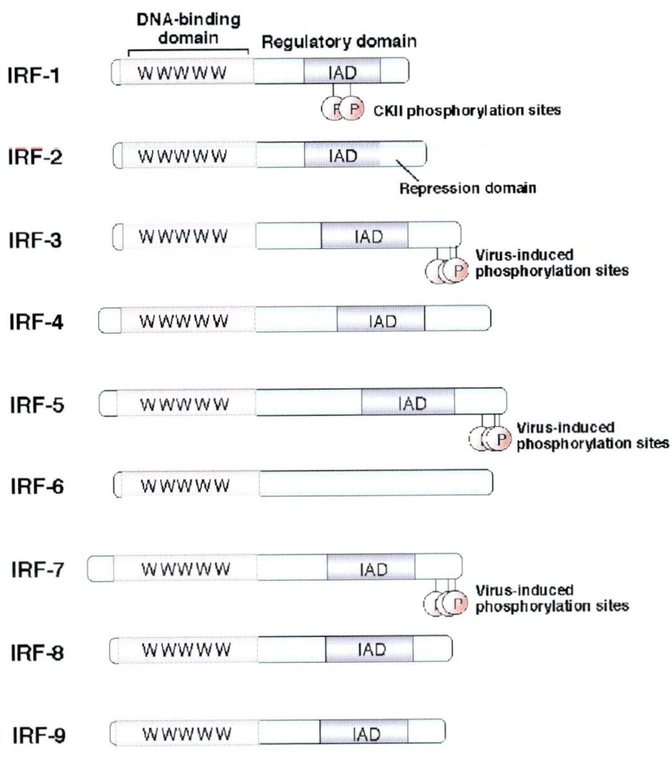

Fig. 1. IRF family of transcription factors. The interferon regulatory factors (IRFs) constitute a family of transcription factors, which posses a novel helix–turn–helix DNA binding motif that is characteristic in spatially conserved tryptophan residues. Following the initial identification of two structurally related members, IRF-1 and IRF-2 [25], many other IRF family members have been identified, and the family is now extended to nine members. In addition, virally encoded IRFs, termed vIRFs, have been identified in human herpes virus 8 (HHV8). IRF-1 may be a prototypical example of a transcription factor that can selectively modulate different sets of genes involved in host defense, depending on the cell type and/or nature of cellular stimuli, so as to evoke appropriate responses. On the other hand, IRF-2 functions as a negative regulator (attenuator) of IFN signaling (see text). IRF-9 is an integral member of the transcription factor ISGF3 complex, therefore, critical for IFN gene induction (see text). More recently, much attention has also been focused on other IRF members, and their roles are becoming clearer. In particular, two closely related members, IRF-3 and IRF7, appear to be critical for the induction of *interferon-α/β (IFN-α/β)* genes, as described in this and other papers [29,30]. Moreover, the critical role of IRF-5 in the TLR-induced expression of proinflammatory cytokines has recently been reported [43].

transcriptional and signaling regulations in the IFN-α/β system has rapidly expanded over the past few years, particularly in the context of TLR signaling. The availability of newly generated mice deficient in one or two of the IRF family members has led to a better understanding of the transcriptional induction of *IFN-α/β* genes by viruses or by ligands of the TLR9 subfamily, wherein IRF-7 functions as the master regulator in normal cells as well as in the "professional" IFN-producing pDCs.

2. IFN signaling and the classical pathway of IFN-α/β induction

The IFN-α/β signaling and pathway have been reviewed in depth elsewhere. In brief, all IFN-α/β species interact with the same receptor complex, termed the IFN-α/β receptor (IFNAR), which consists of at least two subunits, IFNAR1 and IFNAR2. These receptor components are associated with the Janus family of protein tyrosine kinases (Jak kinases), Tyk2 and Jak1, and the binding of IFN-α/β to IFNAR results in the cross-activation of these Jak kinases, which then phosphorylate IFNAR1, the signal transducer and activator of transcription-1 (Stat1) and Stat2. These Stats recruited to the phosporylated IFNAR1 form two distinct transcriptional activator complexes, namely, IFN-α-activated factor (AAF) and IFN-stimulated gene factor 3 (ISGF3). ISGF3, the major transcriptional activator in IFN-α/β signaling, is a heterotrimeric complex of Stat1, Stat2 and IRF-9, and it binds to specific DNA sequences, named the IFN-stimulated response element (ISRE). IFN signaling results in the transcriptional induction of numerous target genes, which include genes critical for the induction of *IFN-α/β* genes, namely, IRF-7, TLR3, TLR7 and dsRNA-recognition molecule retinoic acid-inducible gene I (RIG-I) [17–20].

The promoter region of the *IFN-β* gene contains at least four regulatory *cis*-elements: the positive regulatory domains (PRDs) I, II, III and IV [21–23]. The PRD I and PRD III elements are activated by members of the IRF family [15,16,22,24,25]. On the other hand, PRD II and PRD IV elements, as yet not identified in the IFN-α promoters, are activated by NF-κB and ATF-2/c-Jun, respectively [23,26]. As for the promoter region of *IFN-α* genes, PRD I-and III-like elements (PRD-LEs) that bind to IRFs have been identified [27,28].

In addition to *Irf3*-deficient mice (*Irf3*$^{-/-}$ mice) generated several years ago [29], *Irf7*-deficient mice (*Irf7*$^{-/-}$ mice) have recently been generated [30], allowing the rigorous assessment of the contribution of both transcription factors to *IFN-α/β* gene induction. In MEFs from *Irf7*$^{-/-}$ mice, *IFN-α/β* mRNA induction by viruses [vesicular stomatitis virus (VSV), herpes simplex virus-1 (HSV-1), and encephalomyocarditis virus (EMCV)] is more severely impaired than in *Irf3*$^{-/-}$ MEFs [30]. Consistently, *Irf7*$^{-/-}$ mice are more vulnerable to viral infections than *Irf3*$^{-/-}$ mice, which correlates with a marked decrease in serum IFN level [30]. These results, therefore, finally proved the critical role of the IRF-7-dependent pathway in *IFN-α/β* gene induction in MEFs; IRF-7 plays the major role, functioning even in the absence of IRF-3. IRF-3 also participates in gene induction; however, it contributes little in the absence of IRF-7. It is worth noting that the gene induction is normal in MEFs in the absence of myeloid differentiation primary response gene 88 (MyD88), the adaptor critical for signaling of the TLR9 subfamily [30]. Hence, this MyD88-independent but IRF-7-dependent pathway is referred to as the classical pathway of *IFN-α/β* gene induction, which operates in many cell types for systematic IFN response [30]. Although IRF-5 was also implicated in the transcriptional induction of the *IFN-α/β* genes, we found a normal induction of *IFN-α/β* mRNAs in MEFs from *Irf5*-deficient mice (*Irf5*$^{-/-}$ mice) infected by Newcastle disease virus (NDV) (H. Yanai, unpublished observation; see below).

3. New IFN induction pathway activated by TLR9 subfamily

An exciting direction of IFN-α/β research was set by the discovery of TLRs. Indeed, the activation of many TLRs results in the induction of IFN-α and/or -β, and this induction has received much attention in the context of linking innate and adaptive immunities [12,13,31]. Recently, much attention has been focused on the high-level induction of IFN-α/β upon the activation of TLR9 subfamily members in pDCs [32–34]. Accumulating evidence indeed indicates that certain viruses induce the *IFN-α/β* genes via the activation of the TLR9 subfamily members TLR7, TLR8 and TLR9 [32,35–39]. For example, DNA viruses such as HSV contain a high number of unmethylated CpG motifs in their genome, which activate TLR9 for a robust IFN induction in pDCs [35,36]. Similarly, RNA viruses such as influenza virus or VSV activate TLR7/8 by their genomic, single-stranded RNA (ssRNA) [37–39].

The TLR3- or TLR4-mediated IFN induction involves the Toll/interleukin-1 receptor (TIR)-domain containing adaptor-inducing interferon (TRIF); however, the TLR9 subfamily members exclusively utilize MyD88 as the adaptor for the induction [32,35–39]. It was found that MyD88 interacts with IRF-7 but not with IRF-3 [40,41] in the cytoplasm, and IRF-7 colocalizes with MyD88 in endosomal vesicles [42]. IRF-7 was also found to interact with TRAF6, another adaptor molecule functioning downstream of MyD88 [40,41]. Definitive evidence for the absolute requirement of IRF-7 in *IFN-α/β* gene induction in pDCs via TLR9 subfamily activation has been provided by the analysis of *Irf7*$^{-/-}$ mice [30]. Splenic pDCs derived from *Irf7*$^{-/-}$ mice exhibit a profound defect in the induction of IFN-α/β production when stimulated either by viral infections (HSV and VSV) or by synthetic TLR ligands, such as A/D-type CpG oligodeoxynucleotide (ODN) (CpG-A) and synthetic ssRNA [30]. On the other hand, the induction occurred normally in pDCs from *Irf3*$^{-/-}$ or *Irf5*$^{-/-}$ mice when stimulated by these ligands [30,43]. To clarify further this point, we also examined the IFN-α induction in pDCs from these mutant mice infected by HSV or VSV and found that the induction also occurred normally in these cells (Fig. 2 and Ref. [30]). Therefore, a robust IFN gene induction in pDCs is totally dependent on the activation of IRF-7. As mentioned above, IRF-7 is also essential for IFN induction mediated by the TLR-MyD88-independent cytosolic detection of viruses in fibroblasts (the classical pathway). IRF-7 therefore appears to be the master regulator of the entire IFN-dependent defence mechanism against viral infections [30]. It has been reported that the high-level IFN induction in pDCs may be due to an increased expression level of IRF-7 in these cells relative to other cell types [30,44]. In this regard, we have recently examined IFN-α induction in pDCs from *Irf2*$^{-/-}$ mice. IRF-2 is known to function as the negative regulator (transcriptional attenuator; [45]) of the IFN-ISGF3 pathway and the loss of IRF-2 results in the upregulation of the IFN-inducible genes. Indeed, IRF-7 mRNA expression levels are markedly upregulated in splenic cells [45]. Interestingly, IFN-α

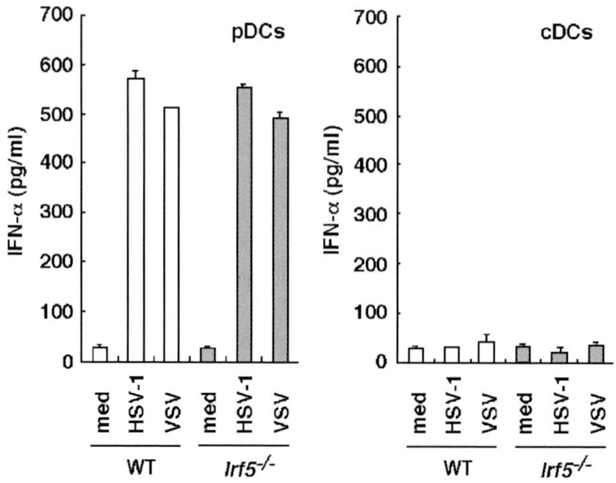

Fig. 2. IFN-α induction in *Irf-5*$^{-/-}$ DC subsets by DNA and RNA viruses. The preparation of splenic pDCs and cDCs were described in [30]. WT and *Irf-5*$^{-/-}$ DCs were infected with 10 MOI of HSV-1 or VSV for 24 h. IFN-α induction levels were measured by ELISA. Results shown are the means (± S.D.) of triplicate determinations.

induction increased in *Irf2*$^{-/-}$ pDCs (Fig. 3); this observation is, therefore, interpreted that the absence of this factor results in an enhanced IFN signaling and IRF-7 induction, which lead to the enhancement of the IRF-7-dependent IFN induction pathway. Interestingly, however, the high-level IFN induction did not occur in cDCs from *Irf2*$^{-/-}$ mice (Fig. 3), suggesting that the upregulation of IRF-7 expression per se does not explain the pDCs' ability to produce IFNs in response to TLR9 stimulation (see below).

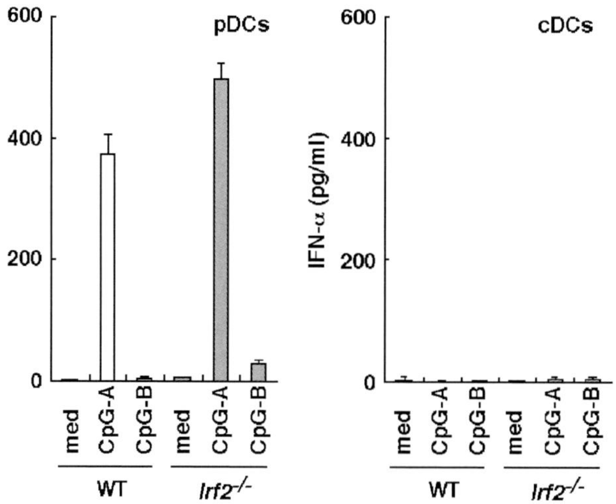

Fig. 3. IFN-α induction in *Irf-2*$^{-/-}$ DC subsets in response to CpG-A ODN. WT and *Irf-2*$^{-/-}$ DCs were stimulated with 3 μM of CpG-A or 0.3 μM of CpG-B for 24 h. IFN-α induction levels were measured by ELISA. Note that robust IFN-α induction dose not occur in *Irf-2*$^{-/-}$ DCs, but the induction was further enhanced in *Irf-2*$^{-/-}$ pDCs compared with wild-type pDCs, when stimulated by CpG-A.

The mutational studies of MyD88 revealed that the death domain of MyD88 is responsible for MyD88 interaction with IRF-7. The death domain also interacts with the interleukin-1 receptor-associated serine/threonine kinase (IRAK) family of serine/threonine kinases, the signal transducer between MyD88 and the tumor necrosis factor receptor-associated factor 6 (TRAF6), suggesting the potential involvement of IRAKs in the IRF-7 pathway [31,46,47]. Indeed, pDCs derived from *Irak4*-deficient mice have a defect in IFN-α production [40], and it has been shown that IRAK1 directly phosphorylates IRF-7 [48]. Furthermore, *Irak4*$^{-/-}$ or *Irak1*$^{-/-}$ pDCs exhibit a severe impairment of IFN-α induction [48] when stimulated by ligands for TLR7 or TLR9, collectively suggesting that IRAK4 may act upstream of IRAK1 in the signaling and these IRAKs are critical for the activation of IRF-7.

4. Spatiotemporal regulation of TLR9 signaling pathway

Although the above results indicate the essential role in the TLR9-MyD88-IRAK-IRF-7 pathway for the robust IFN induction, it remained mysterious how and why pDCs, but not other cell types such as conventional DCs (cDCs) achieve the activation of this pathway. In this context, we have recently demonstrated that the TLR9 ligand CpG-A is retained for long periods in the endosomal vesicles of pDCs, where it colocalizes with IRF-7 that interacts therein with MyD88 [42]. In contrast, CpG-A is rapidly transferred to lysosomal vesicles in cDCs [42]. The importance of this spatiotemporal regulation is underscored by the observation that cDCs too can produce large amounts of IFN in TLR9-dependent manner, when CpG-A is manipulated to undergo endosomal trafficking similar to that in pDCs [42]. Thus, the endosomal persistence of MyD88-IRF-7 signaling, rather than the basal expression levels of IRF-7 mRNA, critically determines the unique ability of pDCs to produce large amounts of IFN-α/β. Consistently, the robust IFN induction does not occur in cDCs from *Irf2*$^{-/-}$ mice expressing IRF-7 at a higher level than wild-type cDCs (Fig. 3). This ingenious spatiotemporal regulation of signaling in pDCs may represent a distinct response to pathogen-associated nucleic acids that could be exploited for the manipulation of immune responses.

5. Positive feedback regulation of IRF-7-mediated IFN induction in classical and TLR9-MyD88-dependent pathways

We have proposed the positive feedback model for the IFN gene induction in MEFs and other cell types such as cDCs [18,29,30]: IRF-7, expressed at low levels in unstimulated cells, is critical for activating the initial phase of gene induction; this induction indeed occurs even in the absence of IRF-3. Although IRF-3 also participates in this pathway, it perhaps needs to interact with IRF-7 for its full function. In other words, the homodimer of IRF-7 or the heterodimer of IRF-7 and IRF-3, rather than the IRF-3 homodimer, is perhaps very critical for inducing IFN-α/β in MEFs infected by viruses. Once the initial activation of IFN genes is achieved by IRF-7 (and IRF-3), the positive feedback regulation becomes fully operational, wherein IFN-induced IRF-7 fully participates (Fig. 4, upper panel). This reciprocal coupling of IFN gene induction and IFN signaling ensures the efficient IFN induction to evoke robust antiviral immune responses [30]. In pDCs, a similar mechanism operates in that IRF-7 induction by IFN signaling (mediated by ISGF3 and attenuated by

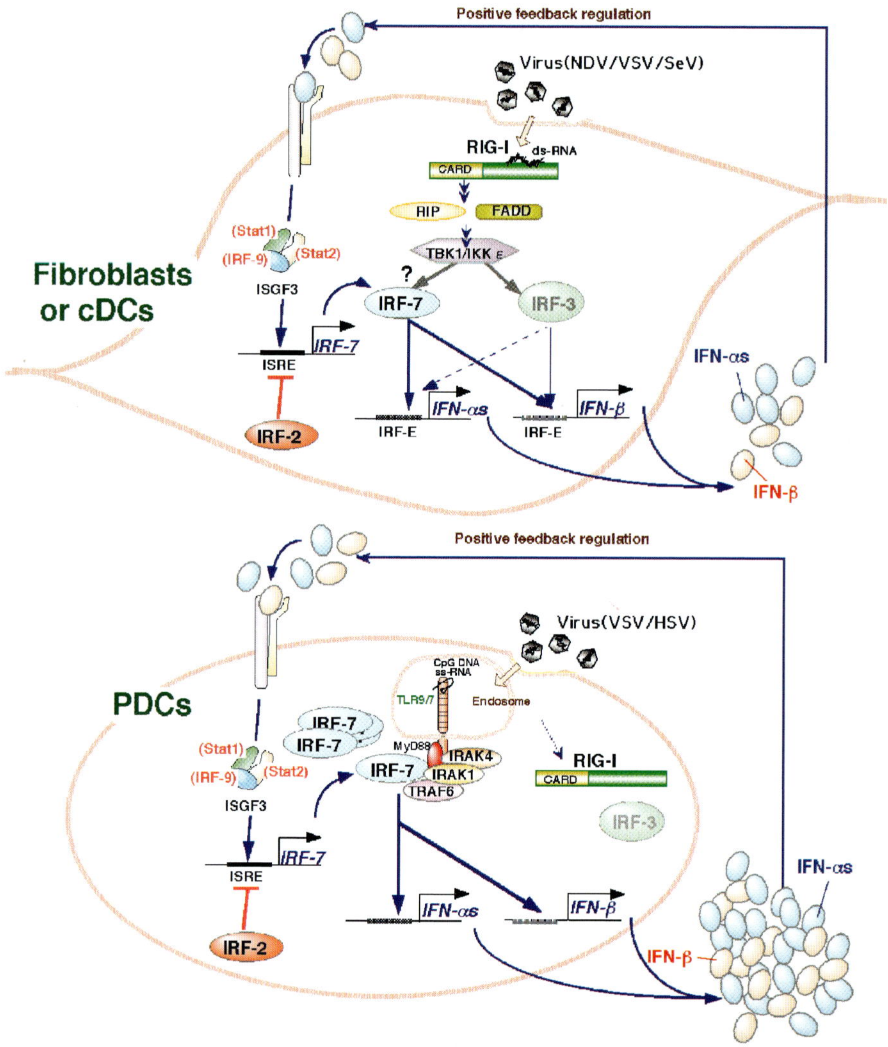

Fig. 4. *IFN-α/β* gene induction; the classical pathway and TLR9-MyD88 pathway. In most cell types, such as fibroblasts and conventional dendritic cells (cDCs), the classical pathway is operational, wherein IRF-7 plays a pivotal role in both the first and second phase of IFN induction (upper panel). In addition, as the crucial components of the cytosolic virus detection system, RIG-I and TBK1 were recently identified [20]. The interaction of the helicase domain of RIG-I with viral RNA or dsRNA may induce protein–protein interactions between the RIG-I CARD domain and other unknown CARD-containing adaptor proteins, resulting in the activation of TBK1. In addition, FADD and RIP1 have also been implicated in this activation pathway, but it remains to be clarified how these factors precisely contribute to the TBK1 activation [52]. Activated TBK1 induces the phosphorylation of the specific serine residues of IRF-3 and IRF-7, resulting in the homodimerization of IRF-7 or the heterodimerization of IRF-7 and IRF-3. These dimers then translocate to the nucleus and activate the *IFN-α/β* genes. IRF-7 and RIG-I are induced by IFN signaling, which is an essential aspect for the amplification of IFN-α/β signaling. In pDCs, which is specialized for the high-level IFN induction (lower panel), IRF-7 directly binds to MyD88. IRF-7 is activated by IRAK4, IRAK1 and TRAF6 for a robust IFN-α/β induction. The newly identified MyD88-IRF-7 signaling pathway is under spatiotemporal regulation, and this signaling occurs in endosomes in pDCs for a long period, whereas in cDCs, the endosomal signaling does not occur unless the TLR9 ligand is manipulated for endosomal retention (together with the TLR9 receptor) (see [42] for details).

IRF-2; Fig. 3) is essential for achieving the high-level IFN induction. Unlike the classical pathway, IRF-3 is not involved in this TLR9 pathway of IFN induction (Fig. 4, lower panel).

6. Future prospects

The series of recent studies carried out by us and many others have largely uncovered the mechanisms of IFN-α/β induction in distinct cell types infected by viruses or activated by TLR ligands. Although not mentioned here, the MyD-88-independent, IRF-3-dependent pathway of IFN induction also operates for the signaling of TLRs other than those of the TLR9 subfamily [49–51]. It is possible that we will see many more mechanisms of sensing viral or host components, such as nucleic acids, that also evoke IFN induction. How pDCs acquired the spatiotemporal signaling mechanism for massive IFN production will also be a very interesting issue. Because of the space limitation, the mechanisms underlying the activation of IRF-3 and IRF-7 have not been touched upon in this article, but the activation of these factors by phosphorylation has been much studied, and we anticipate to learn more about how these factors become activated via other mechanisms [52].

In contrast to the beneficial aspects of the IFN system on the host defence against viral infection or oncogenesis, accumulating evidence also suggests that an aberrant activation of immune systems by high levels of IFN-α/β contributes to the development of autoimmune diseases, such as systemic lupus erythematosus (SLE) [53,54]. An aberrant activation of the MyD88-IRF-7 pathway might be responsible for pathogenesis of this disease. In this context, it is interesting that the TLR9-MyD88-IRF-7 signaling pathway is under spatiotemporal regulation, and that in patients with SLE, a complex(es) of anti-DNA antibodies and DNA is present and it binds to and enters into the endosomes of pDCs via Fc receptor-mediated endocytosis [55]. A further understanding of the IRF-IFN system should provide important insights into improving therapeutic interventions for numerous diseases associated with infection and immunity.

Acknowledgements

This work was supported in part by a grant for Advanced Research on Cancer and Grant-in-Aid 16017220 for Scientific Research on Priority Areas from the Ministry of Education, Culture, Sports, Science, and Technology of Japan and a grant of the Uehara Memorial Foundation. TM was supported by an Ishidu Shun Memorial Scholorship. We thank our colleagues, particularly Dr. Y. Ohba for stimulatory discussions.

References

[1] T. Taniguchi, et al., Human leukocyte and fibroblast interferons are structurally related, Nature 285 (1980) 547–549.

[2] S. Pestka, et al., Interferons and their actions, Annu. Rev. Biochem. 56 (1987) 727–777.

[3] J. Vilcek, G.S. Sen, in: D.M. Fields, P.M. Knipe, P.M. Howley (Eds.), Fields Virology, Third edition, Lippincott-Raven, Philadelphia, 1996, pp. 375–399.

[4] G.R. Stark, et al., How cells respond to interferons, Annu. Rev. Biochem. 67 (1998) 227–264.

[5] D.E. Levy, A. Garcia-Sastre, The virus battles: IFN induction of the antiviral state and mechanisms of viral evasion, Cytokine Growth Factor Rev. 12 (2001) 143–156.
[6] M.G. Katze, I.M. He, B.R. Gale Jr., Viruses and interferon: a fight for supremacy, Nat. Rev., Immunol. 2 (2002) 675–687.
[7] S. Pestka, C.D. Krause, M.R. Walter, Interferons, interferon-like cytokines, and their receptors, Immunol. Rev. 202 (2004) 8–32.
[8] T. Taniguchi, A. Takaoka, A weak signal for strong responses: interferon-α/β revisited, Nat. Rev., Mol. Cell Biol. 2 (2001) 378–386.
[9] Q. Lin, C. Dong, M.D. Cooper, Impairment of T and B cell development by treatment with a type I interferon, J. Exp. Med. 187 (1998) 79–87.
[10] K. Honda, T. Mizutani, T. Taniguchi, Negative regulation of IFN-alpha/beta signaling by IFN regulatory factor 2 for homeostatic development of dendritic cells, Proc. Natl. Acad. Sci. U. S. A. 101 (2004) 2416–2421.
[11] A. Takaoka, et al., Integration of interferon-α/β signalling to p53 responses in tumour suppression and antiviral defence, Nature 424 (2003) 516–523.
[12] C.A. Biron, Interferons α and β as immune regulators-a new look, Immunity 14 (2001) 661–664.
[13] A. Le Bon, D.F. Tough, Links between innate and adaptive immunity via type I interferon, Curr. Opin. Immunol. 14 (2002) 432–436.
[14] A. Iwasaki, R. Medzhitov, Toll-like receptor control of the adaptive immune responses, Nat. Immunol. 5 (2004) 987–995.
[15] T. Taniguchi, et al., IRF family of transcription factors as regulators of host defense, Annu. Rev. Immunol. 19 (2001) 623–655.
[16] Y. Mamane, et al., Interferon regulatory factors: the next generation, Gene 237 (1999) 1–14.
[17] I. Marie, J.E. Durbin, D.E. Levy, Differential viral induction of distinct interferon-a genes by positive feedback through interferon regulatory factor-7, EMBO J. 17 (1998) 6660–6669.
[18] M. Sato, et al., Positive feedback regulation of type I IFN genes by the IFN-inducible transcription factor IRF-7, FEBS Lett. 441 (1998) 106–110.
[19] M. Miettinen, et al., IFNs activate toll-like receptor gene expression in viral infections, Genes Immun. 2 (2001) 349–355.
[20] M. Yoneyama, et al., The RNA helicase RIG-I has an essential function in double-stranded RNA-induced innate antiviral responses, Nat. Immunol. 5 (2004) 730–737.
[21] S. Goodbourn, T. Maniatis, Overlapping positive and negative regulatory domains of the human β-interferon gene, Proc. Natl. Acad. Sci. U. S. A. 85 (1988) 1447–1451.
[22] J.F. Leblanc, et al., Synergism between distinct enhanson domains in viral induction of the human beta interferon gene, Mol. Cell. Biol. 10 (1990) 3987–3993.
[23] D.W. Du, T. Maniatis, An ATF/CREB binding site is required for virus induction of the human interferon beta gene [corrected], Proc. Natl. Acad. Sci. U. S. A. 89 (1992) 2150–2154.
[24] T. Fujita, et al., Interferon-beta gene regulation: tandemly repeated sequences of a synthetic 6 bp oligomer function as a virus-inducible enhancer, Cell 49 (1987) 357–367.
[25] M. Miyamoto, et al., Regulated expression of a gene encoding a nuclear factor, IRF-1, that specifically binds to IFN-β gene regulatory elements, Cell 54 (1988) 903–913.
[26] W.M. Chu, et al., JNK2 and IKKbeta are required for activating the innate response to viral infection, Immunity 11 (1999) 721–731.
[27] J. Ryals, et al., A 46-nucleotide promoter segment from an IFN-alpha gene renders an unrelated promoter inducible by virus, Cell 41 (1985) 497–507.
[28] J. Braganca, et al., Synergism between multiple virus-induced factor-binding elements involved in the differential expression of interferon α genes, J. Biol. Chem. 272 (1997) 22154–22162.
[29] M. Sato, et al., Distinct and essential roles of transcription factors IRF-3 and IRF-7 in response to viruses for IFN-α/β gene induction, Immunity 13 (2000) 539–548.
[30] K. Honda, et al., IRF-7 is the master regulator of type-I interferon-dependent immune responses, Nature 434 (2005) 772–777.
[31] K. Takeda, S. Akira, Toll-like receptors in innate immunity, Int. Immunol. 17 (2005) 1–14.
[32] H. Wagner, The immunobiology of the TLR9 subfamily, Trends Immunol. 25 (2004) 381–386.

[33] A.M. Krieg, CpG motifs in bacterial DNA and their immune effects, Annu. Rev. Immunol. 20 (2002) 709–760.
[34] M. Colonna, G. Trinchieri, Y.J. Liu, Plasmacytoid dendritic cells in immunity, Nat. Immunol. 5 (2004) 1219–1226.
[35] J. Lund, et al., Toll-like receptor 9-mediated recognition of Herpes simplex virus-2 by plasmacytoid dendritic cells, J. Exp. Med. 198 (2003) 513–520.
[36] A. Krug, et al., Herpes simplex virus type 1 activates murine natural interferon-producing cells through toll-like receptor 9, Blood 103 (2004) 1433–1437.
[37] S.S. Diebold, et al., Innate antiviral responses by means of TLR7-mediated recognition of single-stranded RNA, Science 303 (2004) 1529–1531.
[38] F. Heil, et al., Species-specific recognition of single-stranded RNA via toll-like receptor 7 and 8, Science 303 (2004) 1526–1529.
[39] J.M. Lund, et al., Recognition of single-stranded RNA viruses by Toll-like receptor 7, Proc. Natl. Acad. Sci. U. S. A. 101 (2004) 5598–5603.
[40] K. Honda, et al., Role of a transductional-transcriptional processor complex involving MyD88 and IRF-7 in Toll-like receptor signaling, Proc. Natl. Acad. Sci. U. S. A. 101 (2004) 15416–15421.
[41] T. Kawai, et al., Interferon-α induction through Toll-like receptors involves a direct interaction of IRF7 with MyD88 and TRAF6, Nat. Immunol. 5 (2004) 1061–1068.
[42] K. Honda, et al., Spatiotemporal regulation of MyD88-IRF-7 signalling for robust type-I interferon induction, Nature 434 (2005) 1035–1040.
[43] A. Takaoka, et al., Integral role of IRF-5 in the gene induction programme activated by Toll-like receptors, Nature 434 (2005) 243–249.
[44] A. Izaguirre, et al., Comparative analysis of IRF and IFN-alpha expression in human plasmacytoid and monocyte-derived dendritic cells, J. Leukoc. Biol. 74 (2003) 1125–1138.
[45] S. Hida, et al., CD8(+) T cell-mediated skin disease in mice lacking IRF-2, the transcriptional attenuator of interferon-α/β signaling, Immunity 13 (2000) 643–655.
[46] R. Medzhitov, Toll-like receptors and innate immunity, Nat. Rev., Immunol. 1 (2001) 135–145.
[47] N. Suzuki, et al., Severe impairment of interleukin-1 and Toll-like receptor signalling in mice lacking IRAK-4, Nature 416 (2002) 750–756.
[48] S. Uematsu, et al., Interleukin-1 receptor-associated kinase-1 plays an essential role for Toll-like receptor (TLR)7- and TLR9-mediated interferon-α induction, J. Exp. Med. 201 (2005) 915–923.
[49] H. Hemmi, et al., The roles of two IkappaB kinase-related kinases in lipopolysaccharide and double stranded RNA signaling and viral infection, J. Exp. Med. 199 (2004) 1641–1650.
[50] K. Hoebe, et al., Identification of Lps2 as a key transducer of MyD88-independent TIR signalling, Nature 424 (2003) 743–748.
[51] M. Sasai, et al., Cutting Edge: NF-kappaB-activating kinase-associated protein 1 participates in TLR3/Toll-IL-1 homology domain-containing adapter molecule-1-mediated IFN regulatory factor 3 activation, J. Immunol. 174 (2005) 27–30.
[52] K. Honda, et al., Regulation of type I interferon induction: a current View. Int. Immunol. (in press).
[53] P. Blanco, et al., Induction of dendritic cell differentiation by IFN-alpha in systemic lupus erythematosus, Science 294 (2001) 1540–1543.
[54] L. Ronnblom, G.V. Alm, Systemic lupus erythematosus and the type I interferon system, Arthritis Res. Ther. 5 (2003) 68–75.
[55] U. Bave, et al., Fc gamma RIIa is expressed on natural IFN-alpha-producing cells (plasmacytoid dendritic cells) and is required for the IFN-alpha production induced by apoptotic cells combined with lupus IgG, J. Immunol. 171 (2003) 3296–3302.

International Congress Series 1285 (2005) 114–120

www.ics-elsevier.com

Regulatory role of phosphoinositide 3-kinase in immune response

Shigeo Koyasu [a,b,*], Shigeori Nagai [a,b], Masashi Ohtani [a,b], Taro Fukao [a], Yukiko Baba [a,b], Mari Fujiwara [a,b], Satoshi Matsuda [a,b]

[a] *Department of Microbiology and Immunology, Keio University School of Medicine, Japan*
[b] *Core Research for Evolutional Science and Technology, Japan Science and Technology Agency, Japan*

Abstract. We have previously shown that phosphoinositide 3-kinase (PI3K) activity is important in the balance between Th1 and Th2 responses. Lack of PI3K resulted in the impaired host immune response against nematode infection due to decreased Th2 responses. In contrast, PI3K deficiency enhanced Th1 responses and increased the host immune response against *Leishmania major* infection. Studies on the regulatory mechanisms of Th1/Th2 induction by PI3K have revealed that PI3K negatively regulates production of interleukin (IL)-12, a crucial cytokine for Th1 induction, from dendritic cells (DCs). Numerous stimuli inducing IL-12 production concomitantly activate PI3K in DCs, and both PI3K$^{-/-}$ and PI3K inhibitor-treated DCs demonstrated increased IL-12 production. Our findings indicate the presence of negative feedback mechanisms for IL-12 production during DC activation that likely contribute to the prevention of excessive Th1 polarization causing undesired immune responses. This novel mechanism at the same time highlights the importance of negative regulatory signaling and raises possible therapeutic strategies targeting such signal transduction cascades in innate immune system.

Keywords: Phosphatidylinositol-(3,4,5)-trisphosphate; Interleukin-12; Pten; *Strongyloides venezuelensis*; *Leishmania major*

1. Introduction

Innate immunity induced by microbial infection is triggered by stimulation of macrophages and dendritic cells (DCs) through toll-like receptors (TLRs) [1,2].

* Corresponding author. Department of Microbiology and Immunology, Keio University School of Medicine, Japan. Tel.: +81 3 5363 3768; fax: +81 3 5361 7658.

E-mail address: koyasu@sc.itc.keio.ac.jp (S. Koyasu).

doi:10.1016/j.ics.2005.08.050

Stimulation through TLRs by their ligands such as lipopolysaccharide (LPS) (endotoxin) and peptidoglycan (PGN) results in the production of various cytokines including interleukin (IL)-12 [1–6]. IL-12 stimulates natural killer cells, $CD8^+$ T cells, γδT cells, DCs and macrophages to produce interferon-γ (IFN-γ), which activates microbicidal activity of macrophages and plays an important role in limiting microbial growth during the innate immune response [3,7]. IL-12 is also a critical cytokine in antigen specific Th1 responses [4–6]. The resultant inflammatory responses are essential for the eradication of infectious microorganisms. A combination of innate immunity and effective induction of Th1 response is particularly critical in immune response against intracellular microorganisms.

Although the importance of DC-derived IL-12 is apparent in both innate and adaptive immunity, IL-12 may also be harmful if its expression is dysregulated. Exaggeration of IL-12 production may cause endotoxin shock-like syndrome or gastrointestinal damage owing to enhanced sensitization to local microbial agents [8,9]. Moreover, hyper-production of IL-12 results in strong cellular immunity through enhanced Th1 cell induction, which often leads to organ-specific autoimmune diseases [8,9]. Because of the importance of proper regulation of IL-12 production in the immune system, many studies have focused on the regulation of IL-12 production and proposed several potential mechanisms. An anti-inflammatory cytokine IL-10 blocks IL-12 production by DCs in response to second microbial stimulation, resulting in a tolerant status of DCs or “DC paralysis” [10,11]. Another mechanism called “DC exhaustion” may also be important in terms of IL-12 limitation [12]. Chemoattractants often suppress IL-12 production by DC and this effect is probably mediated through Gi protein signaling [13,14].

Furthermore, several intracellular signaling molecules are known to downregulate TLR signaling. Those include IRAK-M and SOCS-1 that act as dominant-negative molecules downstream of TLR signaling [15–17]. Enhanced production of pro-inflammatory cytokines including IL-12 was observed in IRAK-M-deficient macrophages, indicating that IRAK-M is a negative regulator of TLR signaling [15]. SOCS-1 deficiency also causes hyper-production of pro-inflammatory cytokines from macrophages [16,17]. Although this SOCS-1-dependent negative regulation is reportedly specific in TLR4 signaling [16,17], this is also a novel negative regulatory machinery for TLR-mediated signaling.

We have been interested in the role of a lipid kinase, phosphoinositide 3-kinase (PI3K) in the immune system and have shown that PI3K activity negatively regulates TLR signaling as well [18]. Here, we discuss the mechanism and significance of such PI3K-mediated negative regulation of IL-12 production by DCs.

2. The balance of Th1 and Th2 responses in $PI3K^{-/-}$ mice

To examine the role of PI3K in the immune system, we have established mice lacking the p85α regulatory subunit of class I_A PI3K ($PI3K^{-/-}$ mice) [19,20]. $PI3K^{-/-}$ mice were impaired in the development and function of B lymphocyte without apparent defects in T lymphocyte [20–22]. Interestingly, these mice lack gastrointestinal mast cells and are more sensitive to bacterial peritonitis than wild type mice [23]. Adoptive transfer of bone marrow-derived culture mast cells (BMMCs) prepared with IL-3 was able to restore bacterial clearance in the peritoneal cavity to a level similar to that of wild type mice. Since mast cells also play an important role in protection against intestinal parasite infection, we examined the immune response of PI3K$^{-/-}$ mice against an intestinal nematode, *Strongyloides venezuelensis* [23]. As expected, PI3K$^{-/-}$ mice showed impaired clearance of nematode. Unlike bacterial peritonitis, adoptive transfer of BMMCs was unable to restore immunity against *S. venezuelensis* unless BMMCs were cultivated with a combination of IL-4 and IL-10 before transfer. These results suggest that defective immune response to the nematode in PI3K$^{-/-}$ mice may also be due to impaired Th2 induction. In fact, production of Th2 cytokines from mesenteric lymph node cells upon secondary response was significantly impaired in PI3K$^{-/-}$ mice [23].

We then examined whether Th1 response was also affected by the lack of PI3K. We found that PI3K$^{-/-}$ mice on a BALB/c background demonstrated enhanced Th1 response and resolved *Leishmania major* infection, while wild type BALB/c mice elicited a strong Th2 response and succumbed to *L. major* infection as expected [18]. These observations indicate the importance of class I_A PI3K in the regulation of Th1 and Th2 responses in vivo. PI3K positively regulates Th2 response and suppress Th1 response.

3. PI3K-mediated negative feedback regulation of IL-12 production in DCs

In in vitro experiments, we were unable to observe the difference in Th1 and Th2 induction between wild type and PI3K$^{-/-}$ T lymphocytes, suggesting that PI3K activity in cells other than T lymphocytes is critical for the regulation of Th1 and Th2 responses. To this end, we examined the production of IL-12 from DCs, as IL-12 is crucial for Th1 induction. We then demonstrated increased production of IL-12 in splenic and bone marrow-derived DCs (BMDCs) from PI3K$^{-/-}$ mice [18]. Furthermore, a treatment with wortmannin, a specific inhibitor of PI3Ks also increased IL-12 synthesis by wild type DCs in vitro, supporting the above observations [18]. Such augmentation of IL-12 production by inhibiting PI3K is regulated at the transcriptional level as expression of mRNAs for both p35 and p40 subunits of IL-12 is increased in the presence of wortmannin. A similar observation was reported by others in macrophages, which produced more pro-inflammatory cytokines in the presence of PI3K inhibitors [24]. Overproduction of IL-12 by DCs in the absence of PI3K likely results in skewed Th1 response in PI3K$^{-/-}$ mice. Therefore, PI3K probably plays a critical negative regulatory role during induction of Th1 immune response by suppressing the production of IL-12 from DCs (Fig. 1).

A lipid phosphatase Pten counteracts with PI3K by removing the phosphate residue on the 3′ position of inositol ring [25]. To confirm that the product of PI3K is the mediator

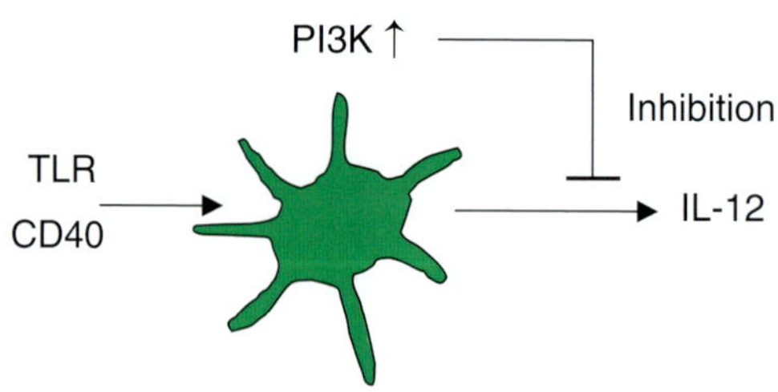

Fig. 1. PI3K-mediated negative feedback regulation of IL-12 production by DCs.

regulating IL-12 expression, we next examined the role of Pten. To this end, we prepared BMDCs by cultivation with GM-CSF of bone marrow cells from $Pten^{flox}$ mice [26] crossed with LysMCre mice [27]. Resulting BMDCs lacked Pten expression and produced lower amounts of IL-12 when stimulated with LPS than control BMDCs (unpublished). These results strongly indicate that the class I_A PI3K-Pten pathways regulating phosphatidylinositol-(3,4,5)-trisphosphate play important role in the IL-12 expression in DCs. Lack of PI3K or Pten did not significantly affect the production of IL-10 from DCs, indicating that the PI3K-Pten pathways controls IL-12 production by DCs independent of IL-10. Since most activators of DCs including LPS, PGN, CpG oligodeoxynucleotide, CD40L and RANKL that induce IL-12 production simultaneously stimulate PI3K [18,28–31], PI3K-mediated signaling pathway can actually work as a negative feedback machinery in the regulation of IL-12 production.

4. Mechanism of PI3K-mediated negative feedback regulation of IL-12

Signaling pathways downstream of TLR have been studied extensively [1,2]. There are at least two pathways, namely MyD88-dependent and-independent pathways. MyD88-dependent pathway involves TIRAP, IRAK and TRAF6, and strongly activates NF-κB pathways. On the other hand, MyD88-independent pathway utilizes TRIF, TBK1 and IRF family members, and is critical for the activation of type I interferon genes. Signal transduction mechanism(s) that activates PI3K under TLRs is still unclear. It has been demonstrated that PI3K activation downstream of TLR2 is mediated through Rac1-dependent manner [29]. On the other hand, it has been reported that TLR4 stimulation activates PI3K pathway downstream of TRAF6 with the aid of receptor interacting protein (RIP) [32]. It is unknown at present if these pathways are also operative in other TLR family members. Since PI3K activation seems to occur under triggering of many TLR members [18], it is likely that some common signaling pathway(s) for TLR-mediated activation of PI3K is present.

It is also important to study how positive and negative (PI3K) pathways are reciprocally controlled. It has been known that NF-κB and p38 MAPK pathways are involved in the activation of both IL-12 p35 and p40 gene transcription [11,33]. It has been shown that PI3K-Akt pathway also suppresses both MAPKs and NF-κB cascades, resulting in decreased production of TNF-α in macrophages [24]. However, there are several reports demonstrating positive regulation of NF-κB transactivation by PI3K [29,34]. Since NF-κB activation is required for the transcription of both IL-12 p35 and p40 [1,6,31], hyper-expression of IL-12 by PI3K inhibition discussed above is definitely inconsistent with such reports. Although more careful study thus should be performed to elucidate the entire mechanism, there are some possibilities to resolve such enigma. According to the above report [24], PI3K inhibition can augment the phosphorylation and degradation of IκBα, which result in nuclear localization of NF-κB protein. On the other hand, NF-κB transactivation by the PI3K cascade in TLR2-mediated signaling is independent on IκBα degradation and dependent on p65 phosphorylation by PI3K pathway [29]. These different functional points of PI3K cascade on NF-κB activation may give some lights on the paradoxical questions. Other possibilities should also be considered [35]; those include

GSK3β and mTOR pathways downstream of Akt, and these pathways can be involved in the regulation of IL-12 gene activation.

As mentioned earlier, there are other signaling molecules (IRAK-M and SOCS-1) controlling the production of pro-inflammatory cytokines including IL-12 [15–17]. PI3K, IRAK-M and SOCS-1 thus compose negative signaling cascades in TLR signaling essential for suppression of exaggerated inflammation and control of Th1/Th2 balance. However, PI3K-and IRAK-M-or SOCS-1-dependent negative regulatory mechanisms seem to function in different phases of innate immune response. The difference is the temporal property of their activation. IRAK-M and SOCS-1 are induced in response to the first activation of TLRs and then function as negative regulators in the second stimuli of TLR agonists [15–17]. Therefore, IRAK-M and SOCS-1 contributes primarily to the second stimuli, which is critical for endotoxin tolerance. In contrast, PI3K is constitutively expressed in innate immune cells and activated very rapidly in response to the first encounter to pathogens [18,28,29]. PI3K therefore acts as a negative regulator in the early (or first) phase of innate immune response by suppressing some of common signaling pathways downstream of TLRs. The innate immune system has thus a highly sophisticated machinery to maintain a proper magnitude of immune response to protect the host from its harmful edge.

5. Perspectives: PI3K as a therapeutic target

PI3K-mediated negative regulatory machinery of IL-12 production may be an ideal therapeutic target. Increased production of IL-12 and resultant enhancement of Th1 immune response by suppressing PI3K activity in DC would be beneficial in DC based anti-tumor immunotherapy since Th1 response favors to effective anti-tumor immune responses [36]. Furthermore, this strategy may be applicable to the treatment of Th2-dominant chronic allergic diseases such as atopic dermatitis and asthma [37]. Availability of specific inhibitor of PI3K, such as wortmannin and Ly294002, and on-going screening of related drugs may be a great advantage for this aspect [38,39]. On the contrary, invention of drugs that activate PI3K or inhibit Pten and DC-selective drug delivery system may result in the suppression of IL-12 production, and be helpful for therapeutic strategy against Th1-associated symptoms such as inflammatory bowel diseases and other organ specific autoimmune diseases.

Acknowledgement

We thank Drs. T. Yamada, M. Tanabe, T. Ota, T. Takayama, T. Asano, T. Takeuchi, J. Hata, Y. Teracuhi, T. Kadowaki and L. K. Clayton for their collaboration and valuable advice. This work was supported by a Grant-in-Aid for Scientific Research (B) (14370116, 16390146) from the Japan Society for the Promotion of Science, a Grant-in-Aid for Scientific Research on Priority Areas (C) (13226112, 14021110), a National Grant-in-Aid for the Establishment of a High-Tech Research Center in a Private University, a grant for the Promotion of the Advancement of Education and Research in Graduate Schools, and a Scientific Frontier Research Grant from the Ministry of Education, Culture, Sports, Science and Technology, Japan.

References

[1] A. Akira, K. Takeda, Toll-like receptor signalling, Nat. Rev., Immunol. 4 (7) (2004) 499–511.

[2] R. Medzhitov, Toll-like receptors and innate immunity, Nat. Rev., Immunol. 1 (2) (2001) 135–145.

[3] G. Tinchieri, Interleukin-12: a proinflammatory cytokine with immunoregulatory functions that bridge innate resistance and antigen-specific adaptive immunity, Annu. Rev. Immunol. 13 (1995) 251–276.

[4] J. Banchereau, et al., Immunobiology of dendritic cells, Annu. Rev. Immunol. 18 (2000) 767–811.

[5] K. Shortman, Y.J. Liu, Mouse and human dendritic cell subtypes, Nat. Rev., Immunol. 2 (3) (2002) 151–161.

[6] M. Moser, K.M. Murphy, Dendritic cell regulation of TH1-TH2 development, Nat. Immunol. 1 (23) (2000) 199–205.

[7] D.M. Frucht, et al., IFN-γ production by antigen-presenting cells: mechanisms emerge, Trends Immunol. 22 (10) (2001) 556–560.

[8] M.K. Gately, et al., The interleukin-12/interleukin-12-receptor system: role in normal and pathologic immune responses, Annu. Rev. Immunol. 16 (1998) 495–521.

[9] M. Falcone, N. Sarvetnick, Cytokines that regulate autoimmune responses, Curr. Opin. Immunol. 11 (6) (1999) 670–676.

[10] C. Reis e Sousa, et al., Paralysis of dendritic cell IL-12 production by microbial products prevents infection-induced immunopathology, Immunity 11 (5) (1999) 637–647.

[11] L. Zhou, A.A. Nazarian, S.T. Smale, Interleukin-10 inhibits interleukin-12 p40 gene transcription by targeting a late event in the activation pathway, Mol. Cell. Biol. 24 (6) (2004) 2385–2396.

[12] A. Langenkamp, et al., Netics of dendritic cell activation: impact on priming of TH1, TH2 and nonpolarized T cells, Nat. Immunol. 1 (4) (2000) 311–316.

[13] M.C. Braun, E. Lahey, B.L. Kelsall, Selective suppression of IL-12 production by chemoattractants, J. Immunol. 164 (6) (2000) 3009–3017.

[14] J. He, et al., Primary role for Gi protein signaling in the regulation of interleukin 12 production and the induction of T helper cell type 1 responses, J. Exp. Med. 191 (9) (2000) 1605–1610.

[15] K. Kobayashi, et al., IRAK-M is a negative regulator of Toll-like receptor signaling, Cell 110 (2) (2002) 191–202.

[16] I. Kinjyo, et al., SOCS1/JAB is a negative regulator of LPS-induced macrophage activation, Immunity 17 (5) (2002) 583–591.

[17] R. Nakagawa, et al., SOCS-1 participates in negative regulation of LPS responses, Immunity 17 (5) (2002) 677–687.

[18] T. Fukao, et al., Negative feedback regulation of IL-12 production in DCs, Nat. Immunol. 3 (9) (2002) 875–881.

[19] Y. Terauchi, et al., Increased insulin sensitivity and hypoglycaemia in mice lacking the p85α subunit of phosphoinositide 3-kinase, Nat. Genet. 21 (2) (1999) 230–235.

[20] H. Suzuki, et al., Xid-like immunodeficiency in mice with disruption of the p85α subunit of phosphoinositide 3-kinase, Science 283 (5400) (1999) 390–392.

[21] H. Suzuki, et al., PI3K and Btk differentially regulate B cell antigen receptor-mediated signal transduction, Nat. Immunol. 4 (3) (2003) 280–286.

[22] D.A. Fruman, et al., Impaired B cell development and proliferation in absence of phosphoinositide 3-kinase p85α, Science 283 (5400) (1999) 393–397.

[23] T. Fukao, et al., Selective loss of gastrointestinal mast cells and impaired immunity in PI3K-deficient mice, Nat. Immunol. 3 (3) (2002) 295–304.

[24] M. Guha, N. Mackman, The phosphatidylinositol 3-kinase-Akt pathway limits lipopolysaccharide activation of signaling pathways and expression of inflammatory mediators in human monocytic cells, J. Biol. Chem. 277 (35) (2002) 32124–32132.

[25] L.C. Cantley, B.G. Neel, New insights into tumor suppression: PTEN suppresses tumor formation by restraining the phosphoinositide 3-kinase/AKT pathway, Proc. Natl. Acad. Sci. U. S. A. 96 (8) (1999) 4240–4245.

[26] A. Suzuki, et al., T cell-specific loss of Pten leads to defects in central and peripheral tolerance, Immunity 14 (5) (2001) 523–534.

[27] B.E. Clausen, et al., Conditional gene targeting in macrophages and granulocytes using LysMcre mice, Transgenic Res. 8 (4) (1999) 265–277.
[28] P. Herrera-Velit, K.L. Knutson, N.E. Reiner, Phosphatidylinositol 3-kinase-dependent activation of protein kinase C-ζ in bacterial lipopolysaccharide-treated human monocytes, J. Biol. Chem. 272 (26) (1997) 16445–16452.
[29] L. Arbibe, et al., Toll-like receptor 2-mediated NF-κB activation requires a Rac1-dependent pathway, Nat. Immunol. 1 (6) (2000) 533–540.
[30] C.L. Ren, et al., Signal transduction via CD40 involves activation of lyn kinase and phosphatidylinositol-3-kinase, and phosphorylation of phospholipase C γ 2, J. Exp. Med. 179 (2) (1994) 673–680.
[31] B.R. Wong, et al., TRANCE, a TNF family member, activates Akt/PKB through a signaling complex involving TRAF6 and c-Src, Mol. Cell 4 (6) (1999) 1041–1049.
[32] M.S. Vivarelli, et al., RIP links TLR4 to Akt and is essential for cell survival in response to LPS stimulation, J. Exp. Med. 200 (3) (2004) 399–404.
[33] H.T. Lu, et al., Defective IL-12 production in mitogen-activated protein (MAP) kinase kinase 3 (Mkk3)-deficient mice, EMBO J. 18 (7) (1999) 1845–1857.
[34] N. Sizemore, S. Leung, G.R. Stark, Activation of phosphatidylinositol 3-kinase in response to interleukin-1 leads to phosphorylation and activation of the NF-κB p65/RelA subunit, Mol. Cell. Biol. 19 (7) (1999) 4798–4805.
[35] M. Martin, et al., Toll-like receptor-mediated cytokine production is differentially regulated by glycogen synthase kinase 3, Nat. Immunol. 6 (8) (2005) 777–784.
[36] L. Fong, E.G. Engleman, Dendritic cells in cancer immunotherapy, Annu. Rev. Immunol. 18 (2000) 245–273.
[37] M.F. Neurath, S. Finotto, L.H. Glimcher, The role of Th1/Th2 polarization in mucosal immunity, Nat. Med. 8 (6) (2002) 567–573.
[38] R.C. Stein, M.D. Waterfield, PI3-kinase inhibition: a target for drug development?, Mol. Med. Today 6 (2000) 347–357.
[39] C. Sadhu, et al., Essential role of phosphoinositide 3-kinase delta in neutrophil directional movement, J. Immunol. 170 (5) (2003) 2647–2654.

International Congress Series 1285 (2005) 121–129

www.ics-elsevier.com

SOCS genes: Critical regulators of cytokine signaling and immune responses

Akihiko Yoshimura *, Hitomi Nishinakamura, Hiromi Takaki

Division of Molecular and Cellular Immunology, Medical Institute of Bioregulation, Kyushu University, Maidashi, Higashi-ku, Fukuoka 812-8582, Japan

Abstract. Immune and inflammatory systems are controlled by multiple cytokines, including interleukins (ILs) and interferons. Many of these cytokines exert their biological functions through *Janus* tyrosine kinases (JAKs) and STAT transcription factors. The CIS (cytokine-inducible SH2 protein) and SOCS (suppressors of cytokine signaling) are a family of intracellular proteins, several of which have emerged as key physiological regulators of cytokine-mediated homeostasis, including innate and adaptive immunity. We investigated the roles of suppressors of cytokine signaling (SOCSs) in regulating dendritic cell (DC) maturation and function. We showed that SOCS1-deficient DCs induced stronger Th1-type responses both in vitro and in vivo. SOCS1-deficient DCs induced higher interferon-γ (IFNγ) production from naive T cells than wild-type DCs in vitro. Lymph node T cells also produced higher amount of IFNγ when SOCS1-deficient bone marrow-derived (BM) DCs were transferred in vivo. Moreover, SOCS1$^{-/-}$ BMDCs raised more effective anti-tumor immunity than wild-type BMDCs. On the other hand, SOCS3-deficeint BMDCs expressed lower levels of MHC, co-stimulators and CD40 in response to LPS. SOCS3-deficient DCs induced lower T cell responses. Thus, SOCS1 and SOCS3 reciprocally regulate DC maturation. © 2005 Published by Elsevier B.V.

Keywords: Cytokine; Tyrosine kinase; STAT; NF-κB; Toll-like receptor (TLR) family

Abbreviations: IL, interleukin; IFN, interferon; TNF, tumor necrosis factor; IBD, inflammatory bowel diseases; RA, rheumatoid antithesis; LPS, lipopolysaccharide; TLR, toll-like receptor; KIR, kinase inhibitory region; STAT, signal transducers and activators of the transcription family of protein; SOCS, suppressors of cytokine signaling; CIS, cytokine-inducible SH2 protein; SH2, src-homology 2.

* Corresponding author. Tel.: +81 92 642 6823; fax: +81 92 642 6825

E-mail address: yakihiko@bioreg.kyushu-u.ac.jp (A. Yoshimura).

0531-5131/ © 2005 Published by Elsevier B.V.
doi:10.1016/j.ics.2005.07.028

1. Introduction

Cytokines regulate many physiological responses and homeostasis, influencing survival, proliferation, differentiation and functional activity of cells of the immune system, as well as those of most other organ systems. Cytokines, including interleukins, interferons and hemopoietins, activate the JAK kinases (JAK1, JAK2, JAK3 and Tyk2) that associate with their cognate receptors. Activated JAKs phosphorylate the receptor cytoplasmic domains that create docking sites for SH2-containing signaling proteins. Among the substrates of tyrosine phosphorylation are members of the signal transducers and activators of transcription family of proteins (STATs) [1]. For example, IFNγ utilizes JAK1 and JAK2 which mainly activate STAT1, whereas IL-6 binding to the IL-6 receptor α chain and gp130 primarily activates JAK1 and STAT3. Interestingly, the anti-inflammatory cytokine IL-10 also activates STAT3.

Suppressors of cytokine signaling (SOCS) and cytokine-inducible SH2 protein (CIS) are a family of intracellular proteins, several of which have been shown to regulate the responses of immune cells to cytokines [2–4]. The discovery of the SOCS proteins appeared to have defined an important mechanism for the negative regulation of the cytokine–JAK–STAT pathway; however, recent studies using gene-disrupted (KO) mice have unexpectedly revealed profound roles of SOCS proteins in many immunological and pathological processes [5].

There are eight CIS/SOCS family proteins; CIS, SOCS1, SOCS2, SOCS3, SOCS4, SOCS5, SOCS6, and SOCS7; each has a central SH2 domain, an amino-terminal domain of variable length and sequence, and a carboxy-terminal 40-amino-acid module known as the SOCS box. Among them, SOCS1 and SOCS3 have been implicated in immune regulation [5]. Both SOCS1 and SOCS3 can inhibit JAK tyrosine kinase activity since they have the kinase inhibitory region (KIR) in their N-terminal domain, which is proposed to function as a pseudosubstrate [2,5]. While SOCS1 directly binds to the activation loop of JAKs through its SH2 domain, the SOCS3 SH2 domain binds the cytokine receptor (Fig. 3). The SOCS3 SH2 domain has been shown to bind to Y757 of gp130, Y985 of the leptin receptor and Y800 of the IL-12 receptor [5].

Dendritic cells (DCs) are characterized by a high capability for antigen capture and processing, migration to lymphoid organs, and expression of various co-stimulatory molecules for antigen-specific lymphocyte activation. Various DC-derived factors that induce Th-cell-polarization have been identified. Well-documented examples are Th1-cell-polarizing cytokines, such as IL-12, IL-23, IL-27, and type 1 IFNs, as well as Th2-cell-polarizing cytokines such as IL-10 and transforming-growth factor-beta (TGF-β). Among them, IFNγ is an important cytokine that activates macrophage and DC. Recent studies have shown that DCs also produce IFNγ, suggesting the presence of an autocrine-positive feedback pathway for DC activation. It has been proposed that the production of IFNγ by DCs at the time of antigen presentation also causes a strong Th1-cell polarization [6]. In mice, CD8α^+ DCs, which produce large amounts of IL-12 and IFNγ, induce Th1 responses, whereas CD8α^- DCs produce lower amounts of IL-12 and preferentially induce Th2 responses [7]. IFNγ secreting Th1-type T cell and cytotoxic T cell (CTL) responses are necessary for effective anti-tumor immunity. Thus, DCs such as CD8α^+ DCs are suggested to be suitable for vaccination in cancer immunotherapy [8].

In the present study we will focus on the roles of SOCS1 and SOCS3 in DC maturation and activation.

2. SOCS1 and innate immunity

SOCS1-knockout (KO) mice die within 3 weeks after birth with very severe inflammation. SOCS1 deficiency in the hematopoietic compartment is thought to be sufficient to cause a SOCS1-deficient inflammatory disease, since the transfer of SOCS1$^{-/-}$ bone marrow into irradiated Jak3-deficient recipients results in premature lethality. SOCS1$^{-/-}$ rag-2$^{-/-}$ mice do not die prematurely, thus, T and/or NKT cells have been suggested to play essential roles in SOCS1$^{-/-}$ diseases. However, mice lacking the SOCS1 gene, specifically in NKT and T cells, did not develop any of the inflammatory pathologies or neonatal death found in SOCS1$^{-/-}$ mice [9]. This indicates that other hematopoietic cells in addition to T and NKT cells are deeply involved in SOCS1$^{-/-}$ inflammatory diseases. Strong candidates are antigen-presenting cells including macrophages and dendritic cells (DCs).

Bacterial lipopolysaccharide (LPS) triggers innate immune responses in DC and macrophages through Toll-like receptor (TLR) 4. Other bacterial pathogens including proteoglycans and CpG-DNA also activate other TLR family receptors. The regulation of TLR signaling is a key step for inflammation, septic shock and innate/adaptive immunity. SOCS1 and SOCS3 were found to be induced by LPS or CpG-DNA stimulation in macrophages and DCs. SOCS1 has been implicated in the hypo-responsiveness to cytokines such as IFNγ after exposure of macrophages to LPS [10]. Furthermore, SOCS1-deficient mice are found to be more sensitive to LPS shock than wild-type littermates [11,12]. SOCS1$^{-/-}$ mice (pre-disease onset), SOCS1$^{+/-}$ mice and IFN$\gamma^{-/-}$ SOCS1$^{-/-}$ mice, as well as STAT1$^{-/-}$ SOCS1$^{-/-}$ mice, have all been shown to be hyper-responsive to LPS and very sensitive to LPS-induced lethality. Macrophages from these mice produced increased levels of the pro-inflammatory cytokines, such as TNFα and IL-12, as well as nitric oxide (NO), in response to LPS. One important mechanism of the suppression of LPS-induced macrophage activation by SOCS1 is inhibition of IFNβ signaling indirectly activated by LPS [13]. However, a direct effect of SOCS1 on the TLR–NF-κB pathway has been also proposed [11,12]. Ryo et al. showed that direct binding of SOCS1 to the p65 subunit of NF-κB induces proteasomal degradation of p65, which is one potential mechanism of TLR signal suppression by SOCS [14]. Moreover, LPS tolerance was severely impaired in SOCS1$^{-/-}$ mice and SOCS1-deficeint peritoneal macrophages [11,12].

SOCS1-deficient dendritic cells (DCs) are also hyper-activated and may be involved in the pathology found in SOCS1$^{-/-}$ mice [15]. We generated mice in which SOCS1 expression was restored in T and B cells on a SOCS1$^{-/-}$ background (SOCS1$^{-/-}$ Tg mice). In these mice, DCs were abnormally accumulated in the thymus and spleen and produced high levels of BAFF/BLyS and APRIL, resulting in the aberrant expansion of B cells and autoreactive antibody production. SOCS1-deficient DCs efficiently stimulated B cell proliferation in vitro and auto-antibody production in vivo. These results indicate that SOCS1 plays an essential role in normal DC functions and in the suppression of systemic autoimmunity that develops in SOCS1$^{-/-}$ Tg mice [15]. Furthermore, we speculate that SOCS1$^{-/-}$ DCs are important in the onset of SOCS1$^{-/-}$

diseases, since SOCS1-deficient DCs can activate proliferation not only of B but also of allogenic T cells [16].

3. Enhanced IFNγ production from T cells by SOCS1-deficient DCs

To examine the effect of SOCS1 deficiency in DCs for T cell activation, we first assessed mixed leukocyte reaction (MLR) with allogeneic T cells from BALB/c mice and $CD11c^+$ splenic DCs (SPDCs) from SOCS1-deficient mice. To eliminate the growth inhibitory effect of IFNγ from DCs, we performed MLR experiments using DCs from an $IFN\gamma^{-/-}$ background. $IFN\gamma^{-/-}$ $SOCS1^{-/-}$ DCs augmented T cell proliferation, and this effect was dependent on the expression level of SOCS1 in DCs (Fig. 1). The levels of Th1-type cytokines such as IFNγ and IL-2 were much higher in the culture supernatants of T cells co-cultured with $SOCS1^{-/-}$ DCs than those co-cultured with WT-DCs, whereas the level of Th2-type cytokines such as IL-4 and IL-10 was not different in these MLRs. These results indicate that SOCS1-deficient DCs induce stronger Th1-type responses in vitro compared with wild-type DCs.

Next, to assess whether $SOCS1^{-/-}$ DCs strongly initiate Th1 polarization in vivo, BMDCs from WT and $SOCS1^{-/-}$ Tg mice were pulsed with KLH and then transferred into separate footpads of the same C57BL/6 mice. Although the levels of CD80, CD86, and CD40 were similar between WT and $SOCS1^{-/-}$ BMDCs after KLH pulse, class II MHC molecules were significantly upregulated in $SOCS1^{-/-}$ BMDCs regardless of antigen loading (Fig. 2A). The migration rate of CFSE-labeled $SOCS1^{-/-}$ BMDCs to the draining popliteal lymph nodes (LNs) was also identical to that of $SOCS1^{+/+}$ BMDCs and the size of each LNs was indistinguishable 3 days after injection (data not shown), when the DC population is thought to peak. However, 5 days after injection, the popliteal LN on the side in which $SOCS1^{-/-}$ BMDCs were injected was swollen more extensively than that receiving the $SOCS1^{+/+}$ BMDCs injection (Fig. 2B).

Then we examined the antigen-specific response of T cells from these LNs. Single cell suspensions were prepared from the popliteal LNs and cultured in the presence or absence of KLH for 4 days. As shown in Fig. 2C, IFNγ and IL-2 were not strongly induced from

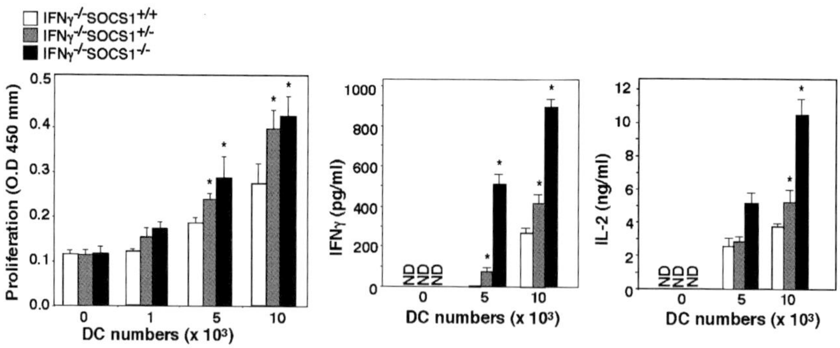

Fig. 1. SOCS1-deficient DCs induce strong Th1 responses in MLR. Proliferative capacity and Th1-type cytokine production of allogeneic T cells from BALB/c mice co-cultured with DCs from spleens of $SOCS1^{+/+}$, $SOCS1^{+/-}$ and $SOCS1^{-/-}$ mice on an $IFN\gamma^{-/-}$ background.

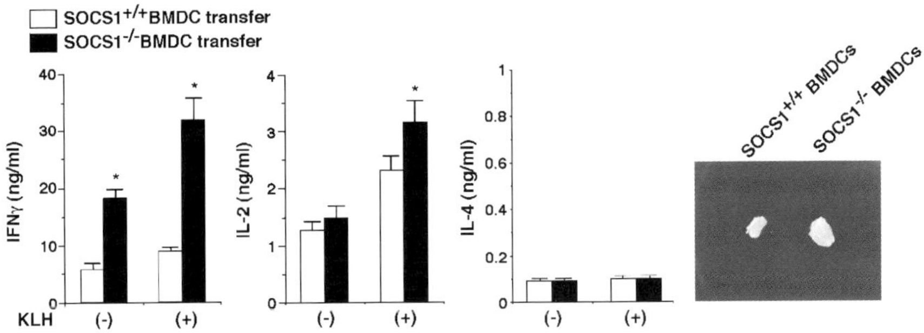

Fig. 2. SOCS1$^{-/-}$ DCs induce Th1-type responses in vivo. KLH-pulsed BMDCs from SOCS1$^{-/-}$ Tg mice and WT littermates were injected into the footpad of C57BL/6 mice. Lymphocytes from the draining lymph node immunized by WT or SOCS1$^{-/-}$ BMDCs for 5 days were cultured for 96 h in the presence or absence of KLH. The concentrations of cytokines were determined by ELISA. Right images represent the draining lymph nodes on 5 days after injections of WT or SOCS1$^{-/-}$ DCs.

KLH-restimulated LN cells by wild-type DC immunization, probably because we used immature BMDCs, while significantly higher levels of these Th1-type cytokines, especially IFNγ, were induced in lymphocytes from the LNs of SOCS1$^{-/-}$ BMDC-immunized side. Th2-type cytokine, IL-4, was not significantly induced in both cases (Fig. 2C). Similar experiments were performed using splenic DCs (SPDCs) from WT and SOCS1$^{-/-}$ Tg mice. Again, the popliteal LN immunized with SOCS1$^{-/-}$ SPDCs were more swollen than that immunized with WT-SPDCs. Lymphocytes from SOCS1$^{-/-}$ SPDC-immunized LN with KLH produced higher amount of IFNγ production than those from WT SPDC-immunized LN (Fig. 2D). However, IL-2 and IL-4 levels were not significantly different. These data suggest that SOCS1-deficient SPDCs could specifically promote IFNγ production from T cells in vivo. These results indicated that SOCS1-deficient DCs induced strong T cell proliferation as well as hyper-Th1 response in vivo.

4. SOCS1$^{-/-}$ DC is a highly potent anti-tumor vaccine

IFNγ-secreting Th1 cells are believed to be critical for long-lasting anti-tumor immunity [16]. Since SOCS1$^{-/-}$ DCs can induce strong Th1-type responses, we examined whether SOCS1 deficiency potentiates the anti-tumor ability of DCs used for therapeutic vaccination against the melanoma, B16 melanoma antigen peptide (TRP2)-loaded BMDCs were injected subcutaneously (s.c.) on days 3 and 10 after injection of B16 melanoma cells (Fig. 3A). Unlike preventive models in which DCs are injected before tumor challenge, normal DCs were not very effective in this therapeutic model. We observed reduction of tumor size and a slight improvement of recipient survival by introduction of WT-BMDCs, but these effects were independent of melanoma antigen (Fig. 3B,C). However, strong reduction of tumor size was observed when the antigen peptide-pulsed SOCS1$^{-/-}$ BMDCs were given (Fig. 3B). The mice immunized with TRP2-pulsed SOCS1$^{-/-}$ BMDCs also survived longer than mice immunized with WT-BMDCs (Fig. 3C). Peptide-unloaded BMDCs were not effective. These data indicate that BMDCs lacking SOCS1 expression represent a strong possibility for creating a powerful vaccine adjuvant for tumor-reactive immunity in vivo.

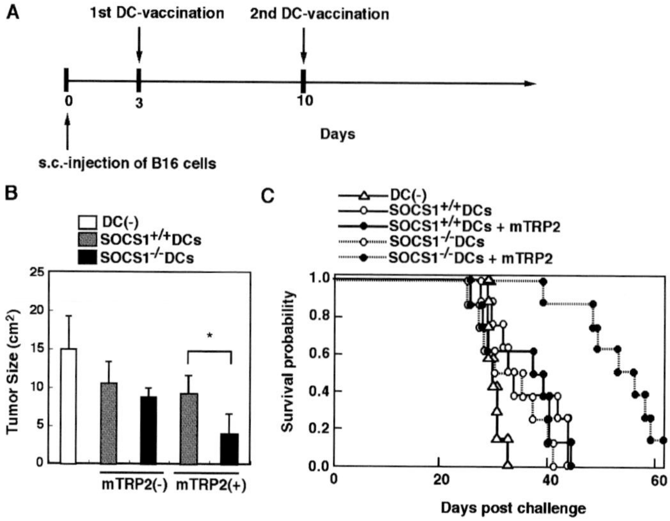

Fig. 3. Analysis of therapeutic immunity against a lethal s.c. challenge with B16 melanoma cells, and induced by vaccination using mTRP2-loaded BMDCs from SOCS1$^{-/-}$ Tg mice and WT littermates ($n=8$). Vaccination schedule (A). Tumor size is assessed by measuring two perpendicular diameters of skin tumor on 26 days after tumor challenge ($n=8$) (B). Kaplan–Meier survival curves are depicted as time after tumor challenge ($n=8$) (C).

In an independent work, Shen et al. reported that silencing the SOCS1 gene using siRNA technology in antigen-presenting DCs strongly enhances antigen-specific anti-tumor immunity [17]. They showed that DCs transfected with SOCS1 siRNA were more responsive to LPS or IFNγ than were DCs with control siRNA, as indicated by enhanced secretion of proinflammatory cytokines, such as IL-6 and TNFα and by enhanced phosphorylation of STAT1, IκB, and JNK, upon stimulation. Antigen (OVA) peptide-pulsed SOCS1-siRNA-treated DCs stimulated OVA-specific cytotoxic T cell proliferation and functioned more strongly than did control DCs. These data indicate that SOCS1-deficient DCs can strongly activate CD4^{+} (helper) and CD8^{+} (cytotoxic) T cells.

4.1. Hyper-expression of IFN-inducible genes in SOCS1$^{-/-}$ DCs

To define the molecular basis for hyper-Th1 skewing by SOCS1$^{-/-}$ DCs, we examined whether SOCS1 affects the adjuvant effect of TLR signaling in DCs. Although the levels of LPS and CpG-ODN-induced upregulation of activation markers and IL-12 production were not altered between WT and SOCS1$^{-/-}$ BMDCs (data not shown), IFNγ production as well as STAT1 activation was more strongly augmented in SOCS1$^{-/-}$ BMDCs compared with WT-BMDCs. It has long been assumed that the only cells producing IFNγ in response to IL-12 are T and NK cells. However, recent studies have shown that DCs also produce IFNγ, which induces strong Th1-cell polarization by an autocrine–paracrine positive feedback pathway during T–DC interaction. Therefore, hyper-production of IFNγ or hyper-activation of IFN signaling in SOCS1$^{-/-}$ DCs may account for hyper-induction of Th1 cells. In consistent with this notion, microarray analysis revealed that IFN-inducible genes were upregulated in SOCS1-deficient BMDCs compared with WT-BMDCs. Furthermore, STAT1 was constitutively tyrosine-phosphorylated in IFNγ$^{-/-}$

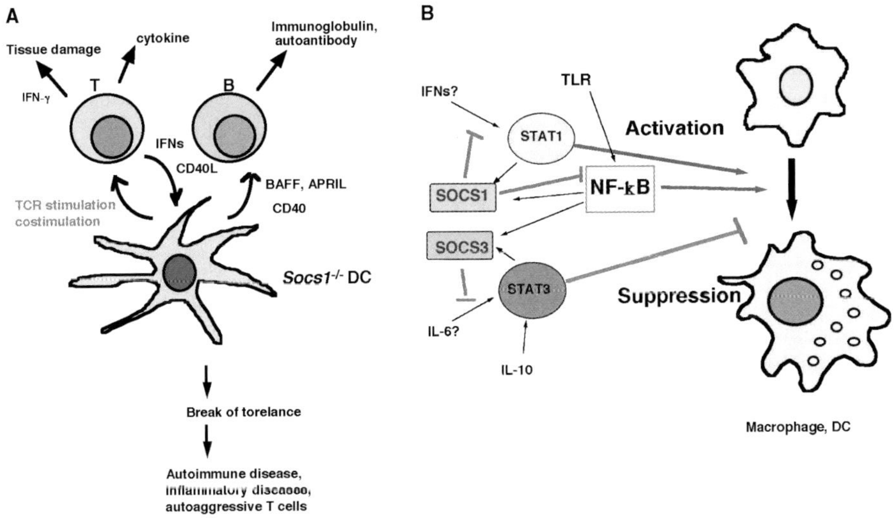

Fig. 4. (A) SOCS1-deficient DCs may disrupt central and peripheral tolerance. SOCS1-deficient dendritic cells (DCs) are hyper-activated and efficiently stimulate B cell proliferation and auto-antibody production as well as T cell proliferation and strong cytokine production. (B) Current simple model of the roles of STAT1, STAT3 and SOCS1, SOCS3 in macrophage and DC activation. SOCS1 suppresses STAT1 (and NF-κB by TLRs) and SOCS3 suppresses STAT3 activated by gp130-related cytokines. STAT1 activates macrophages and DCs, while STAT3 suppresses them, thus, SOCS1 is a negative and SOCS3 is a positive regulator of APCs. It has been known that IL-10 also suppresses macrophage activation through STAT3; however, SOCS3 does not inhibit this pathway since it does not bind to the IL-10 receptor. However, there seems to be a cross-induction of SOCS1 and SOCS3 by STAT1 and STAT3, thus the real situation may be more complicated.

$SOCS1^{-/-}$ BMDCs when they were cultured in GM-CSF. Several genes on the list, such as interferon activating gene 203 and IRF-7, are implicated in Th1 responses. Therefore hyper-activation of the IFNs–STAT1 pathway in DCs could be a mechanism of hyper-induction of Th1 responses in $SOCS1^{-/-}$ DCs.

To define the molecular mechanism of hyper-IFNγ production in $SOCS1^{-/-}$ DCs, we examined the expression of transcription factors, T-bet and Eomes, which are related to regulation of IFNγ expression. As shown in Fig. 4C, T-bet was not detected in both WT and $SOCS1^{-/-}$ BMDCs. However, Eomes expression was only detected in $SOCS1^{-/-}$ BMDCs. These results imply that Eomes may be a key molecule to produce high amount of IFNγ in $SOCS1^{-/-}$ DCs.

5. SOCS1 regulates $CD8a^{+}$ DC differentiation

Mice secondary lymphoid organs have at least three subsets of classical $CD11c^{hi}$ DCs, including $CD8a^{+}$, $CD4^{+}$ and double-negative DCs, as well as a population of $CD11c^{low}$ DCs with plasmacytoid morphology. Among them, $CD8a^{+}$ DCs produce high levels of IL-12 and induce Th1 responses. $CD8a^{+}$ DCs are also able to produce IFNγ upon IL-12 stimulation [18]. DC-derived IFNγ, together with IL-12, may also be important in activation of DCs in an autocrine manner, and lead to Th1 responses. Thus, we examined $CD8a^{+}$ DCs from $SOCS1^{-/-}$ Tg and wild-type mice. The proportion of $CD8a^{+}$ DCs in splenic and LN DCs of SOCS1$^{-/-}$ Tg mice was significantly higher than that from normal C57BL/6 and SOCS1$^{+/+}$ Tg mice. We also compared the expression levels of SOCS1 in wild-type CD8a^{+}, CD4^{+} and double-negative DCs. SOCS1 levels were significantly lower in CD8a^{+} DCs, than those in CD4^{+} and double-negative DCs. Thus, the Th1-skewing nature of CD8a^{+} DCs may be partly explained by the reduced expression of SOCS1.

6. SOCS3 and innate immunity

IL-6 is a pro-inflammatory cytokine that plays a progressive role in many inflammatory diseases, while IL-10 is an immunoregulatory cytokine that has potent anti-inflammatory activity. Although the transcription factor STAT3 is essential for the function of both IL-6 and IL-10, it is not clear how these two cytokines exhibit such contradictory functions. Recently, we demonstrated that at least in macrophages SOCS3 is a key regulator of the divergent action of these two cytokines. In macrophages lacking the SOCS3 gene, or carrying a mutation of the SOCS3 binding site (Y759F) in gp130, not only IL-10, but also IL-6, suppressed LPS-induced TNFα production [19]. SOCS3 protein was strongly induced by both IL-6 and IL-10 in the presence of LPS, but selectively inhibited IL-6 signaling, due to SOCS3 binding the IL-6 receptor, gp130 (Y759), but not the IL-10 receptor [19]. These data indicate that SOCS3 selectively blocks IL-6 signaling, interfering with its ability to inhibit LPS signaling. Consistent with this, mice specifically lacking the SOCS3 gene in macrophages and neutrophils are resistant to acute inflammation as modeled by LPS-shock. This phenotype is the complete opposite to macrophages in STAT3 conditional KO mice that are more sensitive to LPS shock and produce more TNFα in response to LPS [20]. We also found a similar opposite relationship between STAT3 and SOCS3 on DC activation (Matsumura and Yoshimura, unpublished data).

7. Conclusion

SOCS proteins are regulators of cytokine signal transduction and are essential for normal immune physiology, but also appear to contribute to the development of immunological disorders including inflammatory diseases. Recently, accumulated evidence regarding the balance of positive and negative pathways is important for a better understanding of immune systems, and this acquired knowledge will provide new insights assisting the development of novel therapeutic strategies for immunological diseases.

References

[1] J.J. O'Shea, M. Gadina, R.D. Schreiber, Cytokine signaling in 2002: new surprises in the Jak/Stat pathway, Cell 109 (2002) S121–S131.

[2] H. Yasukawa, A. Sasaki, A. Yoshimura, Negative regulation of cytokine signaling pathways, Annu. Rev. Immunol. 18 (2000) 143–164.

[3] W.S. Alexander, Suppressors of cytokine signalling (SOCS) in the immune system, Nat. Rev., Immunol. 2 (2002) 410–416.

[4] A. Yoshimura, et al., Negative regulation of cytokine signaling and immune responses by SOCS proteins, Arthritis Res. Ther. 7 (2005) 100–110.

[5] M. Kubo, T. Hanada, A. Yoshimura, Suppressors of cytokine signaling and immunity, Nat. Immunol. 4 (2003) 1169–1176.

[6] D.M. Frucht, et al., IFN-gamma production by antigen-presenting cells: mechanisms emerge, Trends Immunol. 22 (2001) 556.

[7] B. Pulendran, et al., Developmental pathways of dendritic cells in vivo: distinct function, phenotype, and localization of dendritic cell subsets in FLT3 ligand-treated mice, J. Immunol. 159 (1997) 2222.

[8] R. Maldonado-Lopez, et al., Cytokines regulate the capacity of CD8alpha(+) and CD8alpha(−) dendritic cells to prime Th1/Th2 cells in vivo, J. Immunol. 167 (2001) 4345.

[9] M.M. Chong, et al., Suppressor of cytokine signaling-1 is a critical regulator of interleukin-7-dependent CD8+ T cell differentiation, Immunity 18 (2003) 475–487.

[10] A.H. Dalpke, et al., Suppressors of cytokine signaling (SOCS)-1 and SOCS-3 are induced by CpG-DNA and modulate cytokine responses in APCs, J. Immunol. 166 (2001) 7082–7089.

[11] I. Kinjyo, et al., SOCS1/JAB is a negative regulator of LPS-induced macrophage activation, Immunity 17 (2002) 583–591.

[12] R. Nakagawa, et al., SOCS-1 participates in negative regulation of LPS responses, Immunity 17 (2002) 677–687.

[13] S. Gingras, et al., Re-examination of the role of suppressor of cytokine signaling 1 (SOCS1) in the regulation of toll-like receptor signaling, J. Biol. Chem. 279 (2004) 54702–54707.

[14] A. Ryo, et al., Regulation of NF-kappaB signaling by Pin1-dependent prolyl isomerization and ubiquitin-mediated proteolysis of p65/RelA, Mol. Cell 12 (2003) 1413–1426.

[15] T. Hanada, et al., Suppressor of cytokine signaling-1 is essential for suppressing dendritic cell activation and systemic autoimmunity, Immunity 19 (2003) 437–450.

[16] T. Hanada, et al., Induction of hyper Th1 cell-type immune responses by dendritic cells lacking the suppressor of cytokine signaling-1 gene, J. Immunol. 174 (2005) 4325–4332.

[17] L. Shen, et al., Silencing of SOCS1 enhances antigen presentation by dendritic cells and antigen-specific anti-tumor immunity, Nat. Biotechnol. 22 (2004) 1546–1553.

[18] T. Ohteki, et al., Interleukin 12-dependent interferon gamma production by CD8alpha+ lymphoid dendritic cells, J. Exp. Med. 189 (1999) 1981.

[19] H. Yasukawa, et al., IL-6 induces an anti-inflammatory response in the absence of SOCS3 in macrophages, Nat. Immunol. 4 (2003) 551–556.

[20] K. Takeda, et al., Enhanced Th1 activity and development of chronic enterocolitis in mice devoid of Stat3 in macrophages and neutrophils, Immunity 10 (1999) 39–49.

International Congress Series 1285 (2005) 130–136

www.ics-elsevier.com

Induction of high *Bcl6* expression and its roles in germinal center B cells

E. Arguni [a], N. Tsuruoka [a], M. Arima [a], A. Sakamoto [a], M. Hatano [a,b], T. Tokuhisa [a,*]

[a] *Department of Developmental Genetics [H2], Graduate School of Medicine, Chiba University, Chiba 260-8670, Japan*

[b] *Biomedical Research Center, Chiba University, Chiba 260-8670, Japan*

Abstract. The *Bcl6* proto-oncogene, which encodes a transcriptional repressor, is predominantly expressed in germinal center (GC) B cells. However, inducers of its high expression in GC B cells and a role for Bcl6 in GC B cells were largely unknown. Here we examined transcriptional regulation of the murine *Bcl6* gene. JunD/AP-1 was the major enhancer molecule in GC-derived B lymphoma cells. In addition, we identified the silencer region in the promoter and Bcl6 bound to the silencer region. Activated STATs also bound to the silencer region and competed with Bcl6 for the binding. STAT3 was the major STATs activated in GC B cells. Thus, JunD/AP-1 and STAT3 drive high *Bcl6* expression in GC B cells. Since stimulation of splenic B cells with IL-21 induced high *Bcl6* expression with STAT3 activation and *junD* induction, IL-21 may well be a major inducer for high *Bcl6* expression in GC B cells. IL-21 stimulation of naive B cells induces their apoptosis, and Bcl6-dedicient B cells are more sensitive to IL-21-induced apoptosis. Thus, Bcl6 induced in activated B cells by IL-21 stimulation protects these B cells from the apoptosis, and these B cells may differentiate into GC B cells.

Keywords: Memory; Transcription factors; Enhancer; Promoter; Silencer

1. Introduction

The *Bcl6* gene has been identified from translocation breakpoints of diffuse large cell lymphomas [1] and Bcl6 can function as a sequence specific transcriptional repressor [2,3]. The *Bcl6* gene is ubiquitously expressed in human and mouse tissues, and is predominant in germinal center (GC) B cells of human tonsils [4,5] and mouse

* Corresponding author. Tel.: +81 43 226 2181; fax: +81 43 226 2183.
E-mail address: tokuhisa@faculty.chiba-u.jp (T. Tokuhisa).

doi:10.1016/j.ics.2005.07.026

lymphoid organs [6]. To observe physiological functions of Bcl6, its gene was disrupted in the mouse germ line [7–9]. Although all haematopoietic lineages, including mature lymphocytes, can develop in Bcl6-deficient mice, GC formation is impaired after immunization [9]. GC is a complex cellular microenvironment that directs generation of high affinity memory B cells [10]. Thus, Bcl6 is an important molecule for maintaining physiological immune responses. The promoter region of the human *Bcl6* (*hBcl6*) gene has been reported [11]. Transcriptional start sites of the *hBcl6* gene were identified using mRNA from a human Burkitt's lymphoma cell line, Raji. Nucleotide sequence of the 1.5 kb promoter region contains a TATA box but no CAAT box. Furthermore, a consensus Bcl6-binding sequence was found in the first exon of *hBcl6* gene [12], suggesting that *Bcl6* expression is negatively regulated by Bcl6 itself. However, molecular mechanisms of high *Bcl6* expression are largely unknown.

Expression profiles of this gene are well conserved between humans and mice [6]. However, DNA sequence of the *hBcl6* promoter region identified in Raji cells differs from that of homologous region of the murine *Bcl6* (*mBcl6*) gene. Furthermore, the *mBcl6* database (Celera, Gene ID:12053) indicated that a putative transcriptional start site of the *mBcl6* gene is further downstream of the reported human one, and genomic DNA sequence of the new murine promoter region is quite similar to that of the homologous region of the *hBcl6* gene. Here we show that major transcriptional start sites of the *Bcl6* gene in GC B cells and several cell lines including a GC-derived human B lymphoma line, Ramos, were the further downstream of the reported human one as the *mBcl6* database pointed. The promoter analysis demonstrated that JunD/AP-1 and STAT3 are important transcriptional factors for high *Bcl6* expression in GC B cells. We discuss cytokine signals which induce JunD/AP-1 and activated STAT3 in GC B cells.

2. Materials and methods

Splenic B cells were cultured with LPS (3 μg/ml; Sigma), IL-4 (1000 U/ml), or IL-21 (30 ng/ml; R&D Systems, Inc.) in RPMI1640 supplemented with 10% FCS for 24 h at 37 °C in 5% CO_2.

To analyze the *mBcl6* promoter activity, series of DNA fragment of the putative *mBcl6* promoter region were constructed using standard restriction enzymes and PCR methods. All genomic DNA fragments were inserted into cloning sites of a pGL3-Basic vector carrying the SV40 enhancer and the firefly *Luciferase* reporter gene (Promega). Mutant *Luciferase* constructs were generated by PCR using oligonucleotide primers carrying point mutations (QuikChangeXL Site-Directed Mutagenesis Kit, Stratagene).

Transfection of genes was conducted by electroporation using the Bio-Rad Gene PulserII (Bio-Rad, Hercules, CA). Cells (1×10^7) were resuspended in 0.25 ml of the RPMI1640 medium without FCS. Equimolar amounts of the *Luciferase* reporter plasmids (total 20 μg) and the indicated amount of expression plasmids were added into the cell suspension. For all transfections, pRL-SV40 (1 μg) was added as an internal control for the transfection efficiency. Cells were harvested for the *Luciferase* assay 16–20 h after electroporation. *Luciferase* assay was done using the *Luciferase* Assay Kit (Promega) and standardized using *Luciferase* activity of pRL-SV40.

3. Results

To determine transcriptional start sites of the *mBcl6* gene, we did the rapid amplification of 5′ cDNA ends (5′RACE) analysis with mRNA isolated from FACS-isolated GC B cells or LPS-activated B cells. We identified major transcriptional start sites of the *mBcl6* gene in GC B cells and LPS-activated B cells at +95 and +64, respectively (Fig. 1). An obvious canonical TATA or CCAAT box was not found around these transcriptional start sites. In addition, DNA sequences around the start sites are conserved between mice and humans. We also examined transcriptional start sites of the *hBcl6* gene in GC-derived B lymphoma (Ramos) cells, and the major start site was at +38 in the homologous region of the *hBcl6* gene.

We made reporter constructs containing DNA fragments between −4200 bp and +5 bp, in which the Bcl6-binding sequence was excluded. The deletion from −4200 bp to −472 bp did not change the promoter activity in Ramos cells (data not shown). However, further truncation of the promoter region to −227 bp reduced the activity to less than 10% of the full length (Fig. 2). The region between −367 bp and −227 bp contains two AP-1 sites, an NF-κB site and two Sp1 sites, and we introduced the point mutations into these binding sequences of pBcl6 Luc-472. While a point mutation in the Sp1 sites or the NF-κB site did not modify the activity, mutations of both AP-1 sites reduced the promoter activity to 25% of the original (data not shown), suggesting that these AP-1 sites are important for the full activation of the *mBcl6* promoter in GC B cells.

We examined members of AP-1 family bound to the AP-1-binding sites in Ramos cells and GC B cells, using chromatin immunoprecipitation (ChIP) assays. The DNA region containing the AP-1 sites was detected in the immune complexes precipitated with anti-c-Fos, anti-c-Jun, anti-JunB, or anti-JunD, but not in those with anti-FosB (data not shown). Since the amount of DNA in the complex precipitated with anti-JunD Ab was the largest among these complexes, the binding of JunD/AP-1 to the DNA region in FACS-isolated GC-B cells was examined using ChIP assays. The DNA region was clearly detected in the complexes precipitated with anti-JunD Ab (data not shown). Thus, JunD/AP-1 may be a major enhancer molecule to drive high *Bcl6* expression in GC B cells.

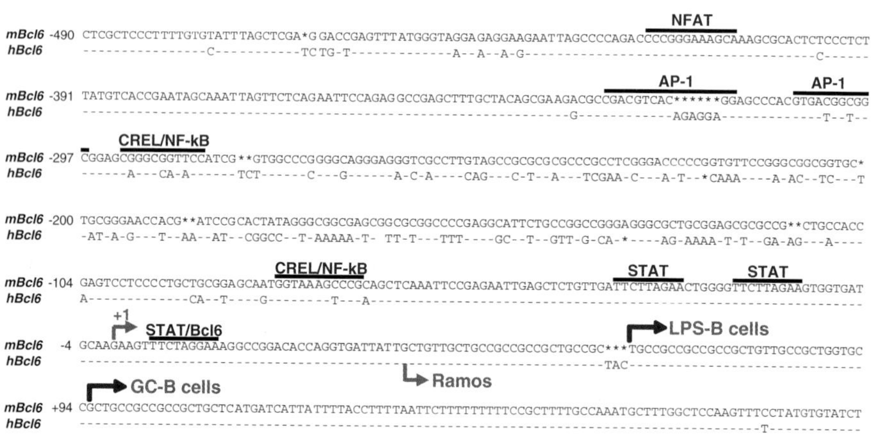

Fig. 1. The promoter region of murine *Bcl6* gene. Nucleotide sequence of the 5′ flanking region of the *mBcl6* gene was compared with that of the *hBcl6* gene. The transcriptional start site of the *mBcl6* gene from the database has been numbered as +1. Consensus sequences for binding of various potential transcriptional factors are noted and underlined.

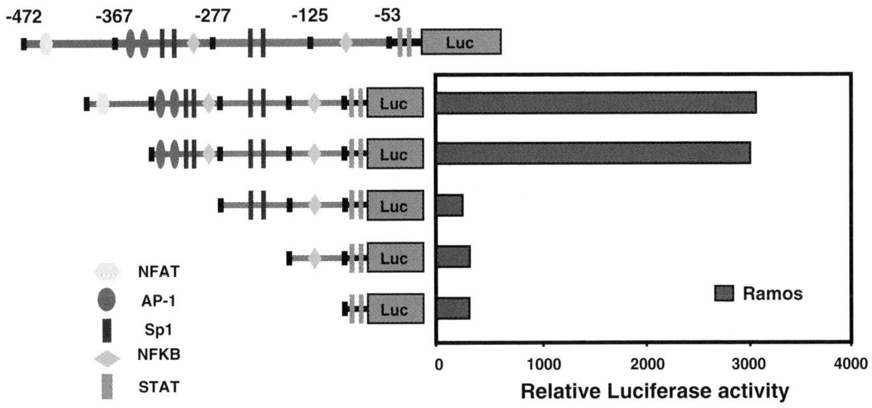

Fig. 2. Positive regulators of the mBcl6 promoter region in a GC-derived B cell line (Ramos). Basal transcriptional activity of serial deletion fragments of pBcl6 Luc-472 was examined in Ramos cells.

Surprisingly, the promoter activity in K562 cells was significantly stronger than that in Ramos cells (data not shown). Since K562 cells do not express the endogenous *hBcl6* gene [4], the strong promoter activity in K562 cells suggested that Bcl6 negatively regulates promoter activity of pBcl6 Luc-472 in Ramos cells. A major transcriptional start site of the *mBcl6* gene in GC B cells is +95, and the region between +1 and +95 contains the Bcl6-binding sequence (+6 to +16) as a silencer element in the *hBcl6* gene [12]. Thus, we extended the 3′ end of pBcl6 Luc-472/+5 to +114 (pBcl6 Luc-472/+114) and introduced the mutation in the Bcl6-binding sequence of pBcl6 Luc-472/+114. Although mutations in two STAT-binding sequences increased its promoter activity 15-fold over the original one, mutations in both the STAT-binding sequences and the Bcl6-binding sequence increased approximately 50-fold of the pBcl6 Luc-472/+114 activity (Fig. 3). These results suggest that Bcl6 binds to the STAT/Bcl6-binding sequences and reduces *Bcl6* expression in GC B cells.

Binding of STATs in GC B cells to the STAT/Bcl6-binding sites was further analyzed using ChIP assays. In GC B cells, STAT3 and a little of STAT5 and STAT6 bound to the STAT/Bcl6-binding sites, suggesting that activated STAT3 induces high *Bcl6* expression in GC B cells by competing with Bcl6 for binding to the STAT/Bcl6-binding sites in the promoter region.

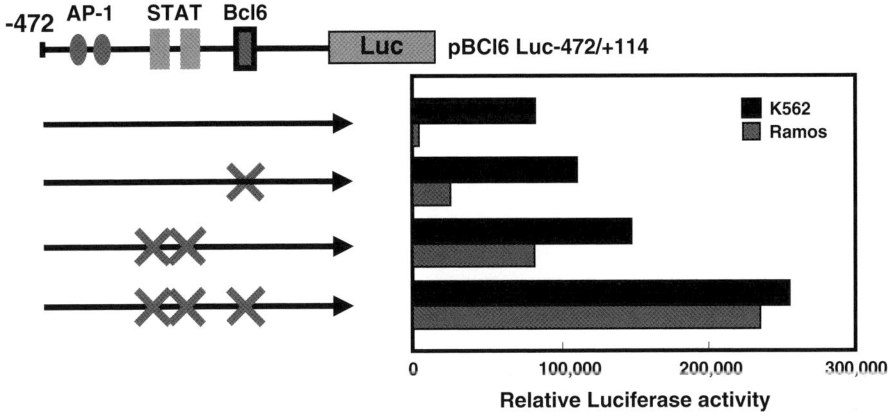

Fig. 3. Autoregulation of the *mBcl6* gene promoter. Basal transcriptional activity of mutated fragments of pBcl6 Luc-472/+114 was examined in K562 and Ramos cells.

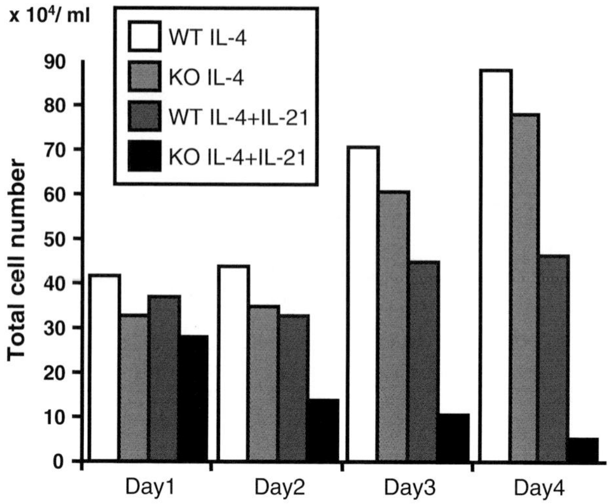

Fig. 4. The role for Bcl6 in protection of B cells from IL-21-induced apoptosis. Splenic B cells were stimulated with LPS+IL-4 in the presence or absence of IL-21. Total live cell numbers were calculated under the microscope.

Since stimulation of B cells with IL-4 [13], IL-6 [14], or IL-21 [15] activates STAT3, we examined *Bcl6* expression in splenic B cells stimulated with these cytokines. *Bcl6* expression was strongly induced in splenic B cells stimulated with IL-4 or IL-21 but not with IL-6 (data not shown). However, costimulation of B cells with IL-4 and IL-21 did not augment *Bcl6* expression. IL-4 or IL-21 stimulation also induced expression of *junD* and *fosB,* but not that of c-*fos*, c-*jun* and *junB* in splenic B cells. We examined activation of STATs in splenic B cells stimulated with IL-4 or IL-21. IL-4 and IL-21 preferentially activated STAT6 and STAT3 within 20 min after stimulation, respectively. Thus, IL-21 is a crucial cytokine to induce JunD/AP-1 and activated STAT3 in GC B cells.

IL-21 induces the apoptosis of splenic B cells, and the activation of B cells with LPS and IL-4 does not prevent IL-21-mediated apoptosis [16]. In order to examine a role for Bcl6 induced in B cells activated with IL-21, splenic B cells from Bcl6-deficient mice were stimulated with LPS+IL-4 in the presence or absence of IL-21. Live cell numbers in splenic B cells stimulated with LPS+IL-4 in the absence of IL-21 were similar between Bcl6-deficient and wild type B cell cultures (Fig. 4). However, the live cell number in Bcl6-deficient B cell cultures in the presence of IL-21 were lower than those in wild type B cell cultures. These results suggest that Bcl6 induced in B cells stimulated with IL-21 protects IL-21-induced apoptosis.

4. Discussion

We identified the promoter region of the *mBcl6* gene. Major start sites (+95 and +64) of *mBcl6* mRNA in GC B cells from immunized mice or in splenic B cells stimulated with LPS were further downstream from that (+1) of the *mBcl6* database, respectively. Since the multiple transcription start sites are a common feature of the genes with a TATA-less promoter [17], these results suggest that the *mBcl6* gene has a TATA-less promoter. Indeed, we found no obvious canonical TATA or CCAAT box around the transcriptional start sites of the *mBcl6* gene. Transcriptional start sites of the genes lacking the TATA box may rely on the GC-rich region that is bound by transcriptional

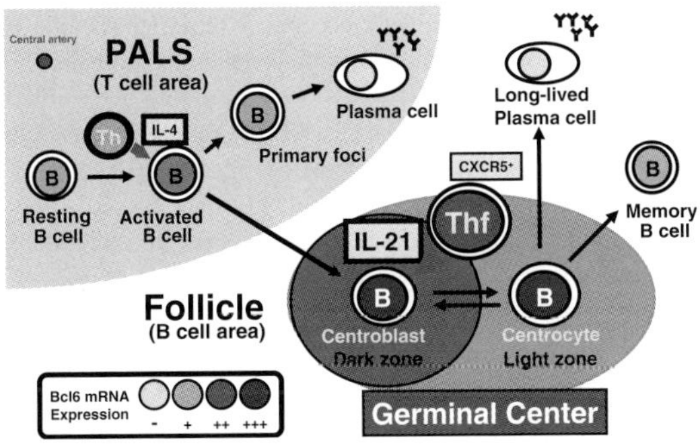

Fig. 5. Germinal center formation in the spleen after immunization. High *Bcl6* expression was induced in germinal center B cells activated with IL-21 derived from CXCR5$^+$ T follicular helper (Thf) cells.

factors [18], and the start sites of *mBcl6* mRNA in GC B cells and LPS-activated B cells are also in the GC-rich region.

JunD/AP-1 and activated STAT3 are crucial factors for high *Bcl6* expression in GC B cells, and stimulation of naive B cells with IL-21 induced high *Bcl6* expression with induction of both JunD/AP-1 and activated STAT3. Thus, IL-21 is important for subsequent differentiation of GC B cells by the induction of Bcl6 expression. Recently, a new major subset of effector T cells that provides help to B cells was identified in lymphoid tissues through expression of the chemokine receptor CXCR5 [19,20]. These T cells, termed T follicular helper (Thf) cells, home to the B cell areas of secondary lymphoid tissue and produce large amounts of IL-21 and Bcl6 [21]. These results strongly suggest that IL-21 derived from Thf cells induces high *Bcl6* expression in GC B cells (Fig. 5).

IL-21 is a recently described type I cytokine produced by Th2 cells that profoundly affects the growth, survival, and functional activation of B, T, and natural killer lymphocytes [15]. Since IL-21 stimulation of splenic B cells induces their apoptosis with an upregulation of Bax [16] and Bax is upregulated in testicular germ cell apoptosis in Bcl6-deficient mice [22], we expected a role for Bcl6 in GC B cells in protection of IL-21-induced apoptosis by preventing Bax expression. Indeed, Bcl6-deficient B cells were much more sensitive to IL-21-induced apoptosis and Bax expression was maintained in those activated B cells 48 h after stimulation (data not shown). Bax is a transcriptional target of p53 [23] and p53 is also a transcriptional target of Bcl6 [24]. Thus, Bcl6 induced in GC B cells stimulated with IL-21 from Thf cells may protect IL-21-induced apoptosis by reducing Bax expression through suppression of p53 expression.

Acknowledgements

We thank H. Satake for technical assistance and K. Yagyu for secretarial assistance. This work was supported by the Uehara Memorial Foundation.

References

[1] K. Offit, et al., t[3;22][q27;q11]: a novel translocation associated with diffuse non-Hodgkin's lymphoma, Blood 74 (1989) 1876–1879.

[2] C. Deweindt, et al., The LAZ3/BCL6 oncogene encodes a sequence-specific transcriptional inhibitor: a novel function for the BTB/POZ domain as an autonomous repressing domain, Cell Growth Differ. 6 (1995) 1495–1503.
[3] P. Dhordain, et al., Corepressor SMRT binds the BTB/POZ repressing domain of the LAZ3/BCL6 oncoprotein, Proc. Natl. Acad. Sci. U. S. A. 94 (1997) 10762–10767.
[4] G. Cattoretti, et al., BCL-6 protein is expressed in germinal-center B cells, Blood 86 (1995) 45–53.
[5] T. Onizuka, et al., BCL-6 gene product, a 92- to 98-kD nuclear phosphoprotein, is highly expressed in germinal center B cells and their neoplastic counterparts, Blood 86 (1995) 28–37.
[6] T. Fukuda, et al., The murine Bcl6 gene is induced in activated lymphocytes as an immediate early gene, Oncogene 11 (1995) 1657–1663.
[7] A.L. Dent, et al., Control of inflammation, cytokine expression, and germinal center formation by BCL-6, Science 276 (1997) 589–592.
[8] B.H. Ye, et al., The BCL-6 proto-oncogene controls germinal-centre formation and Th2-type inflammation, Nat. Genet. 16 (1997) 161–170.
[9] T. Fukuda, et al., Disruption of the Bcl6 gene results in an impaired germinal center formation, J. Exp. Med. 186 (1997) 439–448.
[10] H. Toyama, et al., Memory B cells without somatic hypermutation are generated from Bcl6-deficient B cells, Immunity 17 (2002) 329–339.
[11] K. Ohashi, et al., Characterization of the promoter region of human *BCL-6* gene, Biochem. Biophys. Res. Commun. 214 (1995) 461–467.
[12] M. Kikuchi, et al., Identification of negative regulatory regions within the first exon and intron of the *Bcl6* gene, Oncogene 19 (2000) 4941–4945.
[13] R. Umeshita-Suyama, et al., Characterization of IL-4 and IL-13 signals dependent on the human IL-13 receptor alpha chain 1: redundancy of requirement of tyrosine residue for STAT3 activation, Int. Immunol. 12 (2000) 1499–1509.
[14] J.G. Karras, et al., Signal transducer and activator of transcription-3 [STAT3] is constitutively activated in normal, self-renewing B-1 cells but only inducibly expressed in conventional B lymphocytes, J. Exp. Med. 185 (1997) 1035–1042.
[15] T. Habib, A. Nelson, K. Kaushansky, IL-21: a novel IL-2-family lymphokine that modulates B, T, and natural killer cell responses, J. Allergy Clin. Immunol. 112 (2003) 1033–1045.
[16] D.S. Mehta, et al., IL-21 induces the apoptosis of resting and activated primary B cells, J. Immunol. 170 (2003) 4111–4118.
[17] S.T. Smale, Transcription initiation from TATA-less promoters within eukaryotic protein-coding genes, Biochim. Biophys. Acta 1351 (1997) 73–88.
[18] S. Philipsen, G. Suske, A tale of three fingers: the family of mammalian Sp/XKLF transcription factors, Nucleic Acids Res. 27 (1999) 2991–3000.
[19] P. Schaerli, et al., CXC chemokine receptor 5 expression defines follicular homing T cells with B cell helper function, J. Exp. Med. 192 (2000) 1553–1562.
[20] D. Breitfeld, et al., Follicular B helper T cells express CXC chemokine receptor 5, localize to B cell follicles, and support immunoglobulin production, J. Exp. Med. 192 (2000) 1545–1552.
[21] T. Chtanova, et al., T follicular helper cells express a distinctive transcriptional profile, reflecting their role as non-Th1/Th2 effector cells that provide help for B cells, J. Immunol. 173 (2004) 68–78.
[22] S. Kojima, et al., Disruption of the Bcl6 gene increases testicular germ cell apoptosis in mice, Development 128 (2001) 57–65.
[23] T. Miyashita, J.C. Reed, Tumor suppressor p53 is a direct transcriptional activator of the human bax gene, Cell 80 (1995) 293–299.
[24] R.T. Pha, R. Dalla-Favera, The BCL6 proto-oncogene suppresses p53 expression in germinal-centre B cells, Nature 432 (2004) 635–639.

ELSEVIER

International Congress Series 1285 (2005) 137–144

www.ics-elsevier.com

Chromatin remodeling of the Th2 cytokine gene loci

T. Nakayama [a,*], M. Yamashita [a], M. Kimura [a], A. Hasegawa [a], M. Omori [a], M. Inami [a], S. Motohashi [a], M. Kitajima [a], K. Hashimoto [b], H. Hosokawa [a], R. Shinnakasu [a]

[a] *Department of Immunology, Graduate School of Medicine, Chiba University, Chiba, Japan*

[b] *Department of Life and Environmental Sciences and High Technology Research Center, Chiba Institute of Technology, Narashino, Tsudanuma, Chiba, Japan*

Abstract. Differentiation of naive CD4 T cells into Th2 cells is accompanied by chromatin remodeling including hyperacetylation of histones H3 and H4 in the nucleosomes associated with the IL-4, IL-13 and IL-5 genes. A conserved GATA3 response element (CGRE) containing four GATA consensus sequences was identified 1.6 kbp upstream of the IL-13 gene, corresponding with the 5′ border of the Th2-specific histone hyperacetylation region. The CGRE was shown to bind to GATA3, histone acetyl transferase complexes including CBP/p300, and RNA polymerase II. As for the IL-5 gene locus, CD28 costimulation selectively enhanced histone hyperacetylation through NF-κB activation and subsequent upregulation of GATA3. Chromatin remodeling of type 2 cytokine gene loci occurs also in developing Tc2 cells. IL-4 production and histone hyperacetylation in IL-4-associated nucleosomes in developing Tc2 cells were significantly lower than those of Th2 cells; however, cytokine production and histone hyperacetylation of IL-5 and IL-13 genes were equivalent. Developing Tc2 cells expressed lower GATA3 levels and dramatically increased levels of repressor of GATA (ROG). A ROG response element in the IL-13 gene exon 4 displayed Tc2-specific binding of ROG, HDAC1 and HDAC2. Thus, ROG may confer CD8 T cell-specific repression of histone hyperacetylation and activation of the IL-4 gene locus.

Keywords: Th2; Tc2; ROG; Intergenic transcript; HDAC

1. Introduction

After antigen recognition by T cell receptor (TCR), naive CD4 T cells differentiate into two distinct helper T (Th) cell subsets, Th1 and Th2 cells. Th1 cells produce IFNγ and

* Corresponding author.
E-mail address: tnakayama@faculty.chiba-u.jp (T. Nakayama).

0531-5131/
doi:10.1016/j.ics.2005.08.007

tumor necrosis factor (TNF)β, and initiate cell-mediated immunity against intracellular pathogens. Th2 cells produce IL-4, IL-5 and IL-13, and are involved in humoral immunity and allergic responses. The cytokine environment is crucial in controlling the direction of Th cell differentiation. For Th1 cell differentiation, IL-12-mediated activation of signal transducer and activator of transcription (STAT) 4 is required, while IL-4-mediated STAT6 activation is important for Th2 cell generation. In addition, TCR stimulation events upon encounter with antigens are also indispensable for both Th1 and Th2 cell differentiation. We reported that efficient TCR-mediated activation of the $p56^{lck}$, calcineurin, and Ras-ERK MAPK signaling cascade is crucial for Th2 cell differentiation [1–3]. Recent studies have identified several transcription factors that control Th1/Th2 cell differentiation. Among them, GATA3 appears to be a master transcription factor for Th2 cell differentiation. GATA3 is selectively induced in developing Th2 cells and the ectopic expression of GATA3 induced Th2 cell differentiation even in the absence of IL-4 or STAT6. For Th1 cell differentiation, T-bet was recently identified as a key transcription factor.

CD28 costimulation enhances Th2 responses significantly [4,5]. Upon anti-CD28 mAb stimulation, PI-3 kinase (PI3K) is recruited to CD28 and is activated, and then subsequent activation of NF-κB is induced. It has been reported that GATA3 induction was an outcome of the CD28-induced NF-κB activation in T cells [6,7]. This may be a mechanism by which Th2 responses were enhanced by CD28 costimulation. It is also known that IL-5 production and IL-5-dependent airway inflammation are dependent on NF-κB family members.

Chromatin remodeling of the Th2 cytokine gene loci (IL-4/IL-5/IL-13) occurs during Th2 cell differentiation. A highly conserved 400 bp noncoding sequence 1 (CNS1) was identified, and an important role in coordinate expression of Th2 cytokines was revealed. More recently, a 3′ distal IL-4 enhancer (V_A) containing an inducible DNase I hypersensitive site was identified. Reiner and colleagues reported that demethylation of intron 2 region of the IL-4 gene was associated with cell cycle progression and Th2 cell differentiation. We reported that demethylation of this region is regulated by *polycomb* group genes [8] that are known to regulate transcriptional memory in *Drosophila*.

Hyperacetylation of histone H3 and H4 by histone acetyl transferases (HATs) was suggested to be associated with active chromatin. Recently, we and others have demonstrated that histone hyperacetylation of the Th2 cytokine gene loci occurs in developing Th2 cells in a Th2-specific and STAT6-dependent manner [9–11]. We demonstrated an essential role for GATA3 in the Th2-specific hyperacetylation [9]. We also generated a precise map of the Th2-specific histone hyperacetylation within the IL-13 and IL-4 gene loci, and identified a 71 bp conserved GATA3 response element (CGRE) at 1.6 kbp upstream of the IL-13 locus exon 1. This histone hyperacetylation remodeling process could be a major target for the Th2 master transcription factor GATA3 to induce differentiation towards Th2 cells.

Histone hyperacetylation of another Th2 cytokine gene locus, IL-5, occurs in a Th2-specific STAT6- and GATA3-dependent manner with significantly different kinetics compared to that of the IL-4 and IL-13 genes [9]. The direction of transcription of the IL-5 gene is opposite to that of IL-13 and IL-4. In addition, the RAD50 gene encoding a DNA repair enzyme is located between the IL-5 and IL-13 gene loci. A differential role for GATA3 in the regulation of promoter activity of the IL-5 gene from IL-4 has been suggested. These results encouraged us to explore possible novel molecular mechanisms that would govern histone hyperacetylation of the IL-5 gene locus.

$CD8^+$ cytotoxic T cells (CTLs) secrete type 1 cytokines after TCR stimulation. However, in vitro TCR/CD3 stimulation of $CD8^+$ T cells in the presence of certain cytokines induced CD8 T cells to produce type 2 cytokines. The Tc1/Tc2 terminology was proposed by Sad et al. [12] in analogy to the Th1/Th2 subsets of CD4 T cells. Differences in the profiles of type 2 cytokine production between CD4 T cells and CD8 T cells have been noted. Particularly, the amount of IL-4 produced by type 2 CD8 T cells was reported to be 100-fold less than that by type 2 CD4 T cells. However, a full explanation for the limited production of IL-4 in type 2 CD8 T cells is not yet available.

The unique cytokine production profiles of type 2 CD8 T cells suggest a distinct immunoregulatory role for these cells. In fact, putative unique functions of Tc2 cells in various immune responses and related diseases have been demonstrated. However, the true roles of the type 2 CD8 T cells in the immune responses against microorganisms are still unclear.

2. Materials and methods

2.1. Cell cultures and in vitro T cell differentiation

Splenic CD4 T cells were stained with anti-CD4-FITC, and then, purified using magnetic beads and an Auto-MACS sorter (Miltenyi Biotec), yielding a purity of >98%. Enriched CD4 T cells (1.5×10^6) were stimulated for 2 days with immobilized anti-TCR mAb (H57-597, 3 μg/ml) and soluble anti-CD28 mAb (37.51, 3 μg/ml) in the presence of IL-2 (25 U/ml), IL-12 (100 U/ml), and anti-IL-4 mAb (11B11, 25% culture supernatant) for Th1-skewed conditions. For Th2-skewed conditions, cells were stimulated with immobilized anti-TCR mAb as above but in the presence of IL-2 (25 U/ml), IL-4 (100 U/ml) and anti-IFNγ mAb (R4.6A2, 25% culture supernatant). The cells were then transferred to new dishes and were cultured for another 5 days in the presence of cytokines present in the initial culture. In order to enhance the generation of IL-5-producing cells, stimulation with anti-TCR and anti-CD28 mAbs was performed during the second culture for 5 days. This procedure is slightly different from that used in our previous report [4]. Where indicated Wortmannin (Calbiochem) was added to the culture at the doses of 30 or 300 nM for the first 2 days. In vitro differentiation was then assessed by intracellular cytokine staining with anti-IL-4, anti-IL-5, anti-IL-13 and anti-IFNγ or by ELISA as described [13].

2.2. Chromatin immunoprecipitation (ChIP) assay

The ChIP assay was performed using histone H3 ChIP assay kits (#17-245: Upstate Biotechnology) as described [9]. Anti-GATA3 Ab (H-48: Santa Cruz Biotechnology) was used for precipitation. Where indicated, GFP-positive retrovirus-infected cells were sorted by flow cytometry, and subjected to ChIP assay. Several primer sequences for ChIP assay were described previously [9,13].

3. Results and discussion

Fig. 1 shows the summary of the results of histone hyperacetylation of the IL-13 and IL-4 gene loci. In developing Th2 cells, the expression of GATA3 is induced and GATA3 bounds to the CGRE (conserved GATA3 response element) region. Then, HAT complex and RNAse polymerase II complex are recruited, and induced hyperacetylation of histones downstream of the CGRE region. A long-range histone hyperacetylation in the IL-4 and IL-13 gene loci is detected in developing Th2 cells. Intergenic transcription is also induced at the same region as that with Th2-specific histone hyperacetylation.

The ChIP assay was performed on the IL-5 gene locus and the intergenic region of the IL-5 gene and the RAD50 gene. We detected long-range Th2 specific hyperacetylation in the intergenic region between the IL-5 and RAD50 gene loci, and the levels were increased if anti-CD28 mAb was included in the Th2 cell developing culture. Fig. 2 shows the schematic representation of the levels of histone H3 acetylation.

The levels of histone hyperacetylation and intergenic transcription were not increased in the IL-13 and IL-4 gene loci in the presence of CD28 costimulation. However, the levels of histone hyperacetylation and intergenic transcription were significantly increased in IL-5 gene locus. It is not known the starting site of the histone hyperacetylation and intergenic transcription at the IL-5/RAD50 gene loci. Fig. 3 shows the conserved region between mouse and human. There is a conserved region at 3′ border of hyperacetylatin containing two GATA3 binding motifs. We are now currently investigating the actual levels of GATA3 binding and Pol II binding.

In summary, a series of our investigation indicate that: (i) CD28-costimulation selectively enhanced histone hyperacetylation of the IL-5 gene locus. (ii) The histone hyperacetylation of the IL-5 gene locus appeared to be controlled by NF-κB activation and subsequent upregulation of GATA3. (iii) CD28 costimulation-sensitive histone hyperacetylation and intergenic transcript were observed in the entire intergenic region between the IL-5 and RAD50 gene loci [14].

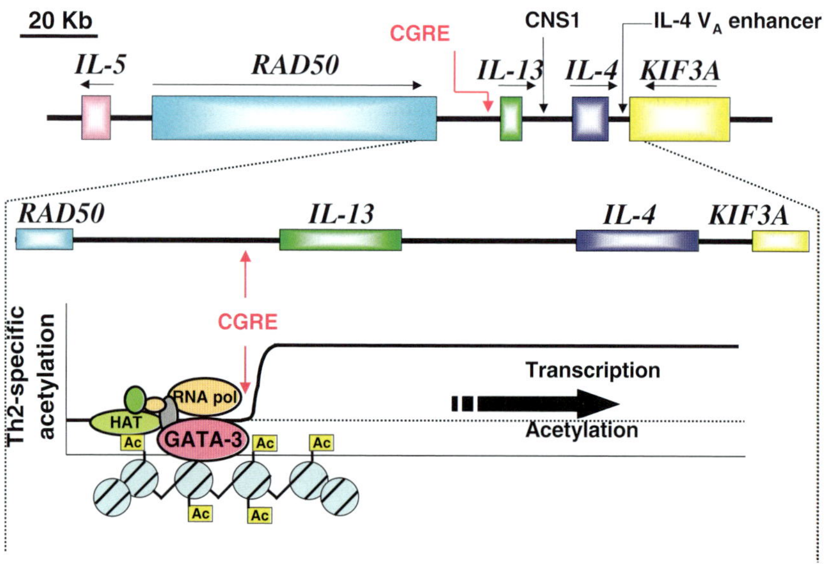

Fig. 1. Schematic representation of histone hyperacetylation of the IL-13 and IL-4 gene loci in developing Th2 cells.

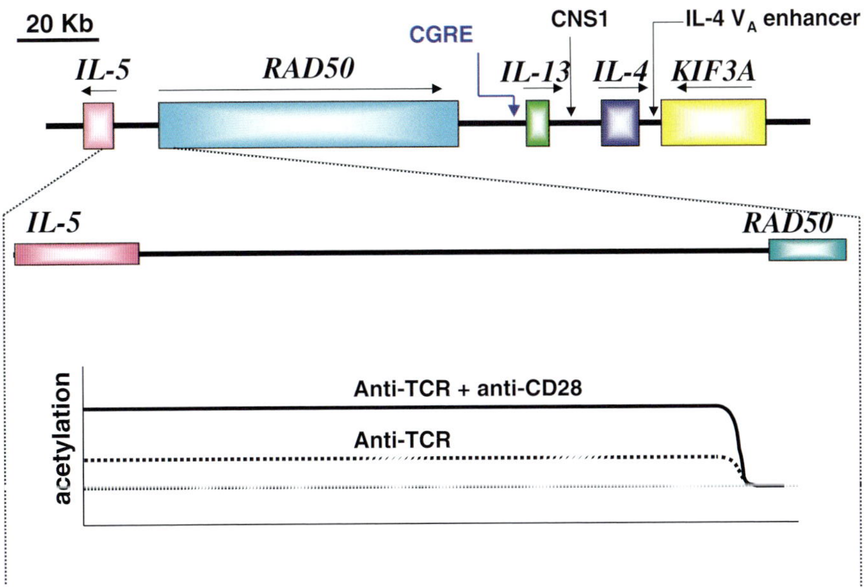

Fig. 2. Schematic representation of histone hyperacetylation of the IL-5 and RAD50 gene loci in developing Th2 cells.

In developing Tc2 cells, the production of IL-4 is known to be selectively decreased with normal production of IL-13 and IL-5. Fig. 4 shows the IFNγ/IL-4 cytokine profiles of the developing Th1, Th2, Tc1 and Tc2 cells. The levels of IL-4 producing cells were significantly reduced in Tc2 cells compared with those of Th2 cells. In addition, developing Tc2 cell population contains IFNγ producing cells, that is not observed in developing Th2 cells.

A schematic representation of possible molecular events underlying GATA3-dependent hyperacetylation within the IL-13 and IL-4 gene loci in developing Th2 and Tc2 cells is shown in Fig. 5. In developing Th2 cells, a GATA3-dependent long-range histone hyperacetylation spanning

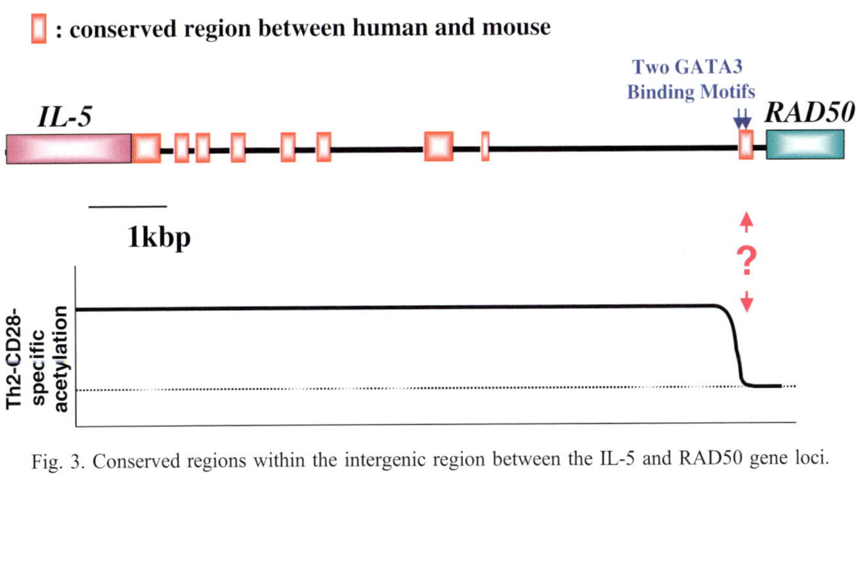

Fig. 3. Conserved regions within the intergenic region between the IL-5 and RAD50 gene loci.

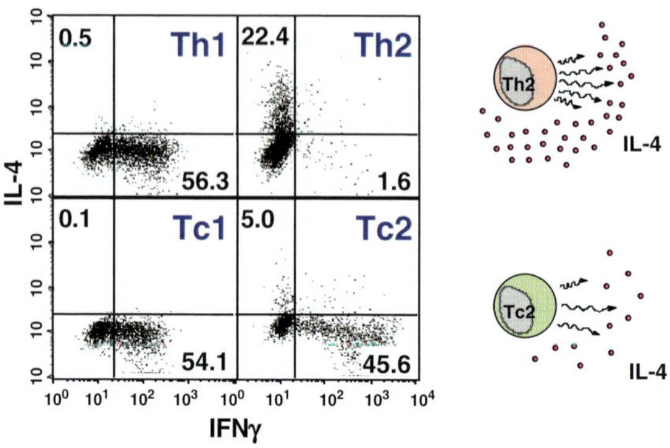

Fig. 4. Limited IL-4 production in CD8 T cells developed under type-2 skewed culture conditions.

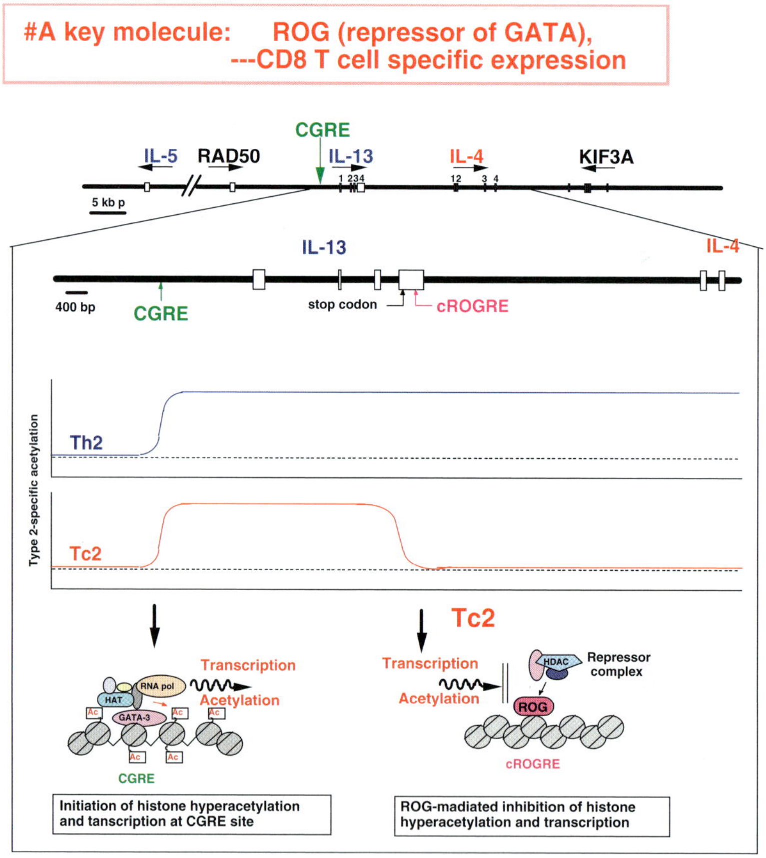

Fig. 5. Schematic representation of possible molecular events underlying GATA3-dependent hyperacetylation within the IL-13 and IL-4 gene loci in developing Th2 and Tc2 cells.

the IL-13 and IL-4 gene loci was demonstrated [9]. We identified a 71 bp conserved GATA response element (CGRE) at 1.6 kbp upstream of the IL-13 locus corresponding with the 5′ border of the Th2-specific histone hyperacetylation region. The CGRE was shown to bind GATA3 and also p300 and RNA polymerase II, and thus, we proposed a crucial role of the CGRE for GATA3-mediated targeting and downstream spreading of core histone hyperacetylation within the IL-13 and IL-4 gene loci [9]. We also detected intergenic transcripts at the region of Th2-specific histone hyperacetylation. It is most likely that histone hyperacetylation initiates at the CGRE site and spreads to a downstream region with transcription. In developing Tc2 cells, the CGRE appears to be also important as evidenced by the fact that the 5′ border of the Th2-specific hyperacetylation region is the same. In addition to the GATA3/CGRE-dependent initiation of acetylation, CD8 T cells seem to possess an additional regulatory mechanism in the histone acetylation events. Activated CD8 T cells but not CD4 T cells expressed a large amount of ROG protein and cROGRE (conserved ROG response element) was able to associate with ROG, HDAC1 and HDAC2 molecules in a Tc2 cell-specific manner. Taken together, it is probable that ROG molecules recruit a putative HDAC complex either directly or by interacting with another molecule and target it to the cROGRE resulting in the repression of histone hyperacetylation that is initiated at the upstream CGRE site. This mechanism appears to be CD8 T cell-specific, and thus, may confer limited production of IL-4 on CD8 T cells to exert distinct immunoregulatory roles from $CD4^+$ Th2 cells by producing a different set of cytokines [13].

Acknowledgements

We thank Ms. Yoko Sawano, Kaoru Sugaya, and Aoi Nakazawa for their secretarial assistance. This work was supported by grants from the Ministry of Education, Culture, Sports, Science and Technology (Japan) (Grants-in-Aid for: Scientific Research in Priority Areas #17016010; Scientific Research B #17390139; Grant-in-Aid for Young Scientists #17790317 and Special Coordination Funds for Promoting Science and technology), the Ministry of Health, Labor and Welfare (Japan), the Program for Promotion of Fundamental Studies in Health Science of the Organization for Pharmaceutical Safety and Research (Japan), The Japan Health Science Foundation, Uehara Memorial Foundation, Mochida Foundation and Kanae Foundation.

References

[1] M. Yamashita, et al., Requirement for $p56^{lck}$ tyrosine kinase activation in T_h subset differentiation, Int. Immunol. 10 (1998) 577–591.

[2] M. Yamashita, et al., T cell antigen receptor-mediated activation of the Ras/mitogen-activated protein kinase pathway controls interleukin 4 receptor function and type-2 helper T cell differentiation, Proc. Natl. Acad. Sci. U. S. A. 96 (3) (1999) 1024–1029.

[3] M. Yamashita, et al., T cell receptor-induced calcineurin activation regulates T helper type 2 cell development by modifying the interleukin 4 receptor signaling complex, J. Exp. Med. 191 (2000) 1869–1879.

[4] M. Kubo, et al., CD28 costimulation accelerates IL-4 receptor sensitivity and IL-4-mediated Th2 differentiation, J. Immunol. 163 (5) (1999) 2432–2442.

[5] I.C. Rulifson, et al., CD28 costimulation promotes the production of Th2 cytokines, J. Immunol. 158 (2) (1997) 658–665.

[6] M. Rodriguez-Palmero, et al., Triggering of T cell proliferation through CD28 induces GATA-3 and promotes T helper type 2 differentiation in vitro and in vivo, Eur. J. Immunol. 29 (12) (1999) 3914–3924.

[7] J. Das, et al., A critical role for NF-κB in *GATA3* expression and T_H2 differentiation in allergic airway inflammation, Nat. Immunol. 2 (1) (2001) 45–50.

[8] M. Kimura, et al., Regulation of Th2 cell differentiation by *mel-18*, a mammalian *polycomb* group gene, Immunity 15 (2) (2001) 275–287.
[9] M. Yamashita, et al., Identification of a conserved GATA3 response element upstream proximal from the interleukin-13 gene locus, J. Biol. Chem. 277 (44) (2002) 42399–42408.
[10] O. Avni, et al., T_H cell differentiation is accompanied by dynamic changes in histone acetylation of cytokine genes, Nat. Immunol. 3 (7) (2002) 643–651.
[11] P.E. Fields, S.T. Kim, R.A. Flavell, Cutting edge: changes in histone acetylation at the *IL*-4 and *IFN-γ* loci accompany Th1/Th2 differentiation, J. Immunol. 169 (2) (2002) 647–650.
[12] S. Sad, R. Marcotte, T.R. Mosmann, Cytokine-induced differentiation of precursor mouse $CD8^+$ T cells into cytotoxic $CD8^+$ T cells secreting Th1 or Th2 cytokines, Immunity 2 (1995) 271–279.
[13] M. Omori, et al., CD8 T cell-specific downregulation of histone hyperacetylation and gene activation of the IL-4 gene locus by ROG, repressor of GATA, Immunity 19 (2) (2003) 281–294.
[14] M. Inami, et al., CD28 costimulation controls histone hyperacetylation of the interleukin 5 gene locus in developing Th2 cells, J. Biol. Chem. 279 (22) (2004) 23123–23133.

International Congress Series 1285 (2005) 145–154

www.ics-elsevier.com

Role of IL-5 in the innate immune system and disease control

Kiyoshi Takatsu*, Byoung-gon Moon, Atsuko Itakura, Yumiko Tsukamoto, Keisuke Horikawa, Masashi Ikutani, Taku Kouro, Satoshi Takaki

Division of Immunology, Department of Immunology and Microbiology, Institute of Medical Science, University of Tokyo, 4-6-1 Shirokanedai, Minato-ku, Tokyo 108, Japan

Abstract. Mature B cells expressing surface IgM as B cell receptor (BCR) consist of two B-cell subpopulations, B-1 and B-2 cells that regulate innate and acquired immunity, respectively. B-1 cells become natural Ig-producing plasma cells in response to natural ligands or self-antigens. Mature B-2 cells proliferate and differentiate into Ig-producing plasma cells under the influence of T helper (Th) cells. Antigen stimulation of B-2 cells induces class switch recombination (CSR) from IgM to other isotypes that is regulated by cytokines and activation-induced cytidine deaminase (AID). IL-5 activates B cells and eosinophils and regulates the innate and acquired immune response. IL-5 stimulates innate B-1 cells and induces the homeostatic proliferation, survival and differentiation of B cells leading to increased secretion of natural antibody. IL-5Rα-deficient mice show the impaired contact sensitivity that is mediated by activated T cells and IgM antibody produced by B-1 cells. IL-5 induces AID and Blimp-1 expression in activated B-2 cells leading to μ to γ1 CSR and IgG1 production. In contrast, IL-4 does not induce μ to γ1 CSR in anti-CD38-activated B-2 cells. Intriguingly, the costimulation of anti-CD38-activated B-2 cells with 8-mercaptoguanosine and IL-4 induces μ to γ1 CSR and IgG1 production, suggesting that unidentified factor(s) is/are required together with AID to complete CSR. We will discuss the role of IL-5 in the innate immune system and disease control, particularly the regulation of contact sensitivity and chronic inflammation through B-1 cell activation and IgM production. © 2005 Elsevier B.V. All rights reserved.

Keywords: B-1; Contact sensitivity; Class switch recombination; AID; Atherosclerosis

* Corresponding author. Tel.: +81 3 5449 5260; fax: +81 3 5449 5407.
E-mail address: takatsuk@ims.u-tokyo.ac.jp (K. Takatsu).

doi:10.1016/j.ics.2005.07.094

1. Introduction

B cell precursors of immunoglobulin (Ig)-secreting cells originate from pluripotent hematopoietic stem cells and differentiate in the fetal liver and, in adult life, in the bone marrow [1,2]. Surface IgM (sIgM)-expressing mature B cells leave the bone marrow and circulate into the peripheral lymphoid organs in which B cells continue their development in the spleen where they are subjected to a round of negative selection [3]. Mature B cells can be activated by antigens under the influence of T helper (Th) cells leading to proliferation and differentiation into antibody-secreting cells (ASCs) [4].

There are two B cell subpopulations, namely B-1 and B-2 cells. B-1 cells differ from conventional B-2 cells in their surface phenotype, anatomical localization, self-replenishing activity, and VH gene usage of IgM [5,6]. B-1 cells constitutively express Mac-1, CD23, and the IL-5Rα chain (IL-5Rα) [7]. B-1 cells are the major source of natural antibody in the IgM, IgG3, and IgA classes [8]. Thus B-1 cells play a critical role in the regulation of the innate immune response.

An efficient B-2 cell response to protein antigens needs interaction with Th cells. Th cells expressing a particular T cell receptor (TCR) recognize the peptide–MHC complex presented on the B cells and become activated. They transiently express CD40 ligand (CD40L) on their surface which interacts with CD40 expressed on B cells to deliver signals for B cell activation and proliferation. Antigen stimulation of sIgM-positive B cells induces genetic events in their IgH gene loci that are essential for the generation of functional diversity in the humoral immune response and essential for efficient antigen elimination. Class switch recombination (CSR) replaces the heavy chain constant region (CH) from Cμ to other CH regions to diversify the effector function of the Ig [9]. The process of CSR is highly regulated by cytokines, B cell activators or both [10,11]. Activation-induced cytidine deaminase (AID) is the essential and sole B cell-specific factor required for CSR [11–14].

IL-5 is a prominent cytokine that induces B-1 cell proliferation and enhances the differentiation of B-1 and B-2 cells into ASCs [15–17]. Transgenic mice carrying the IL-5 gene show an increase in B-1 cell number and enhanced serum IgM, IgA and IgE levels in addition to massive eosinophilia in various tissues [18]. IL-5 can induce μ to γ1 CSR in activated B-2 cells [19]. IL-5 therefore appears to regulate both innate and acquired immunity regarding B cell triggering. We focus on the role of IL-5 in the link between the innate and acquired immune response and disease control.

2. IL-5 and signal transduction

IL-5 is an interdigitating homodimeric glycoprotein that is mainly produced by Th2 cells after stimulation with antigens such as *Mycobacterium tuberculosis*, *Toxocara canis*, or with allergens and by mast cells [17,20]. IL-5 acts on target cells by binding to its specific receptor (IL-5R) that consists of a unique α chain (IL-5Rα) and a common β chain (βc) [21–25]. The βc is a signal-transducing molecule shared with IL-3R and GM-CSFR [26]. The membrane proximal proline-rich sequence (PPXP motif) of the cytoplasmic domain of IL-5Rα and the βc are essential for IL-5-induced signal transduction [22,27–29]. The carboxy-terminal region of IL-5Rα is essential for regulating IL-5-induced CSR [30]). IL-5 stimulation induces the rapid tyrosine phosphorylation of various cellular proteins including the βc, SH2/SH3-containing proteins, Btk, STAT1 and STAT5, PI3K, and MAP kinases leading to the activation of downstream signaling molecules [29,31]. The activation of Jak2 and the STAT5 are essential for IL-5-dependent signal transduction both in B cells and eosinophils [33,34]. The activation of Btk is essential for IL-5 signaling in B cells [32]. A spontaneous Btk mutation (R28C) in mice produces X-linked immunodeficiency (*xid*) [35]. In XID mice the B-1 population is largely absent and B-1 cells are functionally compromised in response to stimulation via the BCR or CD38. XID B cells are hyporesponsive to IL-5, IL-10, and LPS [36–38]. The frequency of IL-5 responsive B cells in XID mice is approximately 100-fold lower than that of wild-type (WT) mice [38]. In IL-5Rα transgenic mice carrying the *xid* gene (XID-5Rα-Tg), B-1 cells do not respond to IL-5 at all [39]. These results demonstrate that the impairment of IL-5 responsiveness in XID B cells is due to an abnormality of IL-5-mediated signaling.

Despite the importance of Btk in B-cell differentiation, the precise function of Btk remains unclear [40]. We isolated a protein called BAM11 that binds to the PH domain of Btk [41]. BAM11 is murine homologue of human LTG19/ENL. The forced expression of BAM11 in IL-5 responsive cells inhibits not only IL-5-induced proliferation but also IL-5-induced Btk activation both in vivo and in vitro. Btk localizes not only in the cytoplasm, but also in the nucleus [41]. The nucleocytoplasmic shuttling of Btk has implications regarding potential targets inside the nucleus. Interestingly, BAM11 has transcriptional co-activation activity that is enhanced by Btk [42]. This "positive–negative mutual regulation system" between BAM11 and Btk may elucidate a novel mechanism on B cell signaling through BCR and IL-5R. The coexpression of TFII-I, another Btk-binding protein together with BAM11 and Btk, further augments BAM11- and Btk-dependent transcriptional co-activation. Furthermore, BAM11 can be co-immunoprecipitated with the INI1/SNF5 protein [42], a member of the SWI/SNF complex. Btk may regulate gene transcription in B cells by activating BAM11 and the SWI/SNF transcriptional complex via TFII-I activation.

3. IL-5 promotes B-1 cell development, homeostasis, and differentiation

The progenitors of B-1 cells are abundant in the fetal omentum and liver but are missing in the bone marrow of adult animals [5]. B-1 cells maintain their number in adult animals by their self-replenishing capacity. These self-replenishing B-1 cells are clearly enriched in the peritoneum in mice, and seen at low frequency in the spleen, but B-1 cells are virtually absent from the lymph nodes, Peyer's patches (PP), and peripheral blood, where most conventional B-2 cells are localized. Consistent with a major role of B-1 cells in IgM production, a number of specificities of natural IgM Ab have been identified in the B-1 repertoire. These include specificities for LPS, phosphorylcholine, *Salmonella* spp., and phosphatidylcholine [5]. The number of IL-5 responsive B-1 cells increases in spontaneously autoimmune NZB and (NZB $\times$ NZW) F1 mice. Coupled with the observation that other autoimmune strains of mice have a higher number of B-1 cells compared with normal mice, B-1 cells are thought to be involved in the development of autoimmune diseases.

IL-5$^{-/-}$ and IL-5R$\alpha^{-/-}$ mice show a severe reduction in the number of B-1 cells in neonates in the peritoneal cavity. B-1 cell numbers return to the normal range in adult life [43,44]. The administration of anti-IL-5 mAb to WT mice, TCR$\delta^{-/-}\beta^{-/-}$ mice, or W/W^{v} mice results in reduction in the total cell number and cell size of B-1 cells to an extent similar to that of IL-5R$\alpha^{-/-}$ mice, while the number and size of B-2 cells do not change. B-1 cell

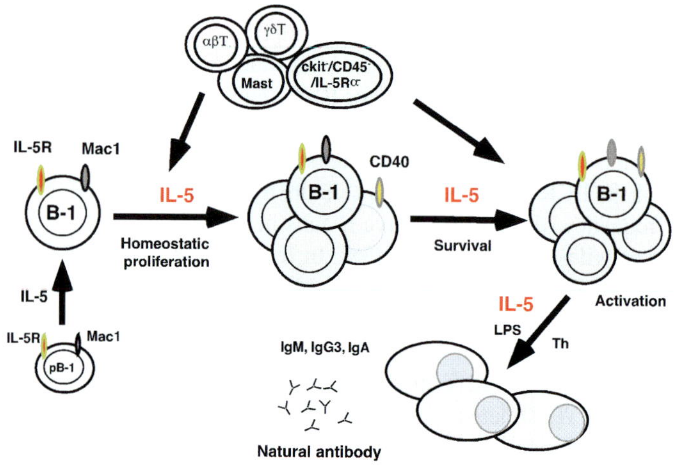

Fig. 1. Schematic illustration of the site of action of IL-5 in the B-1 cell development, homeostatic proliferation, survival, and triggering. IL-5 mRNA is expressed not only Th2 cells and mast cells, but also on non-hematopoietic cells in various tissues.

survival in WT mice and homeostatic proliferation in RAG2-deficient mice are impaired in the absence of IL-5Rα. Significant IL-5 mRNA expression is detectable by RT-PCR in the lungs, spleen, and small intestine of WT mice, RAG-2$^{-/-}$ mice, TCRδ$^{-/-}$β$^{-/-}$ mice, and W/W^{V} mice. IL-5 can be secreted in non-hematopoietic cells in addition to Th2 or mast cells and act on B-1 cells in the mucosal tissues [45]. Mice with selective B-1 cell reduction show a decreased frequency of IgA-producing cells in the LP, and B-1 cell-derived IgA is specific for commensal bacteria [46,47]. In IL-5Rα$^{-/-}$ mice, sIgA^{+} B-1 cells from the effector site are significantly reduced [48], indicating the critical role of the IL-5/IL-5R system in IgA secretion in mucosal tissues.

The B-1 cells of IL-5Rα$^{-/-}$ mice showed defective proliferation and Ig production upon LPS stimulation in vitro, and there are significant differences in serum and fecal IgA levels in LPS-treated WT and IL-5Rα$^{-/-}$ mice [45]. In addition, enhanced IgA production in feces induced by the oral administration of LPS is not observed in IL-5Rα$^{-/-}$ mice. Because the expression levels of TLR4/MD2 on IL-5Rα$^{-/-}$B-1 cells are comparable with those on WT B-1 cells, the IL-5-mediated signaling pathway may couple with the LPS-induced signaling pathway. The IL-5 stimulation of B-1 cells enhances CD40 expression and augments IgM and IgG production after stimulation with CD40L or Th cells. These results illuminate the role of IL-5 in B-1 cell development, homeostatic proliferation and survival and in IgA production in the mucosal tissues in Th-dependent as well as Th-independent manner (Fig. 1).

4. IL-5 enhances IgM and IgG1 production by activated B-2 cells

Signaling through CD40 in combination with Th cell-derived cytokines enhances B cell proliferation and leads to B cell differentiation accompanied CSR and the generation of ASCs. In mice, ASCs formed in vivo can be identified by their high expression of syndecan-1 (CD138) in conjunction with low B220 [49]. Syndecan-1$^+$ cells are shown to display a gene expression profile of plasma cells, with increased expression of the J chain, B lymphocyte-induced maturation protein 1 (Blimp-1) and X-box-binding protein 1 (Xbp-1) mRNA and a reduction in AID, B cell lymphoma 6 (Bcl-6) and Pax5 mRNA [50–52]. Blimp-1 is considered to be a 'master regulator' for plasma cell differentiation [4,51].

CSR to the expression of a particular CH gene isotype is preceded by transcriptional activity at the respective Ig gene locus [3–5]. Cytokines and mitogens are able to rapidly and selectively up-regulate steady-state levels of specific germline CH RNA. CSR between Sμ and another S region 5′ to a CH sequence is mediated by a DNA recombination event that moves the VDJ-segments to a new position upstream of the isotype being expressed. The deleted DNA forms circular structures termed "switch circles" that contain reciprocal recombination products [10]. The involvement of AID has been demonstrated in the regulation or catalysis of the DNA modification step of CSR [13,14].

We examined IL-5-induced CSR using anti-CD38 mAb (αCD38)-activated B-2 cells. The agonistic αCD38 stimulation of mouse splenic B-2 cells induces potent proliferation associated with the significant expression of germline γ1 transcripts, the activation of NF-κB/Rel proteins and enhanced IL-5Rα expression [19,53–55]. IL-5 stimulation does not induce detectable germline γ1 expression by itself. By amplifying deleted circular DNA fragments containing reciprocal junctions, we detected μ to γ1 CSR in IL-5- and αCD38-stimulated B-2 cells [19]. The μ to γ1 CSR is detectable in B-2 cells after four divisions of cell cycle and peaks following five to six division cycles. Intriguingly, IL-4 stimulation does not induce μ to γ1 CSR at all, indicating that IL-5 can induce μ to γ1 DNA recombination independently of IL-4. IL-5 regulates expression of Ig-related genes such as the J chain and Igκ, and genes involved in B cell maturation such as AID and Blimp-1. IL-5-dependent μ–γ1 CSR and IgG1 production are severely impaired in Stat5b$^{-/-}$ B cells. Our data support the notion that Stat5b is essential for IL-5-dependent μ–γ1 CSR and IgG1 secretion, which is schematically illustrated in Fig. 2.

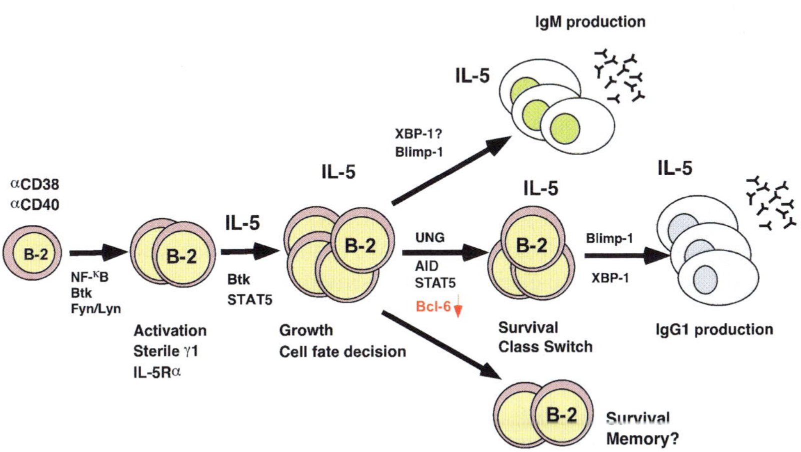

Fig. 2. Schematic illustration of molecules involved in IL-5-induced CSR of μ to γ1 CSR and IgG production by αCD38-activated B-2 cells.

IL-5 potently induces the maturation of activated B-2 cells into IgG- and IgA-producing plasma cells. IL-5 acts on $sIgA^+$ B-2 cells, but not on $sIgA^-$ B cells, to induce IgA production by antigen-primed B-2 cells in PP [56].

Although IL-4, a prominent cytokine for CSR to IgG1 and IgE, does not induce μ to γ1 CSR in αCD38-activated B-2 cells, costimulation of αCD38-activated B cells with 8-mercaptoguanosine (8-SGuo) and IL-4 induces μ to γ1 CSR and IgG1 production. The stimulation of αCD38-activated B cells with 8-SGuo could induce AID expression without showing μ–γ1 CSR and IgG1 production (Y.T. and K.T., unpublished), suggesting the requirement of unidentified factor(s) together with AID to complete μ to γ1 CSR.

IL-5 induces μ to γ1 CSR and IgG1 production in αCD40-activated B-2 cells. Intriguingly, IgG1 production by IL-5-stimulated αCD40-activated B-2 cells is much higher than those produced upon IL-4 stimulation, even though the frequency of IL-5-induced μ to γ1 CSR is much lower than that induced by IL-4. IL-5 should have potent activity to enhance switched B-2 cell maturation to ASCs. Because IL-5 induces increased Blimp-1 expression [34,53], Blimp-1 may lead to enhanced maturation of switched B-2 cells and IgG1 secretion.

5. IL-5 links innate and acquired immunity in regulating immune system and disease

5.1. Contact sensitivity model

Contact sensitivity is a form of delayed-type hypersensitivity that is a classic example of in vivo T cell-mediated immunity. The skin sensitization of mice with a reactive hapten Ag induces contact sensitivity responsiveness. Subsequent challenge at a separate skin site with immunized hapten elicits an inflammatory response in which Ag-specific T cells are recruited locally and mediate Ag-specific inflammation. Askenase and his colleagues described that contact sensitivity being impaired in B cell-deficient mice [57]. They also showed that Ag-specific IgM antibody is required to recruit effector T cells to the site of inflammation. Furthermore, they demonstrated that the activated B-1 cells in the spleen and lymph nodes from Day-1 post-immunized mice are able to reconstitute the defective contact sensitivity response in the B cell-deficient mice [57]. These results clearly indicate the involvement of B-1 cells and Ag-specific IgM antibody in the contact hypersensitivity. Together with their previous evidence, they postulated that the IgM and Ag challenge form local complexes that activate the complement, generating C5a, leading to local vascular activation to recruit the antigen-primed effector T cells that mediate the CS response.

To examine the role of IL-5 in contact sensitivity, we immunized WT and IL-5R$\alpha^{-/-}$ mice with oxazolone (OX) with skin painting. We challenged mice with OX by ear paining 4 days after the sensitization to elicit contact sensitivity and measured ear swelling at 24 h. We found that IL-5R$\alpha^{-/-}$ mice showed impaired contact sensitivity to OX regarding ear swelling, infiltration of inflammatory cells including eosinophils into the inflammatory skin site (A.I. and K.T., unpublished data). The impaired elicitation of contact sensitivity to OX in OX-immunized IL-5R$\alpha^{-/-}$ mice was partially reconstituted by the transfer of lymphoid cells from OX-immunized WT mice. We propose a positive role of IL-5 in contact sensitivity and hypothesize that IL-5 plays role in B-1 cell-mediated Ag-specific IgM production and the induction of eosinophil production (Fig. 3).

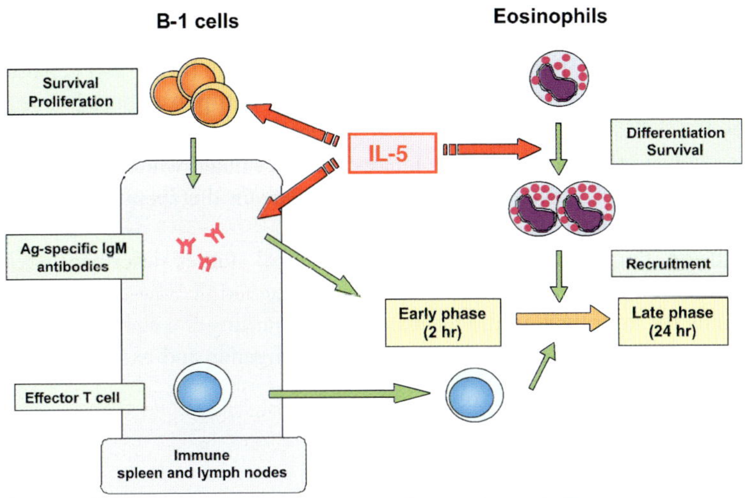

Fig. 3. Hypothetical representation regarding role of IL-5 in the regulation of cutaneous contact sensitivity.

5.2. *Atherosclerotic model*

Atherosclerosis is a chronic inflammatory disease that is caused by the uptake of oxidized LDL (OxLDL) by macrophages on the artery wall, which in turn can form neo-self-determinants recognized by specific innate and adaptive immune responses [58]. During atherogenesis, LDL is oxidized, generating various oxidation-specific neoepitopes, such as malondialdehyde-modified (MDA-modified) LDL (MDA-LDL) or the phosphorylcholine (PC) headgroup of oxidized phospholipids (OxPLs). IL-5 has been detected in human atherosclerotic lesions [59], although it is irregularly expressed. Genetic analysis indicates that EO6, the prototypic IgM anti-OxLDL antibody, is a natural antibody secreted by innate B-1 cells possessing the germline-encoded T15 clonotype [60]. Binder and his colleagues demonstrated that MDA-LDL immunization induces not only MDA-LDL-specific Th2 cells that prominently secrete IL-5, but also an innate T cell independent B-1 response associated with the production of IL-5 leading to the increased secretion of atheroprotective anti-phosphorylcholine T15/EO6 antibody [61]. They also showed using a bone marrow transplant model that IL-5 deficiency leads to decreased titers of T15/EO6 and accelerated atherosclerosis. Their data strongly suggest that IL-5 links acquired and natural immunity specific to the epitopes of OxLDL, providing protection from atherosclerosis, in part by stimulating the expansion of atheroprotective natural IgM specific for OxLDL. Therefore, IL-5 seems to be pivotally involved in the expansion of natural antibodies derived from B-1 cells [61,62].

6. Future perspectives

The successful generation and breeding of mice in whom the genes for IL-5, IL-5Rα, or βc are disrupted indicates that none of these mutations is lethal. Although IgM and IgG levels and B cells in both the B-1 and B-2 lineages are normal in the adult mice, the neonatal IL-5R$\alpha^{-/-}$ mice have up to an 80% reduction in the number of B-1 cells. Because anti-IL-5 treatment induces impairment of mature B-1 cell survival and homeostatic proliferation in WT mice, other signals than IL-5 may play a role together with IL-5 in B-1 cell homeostasis. Although we have demonstrated that IL-5 can induce anti-phosphorylcholine (PC) IgM antibody by B-1 cells, we did not expect Th2 to influence anti-PC antibody responses by B-1 cells that modulate atherosclerosis. It is interesting to evaluate which cell type, Th1, mast cells or others, secretes IL-5 in the lesions. These validate the therapeutic goal of skewing Th responses to atherosclerosis-associated antigens.

In conclusion, the structural, functional, and clinical studies described herein provide insight into the role of IL-5 in innate immune response and disease control and provide a strong impetus for investigating the means of IL-5 regarding linkage between natural and adaptive immunity specific to the epitopes of natural ligands and exogenous antigens.

Acknowledgements

We are grateful to Y. Hitoshi, S. Uehara, and Y. Kikuchi for their helpful discussion. This work was supported in part by a grant from Special Coordination Funds for Promoting Science and Technology and Grant-in-Aid for Scientific Research on Priority Areas from the Ministry of Education, Culture, Sports, Science and Technology, Japan, and Uehara Memorial Foundation.

References

[1] R. Pelayo, et al., Lymphoid progenitors and primary routes to becoming cells of the immune system, Curr. Opin. Immunol. 17 (2005) 100–107.
[2] A.G. Rolink, J. Andersson, F. Melchers, Molecular mechanisms guiding late stages of B-cell development, Immunol. Rev. 197 (2004) 41–50.
[3] J.M. Chung, M. Silverman, J.G. Monroe, Transitional B cells: step by step towards immune competence, Trends Immunol. 24 (2003) 343–349.
[4] M. Shapiro-Shelef, K. Calame, Regulation of plasma-cell development, Nat. Rev., Immunol. 5 (2005) 230–242.
[5] R.R. Hardy, K. Hayakawa, B cell developmental pathway, Annu. Rev. Immunol. 19 (2001) 595–621.
[6] R. Berland, H.H. Wortis, Origins and functions of B-1 cells with notes on the role of CD5, Annu. Rev. Immunol. 20 (2002) 253–300.
[7] Y. Hitoshi, et al., Distribution of IL-5 receptor-positive B cells. Expression of IL-5 receptor on Ly-1(CD5)+ B cells, J. Immunol. 144 (1990) 4218–4225.
[8] S. Fagarasan, N. Watanabe, T. Honjo, Generation, expansion, migration and activation of mouse B1 cells, Immunol. Rev. 176 (2000) 205–215.
[9] T. Honjo, T. Kataoka, Organization of immunoglobulin heavy chain genes and allelic deletion model, Proc. Natl. Acad. Sci. U. S. A. 75 (1978) 2140–2144.
[10] J. Stavnezer, Antibody class switching, Adv. Immunol. 61 (1996) 79–146.
[11] D.D. Dudley, et al., Mechanism and control of V(D)J recombination versus class switch recombination: similarities and differences, Adv. Immunol. 86 (2004) 43–112.
[12] K. Kinoshita, T. Honjo, Linking class-switch recombination with somatic hypermutation, Nat. Rev. MCB 2 (2001) 493–503.
[13] M. Muramatsu, et al., Class switch recombination and hypermutation require activation-induced cytidine deaminase (AID), a potential RNA editing enzyme, Cell 102 (2000) 553–563.
[14] P. Revy, et al., Activation-induced cytidine deaminase (AID) deficiency causes the autosomal recessive form of the Hyper-IgM syndrome (HIGM2). [see comments], Cell 102 (2000) 565–575.

[15] K. Takatsu, et al., T cell-replacing factor (TRF)/interleukin 5 (IL-5): molecular and functional properties, Immunol. Rev. 102 (1988) 107–135.

[16] K. Takatsu, Interleukin 5 and B cell differentiation, Cytokine Growth Factor Rev. 9 (1998) 25–35.

[17] K. Takatsu, S. Takaki, Y. Hitoshi, Interleukin-5 and its receptor system: implications in the immune system and inflammation, Adv. Immunol. 57 (1994) 145–190.

[18] A. Tominaga, et al., Transgenic mice expressing a B cell growth and differentiation factor gene (interleukin-5) develop eosinophilia and autoantibody production, J. Exp. Med. 173 (1991) 429–438.

[19] C. Mizoguchi, et al., IL-5 induces IgG1 isotype switch recombination in mouse CD38-activated sIgD-positive B lymphocytes, J. Immunol. 162 (1999) 2812–2819.

[20] A. Tominaga, et al., Molecular properties and regulation of mRNA expression for murine T cell-replacing factor/IL-5, J. Immunol. 140 (1988) 1175–1181.

[21] S. Mita, et al., Characterization of high-affinity receptors for interleukin 5 on interleukin 5-dependent cell lines, Proc. Natl. Acad. Sci. U. S. A. 86 (1989) 2311–2315.

[22] S. Takaki, et al., Molecular cloning and expression of the murine interleukin-5 receptor, EMBO J. 9 (1990) 4367–4374.

[23] S. Takaki, et al., Identification of the second subunit of the murine interleukin-5 receptor: interleukin-3 receptor-like protein, AIC2B is a component of the high affinity interleukin-5 receptor, EMBO J. 10 (1991) 2833–2838.

[24] Y. Murata, et al., Molecular cloning and expression of the human interleukin 5 receptor, J. Exp. Med. 175 (1992) 341–351.

[25] S. Takaki, et al., Reconstitution of the functional receptors for murine and human interleukin 5, J. Exp. Med. 177 (1993) 1523–1529.

[26] A. Miyajima, et al., Cytokine receptors and signal transduction, Annu. Rev. Immunol. 10 (1992) 295–331.

[27] N. Ogata, et al., JAK2 and JAK1 constitutively associate with an interleukin-5 (IL-5) receptor alpha and betac subunit, respectively, and are activated upon IL-5 stimulation, Blood 91 (1998) 2264–2271.

[28] S. Takaki, et al., A critical cytoplasmic domain of the interleukin-5 (IL-5) receptor alpha chain and its function in IL-5-mediated growth signal transduction [see comments], Mol. Cell. Biol. 14 (1994) 7404–7413.

[29] T. Kouro, et al., Critical residues of cytoplasmic domain of the IL-5 receptor a chain and its function in IL-5-mediated activation of JAK kinase and STAT5, Int. Immunol 8 (1996) 237–246.

[30] B.G. Moon, et al., Functional dissection of the cytoplasmic subregions of the interleukin-5 receptor alpha chain in growth and immunoglobulin G1 switch recombination of B cells, Immunology 102 (2001) 289–300.

[31] K. Pazdrak, et al., The intracellular signal transduction mechanism of interleukin 5 in eosinophils: the involvement of lyn tyrosine kinase and the Ras-Raf-1-MEK-microtubule-associated protein kinase pathway, J. Exp. Med. 181 (1995) 1827–1834.

[32] S. Sato, et al., IL-5 receptor-mediated tyrosine phosphorylation of SH2/SH3-containing proteins and activation of Bruton's tyrosine and Janus 2 kinases, J. Exp. Med. 180 (1994) 2101–2111.

[33] S. Kagami, et al., Both stat5a and stat5b are required for antigen-induced eosinophil and T-cell recruitment into the tissue, Blood 95 (2000) 1370–1377.

[34] K. Horikawa, et al., Essential Role Of Stat5 For IL-5-Dependent Igh Switch Recombination In Mouse B Cells, J. Immunol. 167 (2001) 5018–5026.

[35] D.J. Rawlings, et al., Mutation of unique region of Bruton's tyrosine kinase in immunodeficient XID mice, Science 261 (1993) 358–361.

[36] T. Li, et al., Activation of Bruton's tyrosine kinase (BTK) by a point mutation in its pleckstrin homology (PH) domain, Immunity 2 (1995) 451–460.

[37] Y. Hitoshi, et al., Delayed progression of a murine retrovirus-induced acquired immunodeficiency syndrome in X-linked immunodeficient mice, J. Exp. Med. 177 (1993) 621–626.

[38] Y. Hitoshi, et al., Interleukin-5 receptor positive B cells, but not eosinophils are functionally and numerically influenced in the mice carried with X-linked immunodeficiency, Int. Immunol. 5 (1993) 1183–1190.

[39] M. Koike, et al., Defective IL-5-receptor-mediated signaling in B cells of X-linked immunodeficient mice, Int. Immunol. 7 (1995) 21–30.

[40] J.M. Lindvall, et al., Bruton's tyrosine kinase: cell biology, sequence conservation, mutation spectrum, siRNA modifications, and expression profiling, Immunol. Rev. 203 (2005) 200–215.

[41] Y. Kikuchi, et al., Identification and characterization of a molecule, BAM11, that associates with the pleckstrin homology domain of mouse Btk, Int. Immunol. 12 (2000) 1397–1408.

[42] M. Hirano, et al., Bruton's tyrosine kinase (Btk) enhances transcriptional co-activation activity of BAM11, a Btk-associated molecule of a subunit of SWI/SNF complexes, Int. Immunol. 16 (2004) 747–757.

[43] T. Yoshida, et al., Defective B-1 cell development and impaired immunity against Angiostrongylus cantonensis in IL-5R alpha-deficient mice, Immunity 4 (1996) 483–494.

[44] M. Kopf, et al., IL-5-deficient mice have a developmental defect in CD5+ B-1 cells and lack eosinophilia but have normal antibody and cytotoxic T cell responses, Immunity 4 (1996) 15–24.

[45] B-Y. Moon, et al., The role of IL-5 for mature B-1 cells in homeostatic proliferation, cell survival, and Ig production, J. Immunol. 172 (2004) 6020–6029 (2004).

[46] A.J. Macpherson, et al., A primitive T cell-independent mechanism of intestinal mucosal IgA responses to commensal bacteria, Science 288 (2000) 2222–2226.

[47] S. Fagarasan, et al., Critical roles of activation-induced cytidine deaminase (AID) in the homeostasis of gut flora, Science 298 (2002) 1424–1427.

[48] T. Hiroi, et al., Deficiency of IL-5 receptor alpha-chain selectively influences the development of the common mucosal immune system independent IgA-producing B-1 cell in mucosa-associated tissues, J. Immunol. 162 (1999) 821–828.

[49] L. Kopper, A. Sebestyen, Syndecans and the lymphoid system, Leuk. Lymphoma 38 (2000) 271–281.

[50] M. Busslinger, Transcriptional control of early B cell development, Annu. Rev. Immunol. 22 (2004) 55–79.

[51] A.L. Shaffer, et al., Blimp-1 orchestrates plasma cell differentiation by extinguishing the mature B cell gene expression program, Immunity 17 (2002) 51–62.

[52] A.L. Shaffer, et al., BCL-6 represses genes that function in lymphocyte differentiation, inflammation, and cell cycle control, Immunity 13 (2000) 199–212.

[53] Y. Kikuchi, et al., CD38 ligation induces tyrosine phosphorylation of Bruton tyrosine kinase and enhanced expression of interleukin 5-receptor alpha chain: synergistic effects with interleukin 5, Proc. Natl. Acad. Sci. U. S. A. 92 (1995) 11814–11818.

[54] T. Yasue, et al., A critical role of Lyn and Fyn for B cell responses to CD38 ligation and interleukin 5, Proc. Natl. Acad. Sci. U. S. A. 94 (1997) 10307–10312.

[55] H. Kaku, et al., NF-kappaB is required for CD38-mediated induction of Cγ1 germline transcripts in murine B lymphocytes, Int. Immunol. 14 (2002) 1055–1064.

[56] E. Sonoda, et al., Transforming growth factor beta induces IgA production and acts additively with interleukin 5 for IgA production, J. Exp. Med. 170 (1989) 1415–1420.

[57] R.F. Tsuji, et al., B cell-dependent T cell responses: IgM antibodies are required to elicit contact sensitivity, J. Exp. Med. 196 (2002) 1277–1290.

[58] C.J. Binder, et al., Innate and acquired immunity in atherogenesis, Nat. Med. 8 (2002) 1218–1226.

[59] U. Schönbeck, et al., T(H)2 predominant immune responses prevail in human abdominal aortic aneurysm, Am. J. Pathol. 161 (2002) 499–506.

[60] P.X. Shaw, et al., Natural antibodies with the T15 idiotype may act in atherosclerosis, apoptotic clearance, and protective immunity, J. Clin. Invest. 105 (2000) 1731–1740.

[61] C.J. Binder, et al., IL-5 links adaptive and natural immunity specific for epitopes of oxidized LDL and protects from atherosclerosis, J. Clin. Invest. 114 (2004) 427–437.

[62] A. Daugherty, D.L. Rateri, V.L. King, IL-5 links adaptive and natural immunity in reducing atherosclerotic disease, J. Clin. Invest. 114 (2004) 317–319.

International Congress Series 1285 (2005) 155–159

www.ics-elsevier.com

Vδ1^{+} $\gamma\delta$ T cells producing CC chemokines may bridge a gap between neutrophils and macrophages in innate immunity during *Escherichia coli* infection in mice☆

Y. Yoshikai *, T. Tagawa, K. Shibata, T. Yajima, H. Hara, K. Kishihara

Division of Host Defense, Research Center for Prevention of Infectious Diseases, Medical Institute of Bioregulation, Kyushu University, 3-1-1 Maidashi, Higashi-ku, Fukuoka 812-8582, Japan

Abstract. An influx of neutrophils followed a short time later by an influx of macrophages to the infected site plays a key role in innate immunity against *Escherichia coli* infection. We found in this study that Vδ1$^{-/-}$ mice exhibited impaired accumulation of peritoneal macrophages but not neutrophils and delayed bacterial clearance after intraperitoneal inoculation with *E. coli*. Peritoneal $\gamma\delta$ T cells from *E. coli*-infected wild-type mice produced CCL3/MIP-1α and CCL5/RANTES in response to $\gamma\delta$ T CR triggering in vitro, while such production was not evident in $\gamma\delta$ T cells from *E. coli*-infected Vδ1$^{-/-}$ mice. Neutralization of CCL3/MIP-1α by a specific monoclonal antibody in vivo significantly inhibited the accumulation of macrophages in the peritoneal cavity after *E. coli* infection, resulting in exacerbated bacterial growth in the peritoneal cavity. These results suggest that Vδ1^{+} $\gamma\delta$ T cells bridge a gap between neutrophis and macrophages in innate immunity during *E. coli* infection mediated by production of CC chemokines, enhancing macrophage trafficking to the site of infection. © 2005 Published by Elsevier B.V.

Keywords: Rodent; Bacterial; Chemokines; Cell trafficking; Inflammation

Abbreviations: Vδ1$^{-/-}$ mice, mice deficient in Vδ1 gene; PEC, peritoneal exudate cells; PMN, polymorphonuclear leukocytes.

☆ This work was supported by Uehara Memorial Foundation (Y. Y.).

* Corresponding author. Tel.: +81 92 642 6972; fax: +81 92 642 6973.
E-mail addresses: yoshikai@bioreg.kyushu-ac.jp, nishihit@bioreg.kyushu-u.ac.jp (Y. Yoshikai).

0531-5131/ © 2005 Published by Elsevier B.V.
doi:10.1016/j.ics.2005.07.086

1. Introduction

γδ T cells are present in small numbers in the blood and peripheral lymphoid tissues but are relatively abundant in the epithelia of the epidermis, intestine, uterus, and tongue compared with αβ T cells in mice [1]. Most of the γδ T cell subsets in peripheral lymphoid tissues bear junctionally diverse TCRs, but the γδ T cell subsets in the epithelia, including the Vγ5/Vδ1 subset in the skin and the Vγ6/Vδ1 subset in the tongue and female reproductive tract, bear invariant TCRs [2–4]. These two subsets differentiate in the thymus at the very early stage of ontogeny and bear truly invariant TCRs without junctional diversity [2]. Such characteristics have led to the hypothesis that γδ T cells bearing invariant Vδ1 TCRs represent a more primitive, first line of host defense in innate immunity. In the present study, to elucidate potential roles of invariant Vδ1-bearing γδ T cells in protection against *Escherichia coli* infection, we examined bacterial growth and cellular responses in the peritoneal cavities of mice deficient in the Vδ1 gene (Vδ1$^{-/-}$) following intraperitoneal infection with *E. coli*.

2. Materials and methods

C57BL/6 mice were purchased from SLC Japan (Shizuoka, Japan). Vδ1$^{-/-}$ mice were generated as previously described [5]. Vδ1$^{-/-}$ mice with a C57BL/6 background were backcrossed into C57BL/6 mice more than nine times. Mice were i.p. inoculated with *E. coli* (ATCC26; American Type Culture Collection, Rockville, MD) at a dose of one-fifth the LD_{50} (10^8 CFU/mouse) in 200 μl of PBS on day 0. γδ T cells were positively enriched from peritoneal exudate cells (PEC) by magnetic positive selection using a MACS system and anti-FITC microbeads. Cells were analyzed with a FACSCalibur flow cytometer (BD Biosciences). Tissue culture 96-well plates were incubated for 1 h at 37 °C with 100 μg/ml anti-TCR γδ mAb. The plates were then washed thoroughly and incubated for 1 h at 37 °C with RPMI 1640 medium containing 10% FCS. The γδ T cells (3×10^4 cells/well) were incubated in the 96-well plates for 42 h with or without immobilized anti-TCR γδ mAb in the presence or absence of LPS (10 μg/ml, Sigma). CCL2/MCP-1, CCL3/MIP-1α, CCL5/RANTES and CCL8/Eotaxin levels in the culture supernatants were determined by using an ELISA kit (Genzyme Techne, Minneapolis, MN). Wild-type mice were each injected

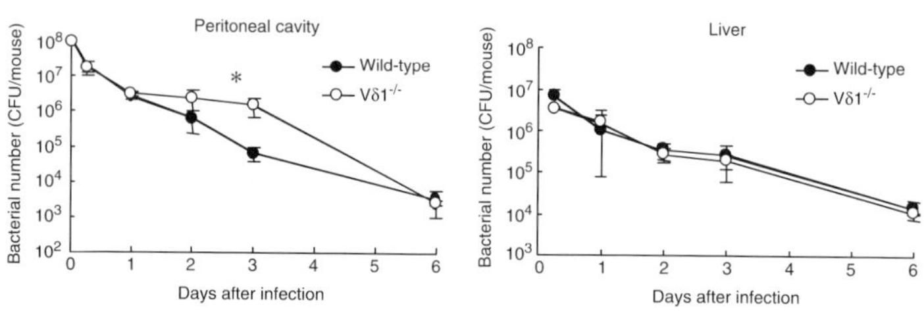

Fig. 1. Kinetics of bacterial growth in the peritoneal cavity and liver after i.p. inoculation with *E. coli*. Wild-type and Vδ1$^{-/-}$ mice were inoculated intraperitoneally with 10^8 CFU of *E. coli* ($0.2 \times$ LD50). Bacterial growth in the peritoneal cavity and liver of each mouse was measured at indicated days after infection. ●, wild-type; ○, Vδ1$^{-/-}$ mice. Day 0 means data from mice without infection (before infection). Each point and vertical bar indicates the mean ± S.D. of 5 mice for each group. The data are representative of three separate experiments. Asterisks indicate significant differences from the values for wild-type mice ($p<0.05$).

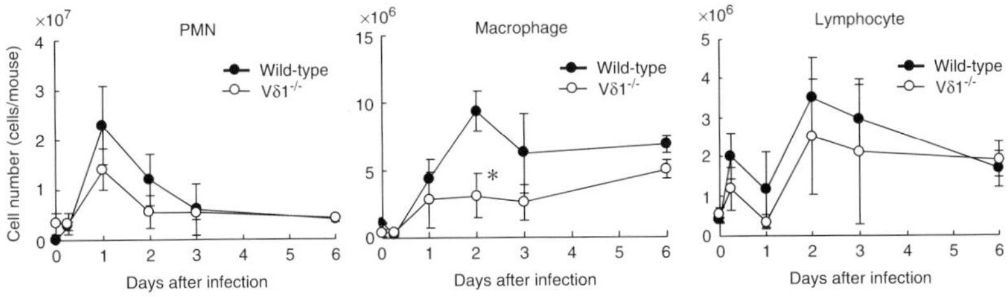

Fig. 2. Kinetics of peritoneal exudate cells after *E. coli* infection. Wild-type and Vδ1$^{-/-}$ mice were inoculated i.p. with 10^8 CFU of *E. coli*. Populations of PEC obtained from wild-type or Vδ1$^{-/-}$ mice at indicated days after *E. coli* infection. PMN, macrophages, and lymphocytes were judged by morphologic characteristics after staining with Giemsa solution. ●, wild-type; ○, Vδ1$^{-/-}$ mice. Each point and vertical bar indicates the mean ± S.D. of 5 mice for each group. The data are representative of three separate experiments. Asterisks indicate significant differences from the values for wild-type mice ($p<0.05$).

i.p. with 100 μg of neutralizing anti-CCL3/MIP-1α polyclonal Ab, anti-CCL5/RANTES mAb or together with both Abs of 100 μg each at 1 h before *E. coli* infection and injected again with 150 μg at 24 h after infection. Control mice were injected with control goat IgG or rat IgG for anti-CCL3/MIP-1αAb or anti-CCL5/RANTES mAb, respectively, or together with both Abs at doses comparable with those used in the experimental animals.

3. Results

Kinetics of bacterial growth was examined in organs of Vδ1$^{-/-}$ mice after i.p. inoculation with *E. coli* at a dose of 10^8 CFU (one-fifth the LD_{50})/mouse. The number of bacteria in the peritoneal cavity in wild-type mice was significantly smaller than that in Vδ1$^{-/-}$ mice on day 3, (Fig. 1, $p<0.05$).

The absolute number of PEC in Vδ1$^{-/-}$ mice was much lower than that of PEC in wild-type mice on day 2 after infection ($p<0.05$). The number of macrophages in the peritoneal cavity was significantly smaller in Vδ1$^{-/-}$ mice than that in wild-type mice on day 2 after infection (Fig. 2, $p<0.05$).

Fig. 3 shows that γδ T cells of wild-type mice produced large amounts of CCL3/MIP-1α and CCL5/RANTES, whereas γδ T cells of Vδ1$^{-/-}$ mice did not produce those chemokines at all upon TCR engagement. The level of CCL3/MIP-1α production in wild-type mice was significantly higher

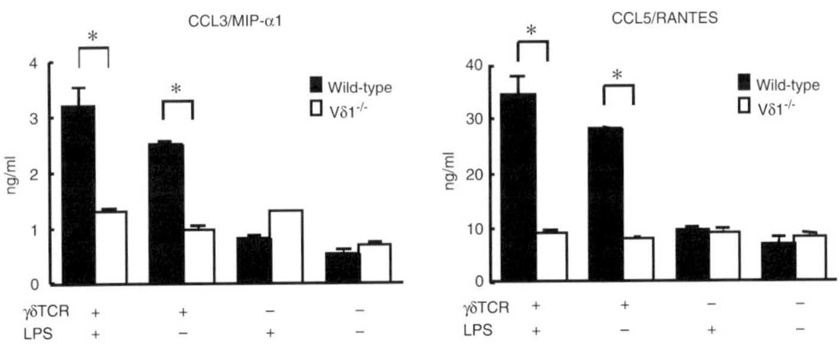

Fig. 3. Production of chemokines by γδ T cells from Vδ1$^{-/-}$ mice infected with *E. coli*. Purified γδ T cells (3×10^4 cells) were cultured in a 96-well culture plate with or without immobilized anti-TCR γδ mAb in the presence or absence of LPS (10 g/ml) for 42 h. Culture supernatants were subjected to ELISAs. The data are representative of three separate experiments and are expressed as the means of triplicates ± S.D. Asterisks indicate significant differences between the values for wild-type mice and Vδ1$^{-/-}$ mice ($p<0.05$).

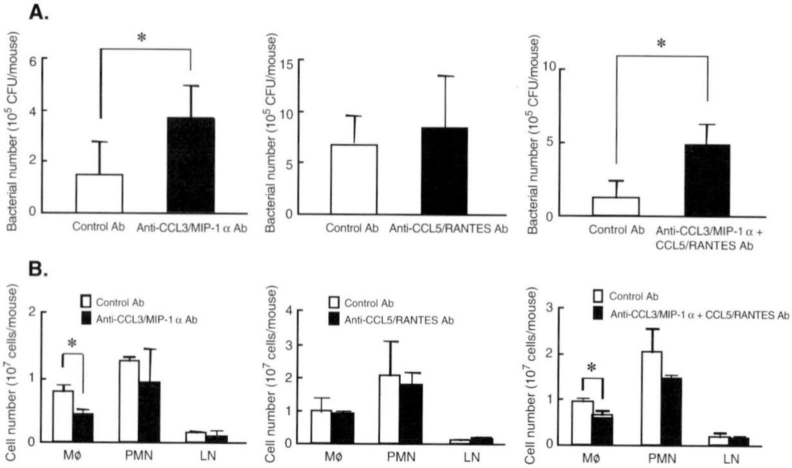

Fig. 4. Effects of chemokine neutralizations on bacterial clearance and cell influx in the peritoneal cavity after *E. coli* infection. Wild-type mice were injected i.p. with 100 μg of neutralizing anti-CCL3/MIP-1α Ab, anti-CCL5/RANTES Ab, both Abs or comparable doses of isotype control Ab at 1 h before *E. coli* challenge and were injected again with 150 μg at 24 h after infection. On day 2 after infection, the numbers of bacteria in the peritoneal cavity (A) and the populations of PEC judged by morphologic characteristics after staining with Giemsa solution (B) were counted. Each column and vertical bar indicates the mean ± S.D. of 3 mice for each group. The data are representative of three separate experiments. Asterisks indicate significant differences between the values for wild-type mice and Vδ$1^{-/-}$ mice ($p<0.05$).

than that of Vδ$1^{-/-}$ mice ($p<0.05$), while CCL5/RANTES level did not differ in Vδ$1^{-/-}$ mice from that in wild-type mice.

As shown in Fig. 4, a significant increase was found in the number of *E. coli* cells in the peritoneal cavities of anti-CCL3/MIP-1α Ab-treated mice compared with that in control Ab-treated mice. Notably, the numbers of Gr-1^+F4/80^+ macrophages in the peritoneal cavities of anti-CCL3/MIP-1α Ab-treated mice were smaller than those in control Ab-treated mice (Fig. 4, $p<0.05$).

4. Discussion

During the course of intraperitoneal infection with *E. coli*, neutrophils are the first cells to migrate from circulation to the peritoneal cavity, with monocytes/macrophages being recruited later. Vδ1^+ γδ T cells play a critical role in second phase of recruitment of monocytes to the infected sites. Thus, Vδ1-bearing γδ T cells, which are thought to be more primitive than other T cells, may bridge a gap between host defense mechanisms by neutroplils and macrophages in innate immunity during *E. coli* infection. In simian immunodeficiency infection, mucosal γδ T cells produced CCL3/MIP-1α, CCL4/MIP-1β and CCL5/RANTES upon TCR triggering [6].

Boismenu et al. reported that a dendritic epidermal T cell line (DECT7-17) bearing invariant Vγ5/Vδ1 TCRs expressed CCL3/MIP-1α, CCL4/MIP-1β and CCL5/RANTES but not CCL2/MCP-1 [7]. Dorner et al. have recently reported that CCL3/MIP-1α, CCL4/MIP-1β, CCL5/RANTES and ATAC/lymphotactin functioned together with IFN-γ as type 1 cytokines [8].

We speculate that Vδ1$^+$ $\gamma\delta$ T cells produce these chemokines together with IFN-γ in response to *E. coli* and are involved in the attraction and activation of macrophages, which consequently eliminate the *E. coli*. The Vγ6/Vδ1 $\gamma\delta$ T cells induced by *E. coli* infection bear truly invariant TCRs, even to the nucleotides in the TCR gene junction [2–4]. The canonical sequence is very simple, with no apparent N-region contribution [2]. Such a characteristic has led to the hypothesis that $\gamma\delta$ T cells represent a preprogrammed T cell subset to recognize a limited set of Ags in *E. coli* or self-Ag induced by *E. coli* infection. At present, the specificity of $\gamma\delta$ T cells remains unknown.

In conclusion, we have shown that Vδ1$^+$ $\gamma\delta$ T cells induced in the peritoneal cavity after *E. coli* infection produce Th1-type chemokines in response to TCR triggering. Vδ1$^+$ $\gamma\delta$ T cells may participate in attraction and activation of macrophages after *E. coli* infection, thus bridging protection mechanisms by neutrophils and macrophages during *E. coli* infection.

Acknowledgements

We thank K. Kaneda for preparing the manuscript and Y. Kobayashi for technical assistance.

References

[1] W. Haas, P. Pereira, S. Tonegawa, Gamma/delta cells, Annu. Rev. Immunol. 11 (1993) 637.

[2] J.J. Lafaille, et al., Junctional sequences of T cell receptor $\gamma\delta$ genes: implications for $\gamma\delta$ T cell lineages and for a novel intermediate of V-(D)-J joining, Cell 59 (1989) 859.

[3] D. Nandi, J.P. Allison, Phenotypic analysis and $\gamma\delta$ T cell receptor repertoire of murine T cells associated with the vaginal epithelium, J. Immunol. 147 (1991) 1773.

[4] K. Heyborne, et al., Evidence that murine Vγ5 and Vγ6 $\gamma\delta$ TCR$^+$ lymphocytes are derived from a common distinct lineage, J. Immunol. 151 (1993) 4523.

[5] H. Hara, et al., Development of dendritic epidermal T cells with a skewed diversity of $\gamma\delta$ TCRs in Vδ1-deficient mice, J. Immunol. 165 (2000) 3695.

[6] T. Lehner, et al., The role of $\gamma\delta$ T cells in generating antiviral factors and β-chemokines in protection against mucosal simian immunodeficiency virus infection, Eur. J. Immunol. 30 (2000) 2245.

[7] R. Boismenu, et al., Chemokine expression by intraepithelial gamma delta T cells. Implications for the recruitment of inflammatory cells to damaged epithelia, J. Immunol. 157 (1996) 985.

[8] B.G. Dorner, et al., MIP-1α, MIP-1β, RANTES, and ATAC/lymphotactin function together with IFN-as “type 1-cytokines”, Proc. Natl. Acad. Sci. U. S. A. 99 (2002) 6181.

International Congress Series 1285 (2005) 160–168

www.ics-elsevier.com

Development and function of IL-10-secreting regulatory T cells: Comparison with naturally occurring $CD4^{+}CD25^{+}$ regulatory T cells

Anne O'Garra *

Division of Immunoregulation, The National Institute for Medical Research (NIMR), NW7 1AA London, United Kingdom

Abstract. Regulatory T cells (Treg) control immune responses to self and nonself Ags. The relationship between Ag-driven IL-10-secreting Treg (IL-10-Treg) and naturally occurring CD4 CD25 Treg is as yet unclear. We show that mouse IL-10-Treg obtained using either in vitro or in vivo regimens of antigenic stimulation did not express the CD4 CD25 Treg-associated transcription factor Foxp3. However, despite the absence of Foxp3 expression, homogeneous populations of IL-10-Treg inhibited the in vitro proliferation of CD4 CD25 T cells with a similar efficiency to that of CD4 CD25 Treg. This inhibition of T cell proliferation by IL-10-Treg was achieved through an IL-10-independent mechanism as seen for CD4 CD25 Treg and was overcome by exogenous IL-2. Both IL-10-Treg and CD4 CD25 Treg were similar in that they produced little to no IL-2. These data show that Foxp3 expression is not a prerequisite for IL-10-Treg activity in vitro or in vivo and suggest that IL-10-Treg and naturally occurring CD4 CD25 Treg may have distinct origins. Thus, these different regulatory populations may have different roles at different stages of the immune response. © 2005 Published by Elsevier B.V.

Keywords: Regulatory T cells (Treg); T helper (Th) cells; Suppression; Regulation; Cytokines

1. Introduction

The immune system evolved to protect the host against the attack of foreign, potentially pathogenic, microorganisms. It does so by recognizing antigens expressed by those microorganisms and mounting an immune response against all cells expressing them, with the ultimate aim of eliminating such cells. Various mechanisms have been reported to

* Tel.: +44 208 816 2508; fax: +44 208 816 2564.
E-mail address: aogarra@nimr.mrc.ac.uk.

doi:10.1016/j.ics.2005.09.009

control and regulate the immune system in order to prevent or minimize reactivity to self-antigens or an over-exuberant response to a pathogen, both of which can result in damage to the host. Deletion of autoreactive cells during T and B cell development allows the immune system to be tolerant of most self-antigens. Peripheral tolerance to self was suggested a number of years ago to result from the induction of anergy in peripheral self-reactive lymphocytes 1. More recently, however, it became clear that avoidance of damage to the host is also achieved by active suppression mediated by regulatory T (Treg) cell populations [2–5].

Treg may be defined as cells that can be shown to inhibit immunopathology or autoimmune disease in vivo. Two major ex vivo derived $CD4^+$ Treg populations have been described to date. Originally, the $CD4^+CD45RB^{low}$ cells (which comprise the compartment of activated $CD4^+$ cells found in normal mice) were found to be able to control the exuberant colitis mediated by the transfer of $CD4^+CD45Rb^{high}$ (naïve) cells [6]. It was later found that control of colitis was achieved by the $CD4^+CD25^+$ subset, which is contained within the $CD4^+CD45RB^{low}$ population (reviewed in [4]). We refer to these $CD4^+CD25^+$ T cells as naturally occurring Treg. They were identified due to their ability to control various manifestations of autoimmunity secondary to neonatal thymectomy [2,3]. Within the $CD4^+CD45RB^{low}$ population, some $CD25^-$ T cells also have regulatory activity [7], but little work has been published in further characterization of this population. More recently, IL-10-producing (IL-10 Treg) and TGF-β-secreting Treg cells were described and shown to have regulatory activity in systems classically used to study the naturally occurring Treg populations. In particular, this novel type of regulatory T cell is able to suppress experimentally induced autoimmune disease and naïve T cell proliferation in vitro and control $CD4^+$ and $CD8^+$ T cell numbers in vivo in lymphopenic hosts [8–12]. It is unclear at this stage whether, or how, these populations are related to each other or to the naturally occurring $CD4^+CD25^+$ Treg with respect to their development and function in the inhibition of the immune response at various levels. This is currently a highly active area of research in immunology, which we review in this perspective.

The original suppressor T cells were first proposed in the early 1970s and thought to cause suppression by secreting antigen-specific suppressor factors, although human regulatory T cells were also described, which suppressed via antigen nonspecific mechanisms. In those early days, the experimental systems used were poorly characterized and, due to the paucity of cell surface markers, lymphocyte subpopulations were difficult to isolate consistently. This field eventually floundered since these cells could not be grown reliably and attempts to clone the putative suppressor factors failed. In addition, the major histocompatibility (MHC) antigen thought to be their restriction element, I–J, was not found as expected in the MHC locus and many suppressor T cell clones were also found not to express a T cell receptor (reviewed in [13]). The concept of immune regulation by specialized T cells remained, however, such that when better cellular and molecular tools became available, the field was reborn. Under a new name, propped by more solid experimental systems and admittedly better data, suppressor T cells are back in business [14]. Regulatory T cells described to date require antigen-specific activation to act, but function through antigen-independent mechanisms.

The $CD4^+CD25^+$ subset is currently the focus of the most intensive research in this area. These cells represent 5–10% of the $CD4^+$ T lymphocytes in healthy adult mice and humans and are thought to perform a specialized role in controlling both the innate and the adaptive immune system [2,3,15]. Although easily identifiable and isolated from unmanipulated mice and humans on the basis of CD25 expression, this chain of the IL-2R is also expressed on activated T cells [2,3,15]. Thus, no characteristic stable surface marker has been described so far. Additional markers expressed by these cells include cytotoxic T-lymphocyte-associated protein 4 (CTLA-4) [16,17] and glucocorticoid-induced TNF receptor (GITR) [18,19], which were initially implicated in the mechanism of Treg action. However, both of these molecules are also expressed by non-regulatory T cells after activation. Secretion of TGF-β and IL-10 is also a common feature of Treg, and the activity of these two cytokines is involved in the ability of this population to control some, but not all, immune responses in vivo [20]. Again, neither TGF-β nor IL-10 secretion is a unique feature of Treg [4].

Recently, the forkhead/winged helix transcription factor Foxp3 was shown to be specifically expressed by $CD25^+$ Treg, as well as by $CD25^-$ T cells with regulatory activity [21–23]. This transcription factor is thought to program the development and function of this subset and, to date, is the most unambiguous marker available to identify naturally occurring Treg. Loss-of-function mutations in this gene, in both humans and mice, caused the absence of Treg (but, importantly, not of other $CD25^+$ activated T cells) and a prominent phenotype that includes autoimmune endocrinopathy, early onset type [1] diabetes, thyroiditis and in some cases severe atopy and food allergy (reviewed in [24,25]). In humans, the disease can be corrected, or at least ameliorated, by bone marrow transplantation [26]. In mice, the hematopoietic component that reverts the disease, or at least prevents it, is the $CD4^+CD25^+$ Treg population [23]. Ectopic expression of Foxp3 as a transgene significantly delayed the onset of the proliferative disease observed in CTLA-4 gene-deleted mice [22]. Furthermore, forced expression of Foxp3 in non-regulatory $CD4^+$T cells caused their acquisition of many properties known to be characteristic of Treg, including inhibition of colitis and gastritis, inhibition of the lymphoproliferative and wasting disease observed in the natural Foxp3 mutant mice, scurfy, and control of the size of the $CD8^+$ T cell compartment in vivo [21,23]. In addition, Foxp3 transduced CD4 T cells could inhibit naïve T cell proliferation in vitro [21,23]. Expression of Foxp3 is thus a reliable marker for naturally occurring Treg, although as discussed below, not all populations displaying regulatory activity express this gene.

It is as yet unclear whether Foxp3 is expressed exclusively at a specific period of development in the thymus, or whether it can be upregulated in the periphery. Induction of Foxp3 in antigen-specific peripheral T lymphocytes would open new therapeutic strategies in the treatment of immunopathologies and could provide a solution to the problem of transplantation tolerance. Some suggestions that Foxp3 can be upregulated on non-regulatory T cells have been reported; however, it is difficult to interpret whether this upregulation was on naturally occurring Treg which have lost the expression of CD25. Whether Foxp3 is the marker that uniquely distinguishes all Treg populations still remains unclear.

$CD4^+CD25^+$ Treg cells protect lymphopenic mice from inflammatory bowel disease [4] and diabetes [27,28] and can also prevent transplant rejection [29,30]. Conversely, a role damaging to the host is their ability to inhibit immune response to tumors [31,32]. IL-10 production by Treg cells contained within the $CD4^{+}CD45RB^{low}$ compartment is essential to protect immunocompromised mice from colitis [33] and from allograft rejection [29] initiated by $CD4^{+}$T cells contained within the $CD45RB^{high}$ compartment. IL-10 and TGF-β have been shown to be important mediators of Treg-mediated suppression of not only colitis [33], but also of autoimmune or allergic pathologies [8,11,34–36]. $CD4^{+}CD25^{+}$ Treg cells inhibit the proliferation and expansion of naïve T cells both in vitro and in vivo [3,7]. However, the in vivo suppression of proliferation [7,10], as already mentioned above, and of wasting disease [7] are IL-10 dependent, in contrast to the inhibition of gastritis [20] and of naïve T cell proliferation in vitro, which are IL-10 independent and thought to require cell–cell contact [3,10,37]. As yet, the mechanisms for this cell-contact-mediated suppression seem to be undefined [3].

2. Antigen-derived IL-10-producing regulatory T cells do not express FOXP3 and do not need FOXP3 for their regulatory function

We and others have shown that regimens of antigen administration that were known to generate anergy/tolerance in vivo, induce the appearance of IL-10-producing T cells [10,34,38–41] Sundstedt et al. have demonstrated that IL-10-producing Treg cells can be induced by repeated intranasal administration of an antigenic peptide of myelin basic protein (MBP) and that these regulatory cells inhibit the proliferation of naïve MBP-specific T cells both in vitro and in vivo. Interestingly, and in keeping with previous findings [7,29,33] using the $CD4^{+}CD25^{+}$ Treg cells, IL-10 mediated the suppression of naïve T cells in vivo [10] but not in vitro [3,10]. To support this, we have shown that naïve $CD4^{+}$T cells can be made to generate in vitro a homogeneous population of IL-10-secreting cells, representative of those in vivo derived populations earlier described [11]. These IL-10 Treg populations show regulatory function to block experimental autoimmune encephalomyelitis (EAE) and their development and function in vivo is IL-10 dependent. However, the inhibition of in vitro T cell proliferation by these IL-10-Treg is not [37]. Thus, it would appear that both types of Treg cells use different mechanisms when they regulate proliferation in vitro or in vivo, and when they control in vivo immune responses and/or pathologies, which may be accompanied by different levels of inflammation [20,33]. In vitro assays used to detect inhibition of naïve T cell proliferation by Treg cells may not reveal a role for IL-10 as a result of the duration of the assay and the type of APC used. In addition, the extent of APC maturation/activation that may occur in vivo may not be reflected in in vitro systems. This is more clearly observed in systems such as the one described by Pasare and Medzhitov, where they showed that TLR ligation of bone marrow derived dendritic cells overcomes the inhibition of naïve T cell proliferation mediated by $CD4^{+}CD25^{+}$ Treg cells. This anti-suppressive action of activated dendritic cells was not fully dissected, but is in part, due to the production of IL-6 [42]. Since IL-10's major effects are to inhibit APC function, including the production of proinflammatory cytokines [43], it is likely that the function of Treg cells is dependent on IL-10 only when cells of the innate immune system are involved and indeed, Treg inhibit innate immunity [15]. In addition, although $CD4^{+}CD25^{+}$ Treg cells can be induced to produce IL-10 and can inhibit colitis, it is clear that IL-10 Treg and other cells, including

Th2 or Th1 cells as well as APC, can also produce IL-10 and control the magnitude of an immune response and thus limit immunopathology [43].

The question remains as to the relationship between these two types of regulatory T cells: the naturally occurring $CD4^{+}CD25^{+}$ Treg cells [2–4] which, depending on the system, may or may not require the suppressive action of IL-10, and the IL-10-producing Treg cells that can be developed under different regimens of antigenic-stimulation, both in vitro [8,11,44] and in vivo [10,34,39,41]. Foxp3-transduced $CD4^{+}CD25^{-}$ T cells after transfer into lymphopenic hosts expressed enhanced levels of IL-10 mRNA, comparable with those of naturally occurring $CD4^{+}CD25^{+}$ Treg cells and higher than the levels found in untransduced cells [23]. Based on these findings, it was suggested that Foxp3 directly upregulates IL-10 production, but it is likely that the cells, besides the expression of Foxp3, require additional signals in vivo for IL-10 gene induction. Taken together these studies did not support a direct relationship between Foxp3 and IL-10 expression. Most recently, we have demonstrated that IL-10 Treg cells obtained using both in vitro and in vivo strategies do not express the transcription factor Foxp3, which distinguishes them from the classic $CD4^{+}CD25^{+}$ Treg cells [37]. Furthermore, we have shown that IL-10 Treg can be obtained in vitro using antigen-specific TCR transgenic T cells not containing naturally occurring Treg cells [11]. Despite their lack of Foxp3 expression, however, as discussed earlier, homogeneous populations of IL-10- Treg cells inhibited the proliferation of naïve $CD4^{+}CD25^{-}$ T cells in vitro with a similar efficiency as $CD4^{+}CD25^{+}$ Treg. It is of note that enhanced IL-10 expression in IL-10 Treg cells was always mirrored by a significant decrease in IL-2 expression, and that IL-2 expression is also absent in Foxp3-expressing $CD4^{+}CD25^{+}$ Treg [22,37]. Foxp3 has been suggested to act as a negative modulator of IL-2 transcription [45], but clearly, this can be achieved in IL-10 Treg by other mechanisms, probably dependent on antigenic stimulation in the presence of immunosuppressive drugs, or secondary to peptide antigen regimens leading to anergy induction [10,11,40,41,46].

What seems to be a prerequisite of the ability of Treg cells to inhibit naïve T cell proliferation in vitro is a lack of IL-2 (and probably IL-4) production, which would support the hypothesis that anergic T cells may regulate naïve T cell proliferation, and thus are active "suppressors" [46] as opposed to working passively. The mechanism(s) whereby Treg cells bring about the cell-contact-dependent inhibition of naïve T cells is as yet unclear. It is of interest that although naturally occurring Treg cells are anergic, they can expand in vivo via mechanisms distinct from that of conventional T cells [7,47,48].

Similarly to $CD4^{+}CD25^{+}$ Treg cells, we showed that the regulatory capacity of IL-10 Treg cells to inhibit naïve CD4+CD25-T cell proliferation in vitro was independent of their intrinsic production of IL-10 and could be overcome by exogenous IL-2 [10,37]. This shows that expression of Foxp3 itself is not always necessary for regulation. We propose that the inhibition of naïve T cell proliferation in vitro represents a first layer of regulation before the innate immune response is activated, when IL-10 becomes involved in the mechanism of suppression [3,49]. This layer of regulation, which is independent of Foxp3 expression, may have as its in vivo equivalent the competition-dependent regulatory activity that can be observed in lymphopenic mice [49] . Inhibition of gastritis mediated by naturally occurring (Foxp3 expressing) Treg [20] is also IL-10 independent, perhaps reflecting low levels of inflammation. In our view, higher layers of regulation of immune responses exist that require production of IL-10 and/or TGF-β. Control of T cell expansion in vivo by $CD4^+CD25^+$ Treg is dependent on IL-10 [7], and the higher inflammation associated with activation of the innate immune response may demand that the regulatory system be notched up. That is why in many in vivo systems, as discussed above, where strong inflammation often induced directly by infectious agents, is the norm, both $CD4^+CD25^+$ Treg cells and IL-10 Treg cells can only inhibit inflammation via IL-10 or TGF-β-dependent mechanisms.

3. Implications for regulatory T cells in control of immune responses to pathogens

Recently, it has been shown that $CD4^+CD25^+$ Treg cells may also regulate the immune response to the pathogen *Leishmania major*, in part through the suppressive action of IL-10 [50]. It had been demonstrated a number of years ago that a Th2 response, observed for example in BALB/c mice infected with *L. major*, was completely incapable of protecting the host. In this system, IL-4 prevented *L. major* clearance by Th1 cells producing IFN γ (reviewed in [51]). Furthermore, regulatory cells within the $CD45Rb^{low}$ compartment were shown to inhibit the clearance of *L. major* by $CD4^+CD45RB^{high}$ T cells via the action of IL-4, but to inhibit wasting disease in the same model via the action of TGF-β. Thus, whilst Th2 cells also produce IL-10 (they are distinguished from Treg because Th2 cells produce in addition IL-4, IL-5 and IL-13) and may contribute to suppression of responses to *L. major* via its action, IL-4 production by Th2 cells can also mediate this suppression in certain models of this disease [6,51]. Anergic IL-10-producing T cells obtained from chronic *Mycobacterium tuberculosis*-infected patients non-reactive to purified protein derivative (PPD), can be made reactive to PPD by the addition of anti-IL-10 antibodies to in vitro cultures and have also been shown to act as Treg cells and inhibit the proliferation of allo-specific $CD4^+$T cells [52].

IL-10 was originally described as a cytokine produced by Th2 cells. However, it soon became clear that this suppressive cytokine was produced by many other cell types including macrophages, B cells and DC (reviewed in [43,53]). We have shown many years ago that IL-10 suppresses the production by DC and macrophages of proinflammatory cytokines such as IL-12, a very important factor in directing Th1 development [43] and yet IL-10 is produced, by macrophages and different populations of DC, albeit in varying levels, and also by Th1 cells [53]. The relative levels of IL-10 and IFN-γ produced by Th1 cells may be an important determinant of the balance between clearance and persistent infection with certain pathogens [43,51,53]. In this regard, IL-10 may also play the important role of feedback regulator to control the pathology associated with an overexuberant, albeit efficacious, Th1 response [54]. Thus, the source of IL-10 during immune responses to pathogens or allergens could be Th1 cells or Th2 cells respectively (reviewed in [43,51,53]), or as more recently suggested, regulatory T cells [35,50,52,55]. Although regulatory T cells were originally implicated in the regulation of autoimmune and/or inflammatory pathologies [2,4,13], it is clear that they may also play a role in regulating the response to infectious pathogens and/or allergens to minimize immune pathology [6,35,50,52,55] (see reviews in [4,24,25,43]).

It is of note, however, that although Th1 and Th2 cells can clearly function as "regulatory" cells by their production of IL-10 (and of IL-4 in the case of Th2 cells) as well as by their ability to reciprocally regulate each other [51], they also mediate effector functions. Such effector functions have not as yet been attributed to the two types of regulatory T cells discussed in this review, as they appear to have no function other than regulation (i.e., suppression) of immune responses.

A number of questions remain to be answered with respect to the development and function of Treg. Firstly, are the naturally occurring $CD4^+CD25^+$ Treg that develop in the thymus, and are Foxp3-dependent mainly important for responses to self antigens and/or antigens encountered in the thymus, or can they also regulate inflammatory pathologies directed against gut flora [4,15]? If so, is the latter achieved by cross-reactivity of $CD4^+CD25^+$ Treg between self and microbial antigens? Secondly, how do naturally occurring $CD4^+CD25^+$ Treg cells expressing Foxp3 compare with the antigen-driven IL-10-producing Treg obtained by in vitro and in vivo regimens of antigenic stimulation? Are these IL-10- Treg long-lived as has been shown for $CD4^+CD25^+$ Treg cells [41,56]? That $CD4^+CD25^+$ Treg cells and possibly other Treg producing IL-10 can regulate immune responses to pathogens and/or T cells with other reactivities has been demonstrated [10,11,50,52]. Whether these IL-10-Treg cells are of the same "lineage" as the naturally occurring Foxp3-dependent $CD4^+CD25^+$ Treg cells, which prevent lymphoproliferative disorders and endocrinopathies, such as diabetes, in mice and humans, seems not to be the case, but is as yet unclear. It still remains to be clarified when each type of Treg develops and plays a role in the regulation of immune pathology. Be it as it may, it is likely that the functional mechanisms involved in regulating immune responses to self antigens are similar to those regulating immune responses to pathogens and other antigens. The molecular mechanisms involved in this regulation appear to depend, however, on the level of inflammation accompanying an immune response. Regardless, these different Treg appear to develop via different mechanisms. A major caveat in the use of Treg in the treatment of inflammatory and autoimmune diseases will be the antigen specificity, since the aim would be to target the pathogenic T cells whilst leaving T cells directed against infectious pathogens and/or tumors undisturbed. Conversely, in the treatment of chronic infectious diseases with antagonists of Treg or their products, it will be important to achieve this without allowing the response of autoreactive T cells.

References

[1] M.K. Jenkins, et al., Induction and maintenance of anergy in mature T cells, Adv. Exp. Med. Biol. 292 (1991) 167–176.

[2] S. Sakaguchi, et al., Immunologic tolerance maintained by $CD25^+CD4^+$ regulatory T cells: their common role in controlling autoimmunity, tumor immunity, and transplantation tolerance, Immunol. Rev. 182 (2001) 18–32.

[3] E.M. Shevach, $CD4^+CD25^+$ suppressor T cells: more questions than answers, Nat. Rev., Immunol. 2 (2002) 389–400.

[4] K.J. Maloy, F. Powrie, Regulatory T cells in the control of immune pathology, Nat. Immunol. 2 (2001) 816–822.

[5] S.P. Cobbold, et al., Regulatory T cells in the induction and maintenance of peripheral transplantation tolerance, Transpl. Int. 16 (2003) 66–75.

[6] F. Powrie, et al., Regulatory interactions between CD45RBhigh and CD45RBlow $CD4^+$ T cells are important for the balance between protective and pathogenic cell-mediated immunity, J. Exp. Med. 179 (1994) 589–600.

[7] O. Annacker, et al., CD25⁺CD4⁺ T cells regulate the expansion of peripheral CD4 T cells through the production of IL-10, J. Immunol. 166 (2001) 3008–3018.
[8] H. Groux, et al., A CD4⁺ T-cell subset inhibits antigen-specific T-cell responses and prevents colitis, Nature 389 (1997) 737–742.
[9] M.G. Roncarolo, et al., Type 1 T regulatory cells, Immunol. Rev. 182 (2001) 68–79.
[10] A. Sundstedt, et al., Role for IL-10 in suppression mediated by peptide-induced regulatory T cells in vivo, J. Immunol. 170 (2003) 1240–1248.
[11] F.J. Barrat, et al., In vitro generation of interleukin 10-producing regulatory CD4(+) T cells is induced by immunosuppressive drugs and inhibited by T helper type 1 (Th1)-and Th2-inducing cytokines, J. Exp. Med. 195 (2002) 603–616.
[12] T. Oida, et al., D4+CD25-T cells that express latency-associated peptide on the surface suppress CD4⁺CD45RBhigh-induced colitis by a TGF-beta-dependent mechanism, J. Immunol. 170 (2003) 2516–2522.
[13] E.M. Shevach, Regulatory T cells in autoimmmunity*, Annu. Rev. Immunol. 18 (2000) 423–449.
[14] E.M. Shevach, Suppressor T cells: rebirth, function and homeostasis, Curr. Biol. 10 (2000) R572–R575.
[15] K.J Maloy, et al., CD4⁺CD25⁺T(R) cells suppress innate immune pathology through cytokine-dependent mechanisms, J. Exp. Med. 197 (2003) 111–119.
[16] S. Read, V. Malmstrom, F. Powrie, Cytotoxic T lymphocyte-associated antigen 4 plays an essential role in the function of CD25(+)CD4(+) regulatory cells that control intestinal inflammation, J. Exp. Med. 192 (2000) 295–302.
[17] T. Takahashi, et al., Immunologic self-tolerance maintained by CD25(+)CD4(+) regulatory T cells constitutively expressing cytotoxic T lymphocyte-associated antigen 4, J. Exp. Med. 192 (2000) 303–310.
[18] J. Shimizu, et al., Stimulation of CD25(+)CD4(+) regulatory T cells through GITR breaks immunological self-tolerance, Nat. Immunol. 3 (2002) 135–142.
[19] R.S. McHugh, et al., CD4(+)CD25(+) immunoregulatory T cells: gene expression analysis reveals a functional role for the glucocorticoid-induced TNF receptor, Immunity 16 (2002) 311–323.
[20] E. Suri-Payer, H. Cantor, Differential cytokine requirements for regulation of autoimmune gastritis and colitis by CD4(+)CD25(+) T cells, J. Autoimmun. 16 (2001) 115–123.
[21] S. Hori, T. Nomura, S. Sakaguchi, Control of regulatory T cell development by the transcription factor Foxp3, Science 299 (2003) 1057–1061.
[22] R. Khattri, et al., An essential role for Scurfin in CD4⁺ CD25⁺T regulatory cells, Nat. Immunol. 4 (2003) 337–342.
[23] J.D. Fontenot, M.A. Gavin, A.Y. Rudensky, Foxp3 programs the development and function of CD4⁺ CD25⁺ regulatory T cells, Nat. Immunol. 4 (2003) 330–336.
[24] F. Ramsdell, Foxp3 and natural regulatory T cells: key to a cell lineage? Immunity 19 (2003) 165–168.
[25] A. O'Garra, P. Vieira, Twenty-first century Foxp3, Nat. Immunol. 4 (2003) 304–306.
[26] O. Baud, et al., Treatment of the immune dysregulation, polyendocrinopathy, enteropathy, X-linked syndrome (IPEX) by allogeneic bone marrow transplantation, N. Engl. J. Med. 344 (2001) 1758–1762.
[27] E.A. Green, Y. Choi, R.A. Flavell, Pancreatic lymph node-derived CD4(+)CD25(+) Treg cells: highly potent regulators of diabetes that require TRANCE-RANK signals, Immunity 16 (2002) 183–191.
[28] B. Salomon, et al., B7/CD28 costimulation is essential for the homeostasis of the CD4⁺CD25⁺ immunoregulatory T cells that control autoimmune diabetes, Immunity 12 (2000) 431–440.
[29] M. Hara, et al., IL-10 is required for regulatory T cells to mediate tolerance to alloantigens in vivo, J. Immunol. 166 (2001) 3789–3796.
[30] C.I. Kingsley, et al., CD25⁺CD4⁺ regulatory T cells prevent graft rejection: CTLA-4-and IL-10-dependent immunoregulation of alloresponses, J. Immunol. 168 (2002) 1080–1086.
[31] J. Shimizu, S. Yamazaki, S. Sakaguchi, Induction of tumor immunity by removing CD25⁺ CD4⁺ T cells: a common basis between tumor immunity and autoimmunity, J. Immunol. 163 (1999) 5211–5218.
[32] D. Golgher, et al., Depletion of CD25⁺regulatory cells uncovers immune responses to shared murine tumor rejection antigens, Eur. J. Immunol. 32 (2002) 3267–3275.
[33] C. Asseman, et al., An essential role for interleukin 10 in the function of regulatory T cells that inhibit intestinal inflammation, J. Exp. Med. 190 (1999) 995–1004.

[34] C. Burkhart, et al., Peptide-induced T cell regulation of experimental autoimmune encephalomyelitis: a role for IL-10, Int. Immunol. 11 (1999) 1625–1634.

[35] O. Akbari, et al., Antigen-specific regulatory T cells develop via the ICOS-ICOS-ligand pathway and inhibit allergen-induced airway hyperreactivity, Nat. Med. 8 (2002) 1024–1032.

[36] X. Zhang, et al., IL-10 is involved in the suppression of experimental autoimmune encephalomyelitis by CD25(+)CD4(+) regulatory T cells, Int. Immunol. 16 (2004) 249–256.

[37] P.L. Vieira, et.al. IL-10 secreting regulatory T cells do not express Foxp3 but have comparable regulatory function to naturally occuring $CD4^{+}CD25^{+}$ regulatory T cells, J. Immunol. (in press).

[38] J. Buer, et al., Interleukin 10 secretion and impaired effector function of major histocompatibility complex class II-restricted T cells anergized in vivo, J. Exp. Med. 187 (1998) 177–183.

[39] C. Pontoux, A. Banz, M. Papiernik, Natural CD4 CD25(+) regulatory T cells control the burst of superantigen-induced cytokine production: the role of IL-10, Int. Immunol. 14 (2002) 233–239.

[40] C. Miller, J.A. Ragheb, R.H. Schwartz, Anergy and cytokine-mediated suppression as distinct superantigen-induced tolerance mechanisms in vivo, J. Exp. Med. 190 (1999) 53–64.

[41] I. Apostolou, et al., Origin of regulatory T cells with known specificity for antigen, Nat. Immunol. 3 (2002) 756–763.

[42] C. Pasare, R. Medzhitov, Toll pathway-dependent blockade of $CD4^{+}CD25^{+}$ T cell-mediated suppression by dendritic cells, Science 299 (2003) 1033–1036.

[43] K.W. Moore, et al., Interleukin-10 and the interleukin-10 receptor, Annu. Rev. Immunol. 19 (2001) 683–765.

[44] H. Jonuleit, et al., Induction of interleukin 10-producing, nonproliferating CD4(+) T cells with regulatory properties by repetitive stimulation with allogeneic immature human dendritic cells, J. Exp. Med. 192 (2000) 1213–1222.

[45] L.A Schubert, et al., Scurfin (FOXP3) acts as a repressor of transcription and regulates T cell activation, J. Biol. Chem. 276 (2001) 37672–37679.

[46] L.S. Taams, et al., Human anergic/suppressive CD4(+)CD25(+) T cells: a highly differentiated and apoptosis-prone population, Eur. J. Immunol. 31 (2001) 1122–1131.

[47] L.S. Walker, et al., Antigen-dependent proliferation of $CD4^{+}CD25^{+}$ regulatory T cells in vivo, J. Exp. Med. 198 (2003) 249–258.

[48] S. Yamazaki, et al., Direct expansion of functional $CD25^{+}CD4^{+}$ regulatory T cells by antigen-processing dendritic cells, J. Exp. Med. 198 (2003) 235–247.

[49] T. Barthlott, G. Kassiotis, B. Stockinger, T cell regulation as a side effect of homeostasis and competition, J. Exp. Med. 197 (2003) 451–460.

[50] Y. Belkaid, et al., $CD4^{+}$ $CD25^{+}$ regulatory T cells control Leishmania major persistence and immunity, Nature 420 (2002) 502–507.

[51] A. Sher, R.L. Coffman, Regulation of immunity to parasites by T cells and T cell-derived cytokines, Annu. Rev. Immunol. 10 (1992) 385–409.

[52] V.A. Boussiotis, et al., IL-10-producing T cells suppress immune responses in anergic tuberculosis patients, J. Clin. Invest. 105 (2000) 1317–1325.

[53] G. Trinchieri, Regulatory role of T cells producing both interferon gamma and interleukin 10 in persistent infection, J. Exp. Med. 194 (2001) F53–F57.

[54] C. Li, I. Corraliza, J. Langhorne, A defect in interleukin-10 leads to enhanced malarial disease in *Plasmodium chabaudi chabaudi* infection in mice, Infect. Immun. 67 (1999) 4435–4442.

[55] P. McGuirk, C. McCann, K.H. Mills, Pathogen-specific T regulatory 1 cells induced in the respiratory tract by a bacterial molecule that stimulates interleukin 10 production by dendritic cells: a novel strategy for evasion of protective T helper type 1 responses by *Bordetella pertussis*, J. Exp. Med. 195 (2002) 221–231.

[56] S. Sakaguchi, et al., Immunologic self-tolerance maintained by activated T cells expressing IL-2 receptor alpha-chains (CD25). Breakdown of a single mechanism of self-tolerance causes various autoimmune diseases, J. Immunol. 155 (1995) 1151–1164.

ELSEVIER

International Congress Series 1285 (2005) 169–176

www.ics-elsevier.com

The dialogue between natural killer cells and dendritic cells

Magali Terme [a], Cédric Ménard [a], Julien Taieb [a], Christophe Borg [a], Koji Maruyama [a], Hiro Wakasugi [b], Laurence Zitvogel [a,*]

[a] *Department of Clinical Biology, ERM 0208, INSERM, Institut Gustave Roussy, 39, rue Camille Desmoulins, 94805 Villejuif, France*

[b] *Division of Pharmacology, Tokyo Cancer Center, Tokyo, Japan*

Abstract. Natural killer (NK) cells play an important role in the early innate response against cancer and infections whereas dendritic cells (DC) are critical in the initiation of adaptive immune responses through their unique antigen presentation capacities. It was discovered in 1999 by Fernandez et al. that DC and NK cells make functional interactions. In vitro, IL-12/IL-18, IL-15 and IFN-α/β production by activated DC enhance NK cell IFN-γ production, proliferation and cytotoxic potential, respectively. Activated NK cells induce DC maturation either directly or in synergy with suboptimal levels of microbial signals. NK cell-induced DC activation is dependent on both TNF-α/IFN-γ secretion and a cell–cell contact. Finally, immature DC appear susceptible to autologous NK cell-mediated cytolysis while mature DC are protected. Thus, the outcome of NK/DC cross-talk is likely to influence both innate and adaptive immune responses. In vivo, NK/DC interactions occur at least in lymphoid organs and promote Th1 differentiation. Thus, DC and NK cells are equipped with complementary sets of receptors that allow the recognition of various pathogenic agents, rendering the cross-talk between the two partners mandatory.

Keywords: Dendritic cells; Natural killer cells; Tumor immunity

1. Introduction

Natural killer (NK) cells are lymphocytes of the innate immune system that are involved in the early defense against foreign cells, as well as autologous cells undergoing various forms of stress, such as microbial infection or tumor transformation. NK cells are cytotoxic, inducing apoptosis of cells recognized as targets. Upon stimulation, they also

* Corresponding author. Tel.: +33 1 42 11 50 41; fax: +33 1 42 60 94.
E-mail address: zitvogel@igr.fr (L. Zitvogel).

0531-5131/ © 2005 Published by Elsevier B.V.
doi:10.1016/j.ics.2005.07.081

secrete large amounts of cytokines including IFN-γ, TNF-α and GM-CSF, and chemokines such as CCL3 (MIP1-α), CCL4 (MIP1-β) and CCL5 (RANTES). NK cells identify their targets through a set of activating or inhibitory receptors that allow them to recognize pathogen-encoded molecules ("non-self-recognition"), self-proteins whose expression is upregulated in transformed or infected cells ("stress-induced self-recognition"), or self-proteins that are expressed by normal cells but downregulated by infected or transformed cells ("missing self-recognition") [1–3]. NK cell activation is controlled by the dynamic balance between these activating and inhibitory signals.

Dendritic cells (DC) are classically defined as the sentinels of the immune system. At an "immature" stage of development, DC continuously sample the antigenic environment in peripheral tissues and migrate at a slow rate to lymph nodes (LN). Under these steady-state conditions, DC express low levels of MHC and costimulatory molecules and their interaction with naïve T cell thus leads to T cell tolerance [4]. By contrast, encounter with microbial products or tissue damage in the periphery initiates DC maturation and their rapid migration to LN. This activation program is in part due to the engagement of a complex set of innate sensors, such as the toll-like receptors (TLR), which are able to recognize molecules and molecular patterns shared by various classes of microbes. Mature DC then express high levels of MHC and costimulatory molecules which allow them to activate naïve T cells.

DC and NK cells thus share the property to recognize pathogens or pathogenic cells while expressing different sets of receptors, suggesting that activation of both cell types in a given pathological situation will depend on their cross-talk. Indeed, in 1999, it was discovered that NK cell effector functions are stimulated through direct contact with activated DC, which led to the novel concept of dendritic cell-activated killers (DAK) [5]. It was subsequently found that DC/NK interaction was bi-directional and complex, as it could result not only in NK cell activation but also in DC maturation or apoptosis, depending on the activation status of both players.

2. The molecular mechanisms of DC/NK interactions

2.1. DAK activity

Original studies by Fernandez et al. showed that in mice with MHC class I-negative tumors adoptively transferred- or Flt3 ligand-expanded DC promoted NK cell-dependent anti-tumor effects. In vitro studies demonstrated a cell-to-cell contact between DC and resting NK cells that results in a substantial increase in both NK cell cytolytic activity and IFN-γ production [5]. Subsequent studies have focused on dissecting the signals involved in DAK activity. Both cytokines and cell–cell contacts are involved.

2.1.1. Role of cytokines

Under conditions of stimulation by various pathogens or by TLR ligands, DC constitute a source of all the cytokines known to trigger NK cell functions such as IL-15, type I interferons, IL-12 and IL-18 (reviewed in [6,7]).

IL-12 production leads to IFN-γ production by NK cells. This has been demonstrated for LPS-stimulated $CD34^+$ derived-DC [8,9], actinobacillus-stimulated monocyte-derived DC [10] or poly(I:C)-stimulated human myeloid DC [11] in humans, or virus-activated plasmacytoid DC (pDC) in mice [12].

IL-18 is known to synergize with IL-12 to induce IFN-γ secretion by various cell types including NK cells. In the case of the NK/DC crosstalk, IL-12/IL-18 secretion by $CD34^+$-derived DC has been shown to enhance NK cell cytotoxicity [13]. Moreover, Andrews et al. found that both IL-18 and $CD8\alpha^+$ DC were essential for NK cell expansion in vivo during MCMV infection [14].

IL-2 is also produced by some mouse DC subsets in vitro and may account for the induction of IFN-γ production by NK cells. This is the case for mouse bone marrow-derived DC (BMDC) cultured with GM-CSF and stimulated with TLR4 ligands such as LPS or *Escherichia coli* bacteria [14]. The role of IL-2 production by mouse DC in DAK activity has been confirmed in vivo in the context of a response to *E. coli* injection [15].

IL-15 is secreted by mouse GM-CSF+IL-4-derived BMDC and promotes in vitro NK cell cytotoxicity and IFN-γ secretion. This effect requires the expression of the IL-15Rα on DC [16], suggesting that murine DC require IL-15Rα to present IL-15 in trans to NK cells during NK cell priming. Ferlazzo et al. recently found that in humans, IL-15 production by monocyte-derived DC or spleen DC induces NK cells to proliferate [17].

IFN-α/β may be produced by distinct DC subsets, although pDC appear specialized in high level secretion of these cytokines in response to viral particles, viral ssRNA, or viral and bacterial unmethylated CpG sequences (reviewed in [17]). Type I interferons are essential for in vitro induction of NK cell cytotoxicity by various DC types in response to different stimuli, such as mouse GM-CSF-derived BMDC stimulated with TLR4 ligands [15], and mouse [12] or human [11] pDC activated by viruses or by TLR7/8/9 ligands.

2.1.2. Role of cell/cell contacts

Optimal NK cell activation by DC also requires direct cell-to-cell contacts, as established in the first study on the NK/DC cross-talk [5]. In another system, MHC class I-related (MIC) A and B expression by IFN-α-stimulated DC were found to be critical for DAK activity [18]. Recently, Borg et al. found that NK and DC form stimulatory synapses involving cytoskeleton rearrangement and lipid raft mobilization in DC [9]. Synapse formation allows the polarized secretion of preassembled stores of IL-12 by DC towards the NK cell, leading to IFN-γ secretion.

2.2. DC maturation induced by NK cells

Piccioli et al. originally found that culture of activated human NK cells with immature monocyte-derived DC, at low NK/DC ratios (1:5), led to an increase in DC cytokine production [19]. Soluble factors such as TNF-α and IFN-γ, as well as cell-to-cell contacts, are required for NK cell-mediated DC activation. IL-2-activated NK cells can also induce maturation of blood pDC and myeloid DC, and synergise with suboptimal concentrations of CpG oligonucleotides to promote strong IFN-α and TNF production by blood pDC. Both effects are dependent on cell-cell contacts, although the receptors/ligands involved have not been identified yet [11]. In the mouse, activated NK cells can trigger TREM2/KARAP (DAP12) signaling in GM-CSF/IL-4-derived BMDC, thereby promoting upregulation of CD86 molecules [20].

Thus, activated NK cells can induce DC maturation either directly or in synergy with suboptimal levels of microbial signals. NK cell-induced DC activation is dependent on both TNF-α/IFN-γ secretion and a cell–cell contact. As shown by Vitale et al. in a human setting [21], the NK cell-mediated DC maturation involving the release of TNF-α by NK cells depends on the triggering of NKp30 and is counter-regulated by KIR and NKG2A inhibitory receptors. In a mouse tumor model, the group of Mocikat has been able to show a critical role for IL-12 produced by endogenous DC following IFNγ secretion by activated NK cells, underscoring a link between innate immunity and cross-priming of CTL [22]. Therefore, NK help might be critical for optimal DC activation and subsequent induction of T cell responses in conditions where inflammation is poor but where NK cell activation could occur through direct recognition of target cells. In particular, this may be relevant to defense against cancer, as discussed below.

2.3. DC killing by NK cells

Whereas low NK/immature DC ratios (1:5) lead to DC maturation, higher NK/immature DC ratios (5:1), result in the killing of immature DC by the autologous NK cells [19,23]. Importantly, immature DC are susceptible to autologous NK cell-mediated cytolysis while mature DC are protected. In vitro, signals delivered by NKp30 are critical for lysis of immature DC [23] while resistance to NK lysis is mediated by upregulation of MHC class I molecules during DC maturation, in particular HLA-E [24]. In vivo, NK-mediated DC elimination has also been observed in different mouse models. Hayakawa et al. reported that immature DC are rapidly eliminated by NK cells via a pathway dependent on the TNF-related apoptosis-inducing ligand (TRAIL) [25]. Similarly, transplantation of alloreactive NK cells has been shown to suppress T cell-mediated graft versus host disease by eliminating host DC [26]. By killing immature DC, NK cells might thus regulate DC homeostasis and thereby the balance between tolerance and immunity. However, it remains to be determined whether DC killing by NK cells might happen in vivo in the absence of DC or NK transfer.

3. Location of the DC/NK cell cross-talk

DC are distributed across all non-lymphoid tissues and include Langerhans cells, interstitial DC (IDC) and monocyte-derived DC. Several DC subsets are also found in secondary lymphoid organs and have been well-defined in the mouse [30]. The CD8α^-DC subset resides in splenic marginal zones [27]. Mature NK cells are found in the circulation and in several tissues. CD56^{dim} and CD56^{bright} have different tissue distributions. CD56^{bright} NK cells express L-selectin and CCR7 and are preferentially localized in LN. By contrast, CD56^{dim} NK cells are poorly represented in LN but comprise 95% of blood NK cells and 85% of spleen NK cells. CD56^{dim} NK cells also express receptors for inflammatory chemokines. They might represent a reservoir of “immature” NK cells that will be activated in case of inflammation [28].

3.1. In secondary lymphoid organs

In the mouse, few NK cells are found in LN but they can be recruited in response to inflammation induced by adjuvant [29], DC injection [20,29] (Terme et al., submitted) or

Leishmania major inoculation [30]. At steady state, NK cells have been reported to reside in the LN outer paracortex in close vicinity to DC near HEV. In contrast to T cells which move rapidly, it has been reported that the majority of NK cells are slow motile cells [30].

In humans, NK cells and DC colocalize in T cell areas of LN, where they might thus interact [16]. Two studies have compared $CD56^{bright}$ with $CD56^{dim}$ NK cells ability to interact with DC. Vitale et al. found that both NK subsets (purified from the blood) upregulate CD69 expression when cultured with mature DC [31]. However, only $CD56^{bright}$ NK cells secrete IFN-γ and proliferate in these cocultures. Ferlazzo et al. reported a similar phenomenon using lymph node or splenic human NK cells [16].

3.2. In non-lymphoid peripheral tissues

Immature DC and NK cells express receptors for inflammatory chemokines. In vitro, both subsets strongly migrate in response to CXCR3, CXCR4 and CCR5 ligands [32]. Hepatic production of CCL3 (MIP1-α, CCR5 ligand) is required for mouse NK cells homing to the liver and effective control of MCMV infection. NK cells may also migrate to inflamed LN and lung in a CXCR3 dependent fashion [29]. DC have been shown to dramatically accumulate in inflamed tissues as well [32]. Thus, DC and NK cells might colocalize in inflamed tissues. Moreover, NK cell secretion of CCL3, CCL4 and CCL5 upon stimulation might favor NK/DC encounter within inflamed tissues. The reverse is likely to be true as DC can secrete pro-inflammatory chemokines as well. Direct contacts between DC and NK cells in vivo have been observed in different systems. $DC\text{-}SIGN^{+}$ decidual APCs were observed in situ to have intimate contact with $CD56^{+}/CD16^{-}/ICAM\text{-}3^{+}$ decidual natural killer cells during human pregnancy [33]. NK/DC interactions were also found in Malassezia-induced atopic skin lesions, and in imatinib mesylate induced-lichenoid dermatitis [34]. $PEN5^{+}$ NK cells can also be found in tissues infiltrated with malignant langherans histiocytosis (LZ et al., unpublished data), suggesting that a dysregulation of the LC/NK cell cross-talk could participate in this chronic inflammation. Both NK cells and DC have been shown to infiltrate tumors but only little evidence of their interaction within the tumors has been described [34].

4. NK-DC interactions in tumors

LN NK cells may have an important role in the initiation of T cell responses by contributing to DC maturation. Indeed, under in vitro conditions where DC are suboptimally activated with type I IFN, NK cells license DC to prime T cell responses [35]. LN NK cells also contribute to skew T cell responses. Indeed, $CD56^{bright}$ NK cells secrete high levels of IFN-γ, TNF-β, IL-10, IL-13 and GM-CSF in response to IL-15/IL-18, IL12/IL-15 or IL-12/IL-18 stimulation which gives them the potential to modulate the type of T cell responses initiated in the LN. This point has been demonstrated by Martin-Fontecha et al. who reported that NK cell recruitment in mouse LN provides early IFN-γ production necessary for Th1 polarization in a model of $CD4^{+}$ T cell response to ovalbumin (OVA). NK cell recruitment into the LN may be induced by footpad injection of LPS activated DC or adjuvants such as R848 or Ribi [29]. NK cell depletion leads to defective Th1 polarization of $CD4^{+}$ T cells activated by LPS-matured OVA-pulsed DC. However, it is not clear whether IFN-γ produced by NK cells is necessary at the level of naïve T cells or at the level of DC presenting the MHC class II/OVA complexes [29]. A recent report assigns a new role for the DC/NK cell cross-talk in immune responses. The authors demonstrate efficient CTL priming and long-term CD8+ T cell memory against A20 tumor antigens in the absence of CD4+ T cell help using CD40−/− mature DC, unpulsed with tumor antigens but capable of NK cell triggering. Their data clearly show that IFNγ was necessary for NK cell activation, activation of endogenous DC and IL-12 production leading to CTL induction (22).

It is assumed that tumor cells are poorly immunogenic and not recognized by the immune system because "danger signals' are missing in vivo. NK cell activation by tumor cells (MHC class I low, TAP deficient or overexpressing NKG2D ligands, CD27 or gp96) has been shown to promote the elicitation of cognate and protective T cell responses against the tumor. In these examples, tumor recognition by NK cells involves receptors that allow them to detect "missing self" and/or "induced-self". In some cases, T-cell mediated tumor rejection was shown to be dependent on DC activation by NK cells [36]. IFN-γ secreted during NK cell-mediated tumor rejection is critical for cytotoxic T lymphocytes (CTL) generation particularly when tumors express CD70 or CD80 and CD86 [37]. However, tumor rejection by CTL following recognition of NKG2D ligands by NK cells does not depend on IFN-γ but requires $CD4^+$ T cell help [38].

Anti-CD40 therapy has been shown to induce substantial NK-mediated anti-tumor and anti-metastatic effects [39]. As CD40 is expressed neither on NK cells nor on the tumor cells used, it was suggested that NK cell activation is mediated by increased cytokine production upon CD40 ligation on DC. Similarly, modulation of the c-kit signaling pathway in DC leads to marked NK cell activation in various strains of mice [34]. Indeed, a 10- to 21-day oral therapy with the c-kit inhibitor imatinib mesylate promotes the selective expansion of $CD69^+$ NK cells and NK-cell-dependent antitumor effects in tumor models resistant to imatinib mesylate in vitro. Nanomolar concentrations of imatinib mesylate are sufficient to endow DC with NK cell stimulatory capacities in vitro without promoting DC maturation. The effect of imatinib mesylate does not depend on IL-12 secretion by DC but requires NK-DC contacts. The capacity of imatinib mesylate to endow DC with NK cell stimulatory capacities has also been shown in patients with gastrointestinal sarcoma (GIST). GIST are tumors displaying the typical features of NK cell sensitivity (TAP1 deficiency, overexpression of MIC and ULBP at mRNA and protein levels) and are lysed as efficiently as K562 cells by NK cells [34]. Up to 50% of patients bearing a GIST and treated with imatinib mesylate acquire enhanced NK cell effector functions. The relevance of NK cell activation for the clinical outcome was suggested by a correlation between the objective responses at 1 year and early NK cell triggering (at 2 months) on a cohort of 42 patients. Importantly, the time to progression was significantly longer in patients exhibiting NK cell activation the first 2 months of therapy [34].

Acknowledgements

L.Z. was supported in part by specific grants from European Union ("ALLOSTEM"), Ligue Nationale contre le Cancer ('Equipes labellisées La Ligue') and institutional grants from INSERM, CNRS and Ministère de l'Enseignement Supérieur et de la Recherche.

References

[1] L. Moretta, A. Moretta, Unravelling natural killer cell function: triggering and inhibitory human NK receptors, EMBO J. 23 (2004) 255–259.

[2] D.H. Raulet, Interplay of natural killer cells and their receptors with the adaptive immune response, Nat. Immunol. 5 (2004) 996–1002.

[3] E. Vivier, C.A. Biron, A pathogen receptor on natural killer cells, Science 296 (2002) 1248–1249.

[4] R.M. Steinman, M.C. Nussenzweig, Inaugural article: avoiding horror autotoxicus: the importance of dendritic cells in peripheral T cell tolerance, Proc. Natl. Acad. Sci. U. S. A. 99 (2002) 351–358.

[5] N.C. Fernandez, et al., Dendritic cells directly trigger NK cell functions: cross-talk relevant in innate anti-tumor immune responses in vivo, Nat. Med. 5 (1999) 405–411.

[6] A. Iwasaki, R. Medzhitov, Toll-like receptor control of the adaptive immune responses, Nat. Immunol. 5 (2004) 987–995.

[7] K.B. Nguyen, et al., Coordinated and distinct roles for IFN-alphabeta, IL-12, and IL-15 regulation of NK cell responses to viral infection, J. Immunol. 169 (2002) 4279–4287.

[8] F. Gerosa, et al., Reciprocal activating interaction between natural killer cells and dendritic cells, J. Exp. Med. 195 (2002) 327–333.

[9] C. Borg, et al., NK cell activation by Dendritic Cells (DC) require the formation of a synapse leading to IL-12 polarization in DC, Blood 104 (2004) 3267–3275.

[10] T. Kikuchi, et al., Dendritic cells stimulated with Actinobacillus actinomycetemcomitans elicit rapid gamma interferon responses by natural killer cells, Infect. Immun. 72 (2004) 5089–5096.

[11] F. Gerosa, et al., The reciprocal interaction of NK cells with plasmacytoid or myeloid dendritic cells profoundly affects innate resistance functions, J. Immunol. (2005) 174.

[12] M. Dalod, et al., Dendritic cell responses to early murine cytomegalovirus infection: subset functional specialization and differential regulation by interferon alpha/beta, J. Exp. Med. 197 (2003) 885–898.

[13] Y. Yu, et al., Enhancement of human cord blood CD34+Cell-Derived NK cell cytotoxicity by dendritic cells, J. Immunol. 166 (2001) 1590–1600.

[14] D.M. Andrews, et al., Functional interactions between dendritic cells and NK cells during viral infection, Nat. Immunol. 4 (2003) 175–181.

[15] F. Granucci, et al., A contribution of mouse dendritic cell-derived IL-2 for NK cell activation, J. Exp. Med. 200 (2004) 287–295.

[16] R. Koka, et al., Cutting edge: murine dendritic cells require IL-15R{alpha} to prime NK cells, J. Immunol. 173 (2004) 3594–3598.

[17] G. Ferlazzo, et al., Distinct roles of IL-12 and IL-15 in human natural killer cell activation by dendritic cells from secondary lymphoid organs, Proc. Natl. Acad. Sci. U. S. A. 101 (2004) 16606–16611.

[18] M. Jinushi, et al., Critical role of MHC class I-related chain A and B expression on IFN-alpha-stimulated dendritic cells in NK cell activation: impairment in chronic hepatitis C virus infection, J. Immunol. 170 (2003) 1249–1256.

[19] D. Piccioli, et al., Contact-dependent stimulation and inhibition of dendritic cells by natural killer cells, J. Exp. Med. 195 (2002) 335–341.

[20] M. Terme, et al., IL-4 confers NK stimulatory capacity to murine dendritic cells: a signaling pathway involving KARAP/DAP12-triggering receptor expressed on myeloid cell 2 molecules, J. Immunol. 172 (2004) 5957–5966.

[21] M. Vitale, et al., NK-dependent DC maturation is mediated by TNFa and IFNg released upon engagement of the NKp30 triggering receptor, Blood 106 (2) (2005) 566–571 (Jul 15).

[22] C. Adam, et al., DC-NK cell cross talk as a novel CD4+ T-cell-independent pathway for antitumor CTL induction, Blood 106 (1) (2005) 338–344 (Jul 1. Electronic publication 2005 Mar 15).

[23] G. Ferlazzo, et al., Human dendritic cells activate resting natural killer (NK) cells and are recognized via the NKp30 receptor by activated NK cells, J. Exp. Med. 195 (2002) 343–351.

[24] M. Della Chiesa, et al., The natural killer cell mediated killing of autologous dendritic cells is confined to a cell subset expressing CD94/NKG2A, but lacking inhibitory killer Ig-like receptors, Eur. J. Immunol. 33 (2003) 1657–1666.

[25] Y. Hayakawa, et al., NK cell TRAIL eliminates immature dendritic cells in vivo and limits dendritic cell vaccination efficacy, J. Immunol. 172 (2004) 123–129.

[26] L. Ruggeri, et al., Effectiveness of donor natural killer cell alloreactivity in mismatched hematopoietic transplants, Science 295 (2002) 2097–2100.
[27] K. Shortman, Y.J. Liu, Mouse and human dendritic cell subtypes, Nat. Rev. Immunol. 2 (2002) 151–161.
[28] G. Ferlazzo, et al., The abundant NK cells in human secondary lymphoid tissues require activation to express killer cell Ig-like receptors and become cytolytic, J. Immunol. 172 (2004) 1455–1462.
[29] A. Martin-Fontecha, et al., Induced recruitment of NK cells to lymph nodes provides IFN-gamma for T(H)1 priming, Nat. Immunol. 5 (2004) 1260–1265.
[30] M. Bajenoff, et al., NK cells are slow motile cells localized in the lymph node outerparacortex where they make contacts with dendritic cells, Pasteur I ed. Paris, 2004, .
[31] M. Vitale, et al., The small subset of CD56brightCD16-natural killer cells is selectively responsible for both cell proliferation and interferon-gamma production upon interaction with dendritic cells, Eur. J. Immunol. 34 (2004) 1715–1722.
[32] S. Sozzani, et al., Chemokines and dendritic cell traffic, J. Clin. Immunol. 20 (2000) 151–160.
[33] U. Kammerer, et al., Unique appearance of proliferating antigen-presenting cells expressing DC-SIGN (CD209) in the decidua of early human pregnancy, Am. J. Pathol. 162 (2003) 887–896.
[34] C. Borg, et al., Novel mode of action of c-kit tyrosine kinase inhibitors leading to NK cell-dependent antitumor effects, J. Clin. Invest. 114 (2004) 379–388.
[35] D. Tosi, et al., Role of cross-talk between IFN-alpha-induced monocyte-derived dendritic cells and NK cells in priming CD8(+) T cell responses against human tumor antigens, J. Immunol. 172 (2004) 5363–5370.
[36] R. Mocikat, et al., Natural killer cells activated by MHC class I(low) targets prime dendritic cells to induce protective CD8 T cell responses, Immunity 19 (2003) 561–569.
[37] J.M. Kelly, et al., Induction of tumor-specific T cell memory by NK cell-mediated tumor rejection, Nat. Immunol. 3 (2002) 83–90 (Electronic publication 2001 Dec 2017).
[38] Y. Hayakawa, et al., Cutting edge: tumor rejection mediated by NKG2D receptor-ligand interaction is dependent upon perforin, J. Immunol. 169 (2002) 5377–5381.
[39] J.G. Turner, et al., Anti-CD40 antibody induces antitumor and antimetastatic effects: the role of NK cells, J. Immunol. 166 (2001) 89–94.

Manipulation of the innate immune system and new strategies for disease control

International Congress Series 1285 (2005) 179–183

www.ics-elsevier.com

Suppression of IgE antibody responses by NKT cells—mechanisms of NKT cell-mediated regulatory function

Satoshi Kojo, Michishige Harada, Ken-ichiro Seino, Masaru Taniguchi *

Laboratory for Immune Regulation, RIKEN Research Center for Allergy and Immunology, Suehiro-cho 1-7-22, Tsurumi, Yokohama, Kanagawa 230-0045, Japan

Abstract. Vα14 natural killer T (NKT) cells exhibit various immune-regulatory properties in vivo. A repeated injection of α-galactosylceramide (α-GalCer) into mice induced suppression of antigen-specific IgE, IgG1 and IgG2a production in vivo. The suppression of antigen specific Ig responses seems to be due to the generation of regulatory DCs producing high IL-10 and low IL-12 by IL-10 derived from Vα14 NKT cells, because repeated α-GalCer stimulation changed cytokine profiles, such as high IL-10 and low IFN-γ production in Vα14 NKT cells. The unique cytokine profile (high IL-10 and low IL-12) in the regulatory DCs appeared to be regulated by upregulation of phosphorylation of extracellular signal-regulated kinase-1/2 and augmented production of $I\kappa B_{NS}$. The regulatory DCs thus induced in turn generated antigen specific Tr1 type regulatory T cells producing IL-10 suppressing Ig responses in an antigen specific fashion. © 2005 Elsevier B.V. All rights reserved.

Keywords: NKT cells; α-Galactosylceramide; IgE; Allergy; Tolerance

1. Introduction

Vα14 natural killer T cells (Vα14 NKT cells) represent a distinct lymphocyte subpopulation characterized by the expression of an invariant antigen receptor α-chain encoded by the Vα14-Jα281 gene segments in mice. The invariant antigen receptors

Abbreviations: α-GalCer, α-galactosylceramide; NKT cell, natural killer T cell; TLR, toll-like receptor; EAE, experimental allergic encephalomyelitis; ACAID; anterior chamber associated immune deviation.

* Corresponding author. Tel.: +81 45 503 7001; fax: +81 45 503 7003.
E-mail address: taniguti@rcai.riken.jp (M. Taniguchi).

0531-5131/
doi:10.1016/j.ics.2005.08.002

recognize glycolipid antigens, including α-galactosylceramide (α-GalCer), presented by CD1d [1,2]. It has been reported that Vα14 NKT cells play a pivotal role in influencing a very diverse group of immune responses [1,2]. Vα14 NKT cells are involved in immune-regulatory responses, such as the maintenance of transplantation tolerance, anterior chamber associated immune deviation (ACAID), and prevention of some autoimmune diseases, i.e., experimental allergic encephalomyelitis (EAE) and type 1 diabetes in NOD mice. However, the mechanisms by which Vα14 NKT cells exert the immune-regulatory functions are poorly understood. A contribution of DCs in the Vα14 NKT cell-mediated regulatory immune responses has been suggested. In fact, treatment of NOD mice with α-GalCer led to increase in the number of CD8α$^-$ DCs in the pancreatic lymph nodes, and adoptive transfer of such DCs could prevent the development of diabetes [3,4]. These data strongly implicate a role of regulatory DCs acting downstream of Vα14 NKT cell activation.

Here, we show that repeated activation of Vα14 NKT cells with α-GalCer significantly suppresses IgE production in vivo, which is mediated by the generation of regulatory DCs producing IL-10 and antigen specific CD4 regulatory T cells (Tr1) producing IL-10.

2. Materials and methods

The materials and methods used in this study are shown in Ref. [5].

3. Results

3.1. Suppression of antibody responses by repeated α-GalCer treatment

Using an IgE model, we first assessed the effect of repeated α-GalCer treatments in antibody production in vivo. Repeated injection of α-GalCer significantly reduced OVA/Alum-induced IgE levels in NKT cell-dependent manner (Fig. 1). This treatment also reduced antigen-specific IgG1 and IgG2a levels (Fig. 1).

3.2. Induction of IL-10 producing DCs by NKT cell activation

To examine whether NKT cell activation rendered DCs to be immune-regulatory, we assessed the alteration of surface phenotypes of splenic DCs after repeated α-GalCer treatment and found that the maturation of DCs was not observed when α-GalCer was repeatedly injected [5]. Rather, expression levels of surface costimulatory molecules in these DCs were significantly lower and almost similar to those of unstimulated DCs [5]. DCs isolated from mice with repeated α-GalCer injection showed enhanced IL-10 production but dramatically reduced levels of IL-12 and also possessed inhibitory activity on various immune responses, such as suppression of EAE, and type I diabetes development and maintenance of transplantation tolerance [5]. Therefore, the DCs generated after repeated α-GalCer stimulation are regulatory ones.

In order to understand the mechanism of the characteristic cytokine production in the regulatory DCs, we first assessed alteration of cytokine productions of Vα14 NKT cells after in vivo α-GalCer treatment. We isolated Vα14 NKT cells from naïve or in vivo α-GalCer treated (3 times) mice and re-stimulated them in vitro with α-GalCer-pulsed fresh DCs. Interestingly, freshly isolated Vα14 NKT cells already possessed large amounts of cytokine mRNAs (i.e., IFN-γ and IL4/IL-10), but did not produce any cytokines without stimulation. However, the α-GalCer treatment of naïve Vα14 NKT cells immediately produced both Th1 and Th2 cytokines, whereas repeated stimulation of α-GalCer reduced the ability of Vα14 NKT cells to produce IFN-γ but

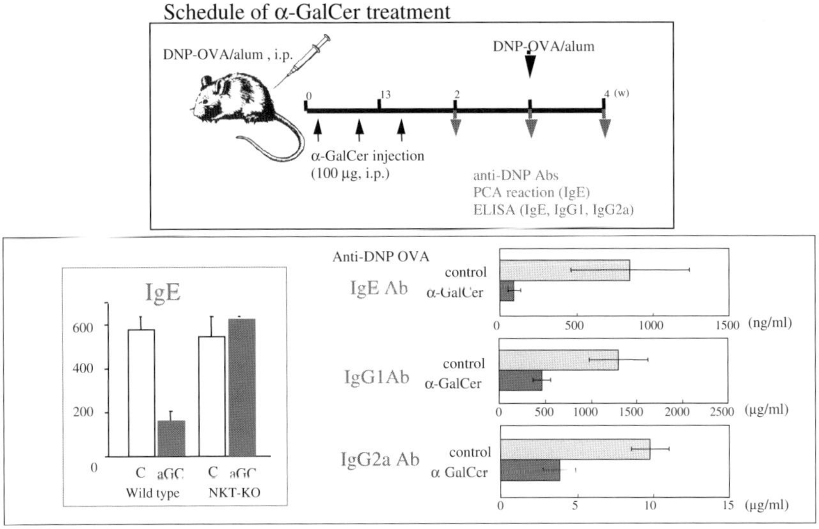

Fig. 1. Suppression of antibody responses by repeated α-GalCer treatment.

not IL-10 (regulatory Vα14 NKT cells) (Fig. 2). In other words, activated, but not naïve, Vα14 NKT cells stop producing IFN-γ but still keep producing IL-10.

The cytokine changes from naïve to activated Vα14 NKT cells are important for initiating the regulatory cascade, because IL-10 from Vα14 NKT cells in the absence of IFN-γ induced regulatory function in naive DCs. In fact, when we co-cultured freshly isolated DCs with regulatory Vα14 NKT cells, IL-10 production by the DCs was augmented upon LPS stimulation, indicating that regulatory Vα14 NKT cells induced the regulatory DCs (Fig. 2). This upregulation of IL-10 production by DCs was completely inhibited by addition of mAb to IL-10 receptor (Fig. 2). We further confirmed by the results that co-culture of naïve DCs with recombinant IL-10 generated the regulatory DCs. These results indicate that the regulatory Vα14 NKT cells generate regulatory DCs in an IL-10 dependent manner.

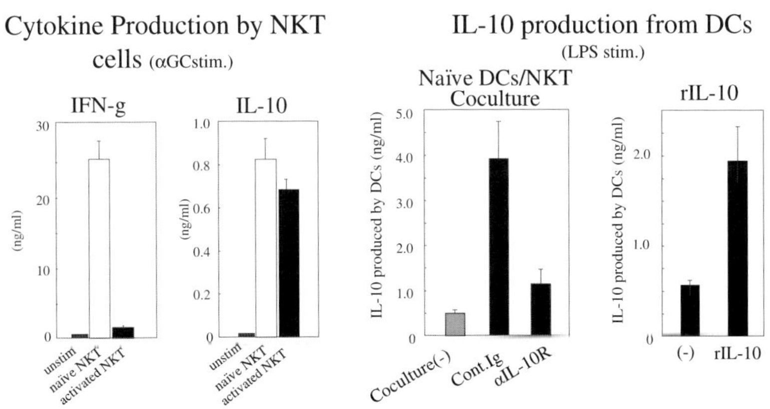

Fig. 2. Changes of cytokine profile in NKT cells and DCs.

3.3. DC subpopulations after in vivo α-GalCer treatment

To investigate the change of DC subpopulations after in vivo α-GalCer treatment, we examined the expression levels of CD8α/CD11b, B220/CD11c, and CD45RB/CD11c on DCs. However, no significant difference was detected among DC subpopulations [5]. We further examined the cytokine profiles in $CD8\alpha^{+}$ and $CD8\alpha^{-}$ DC subpopulations. In DCs from mice with repeated α-GalCer stimulation, IL-10 production of $CD8\alpha^{-}$ DC was upregulated, but IL-12 production of $CD8\alpha^{+}$ DC was downregulated [5].

3.4. Signal molecules responsible for changes in cytokine profiles in the regulatory DCs

In order to understand the molecular events in the regulatory DCs, we examined the molecular changes in the intracellular signaling pathway. By Western blotting analysis, we found that phosphorylation of extracellular signal-regulated kinase (ERK)-1/2, which is known to be important for IL-10 production, but not p38 was more rapidly and strongly induced in the regulatory DCs (Fig. 3). Consistent with the enhanced phosphorylation of ERK-1/2 in the regulatory DCs, IL-10 production from the regulatory DCs was significantly suppressed by a specific inhibitor of ERK-1/2 in a dose-dependent fashion (Fig. 3). This indicates that a signal pathway through ERK-1/2 is responsible for the elevated level of IL-10 production in the regulatory DC.

Then, we analyzed the NF-κB signaling pathway which is known to be important for IL-12 production. The mobility shift assay demonstrated that the nuclear DNA binding of NF-κB after TLR stimulation was significantly inhibited in the regulatory DCs (Fig. 3). However, as shown in Fig. 3, the expression of $I\kappa B_{NS}$, which directly binds NF-κB and inhibits its activity, was dramatically augmented in the regulatory DCs, indicating that induction of $I\kappa B_{NS}$ down-modulates IL-12 production in the regulatory DCs.

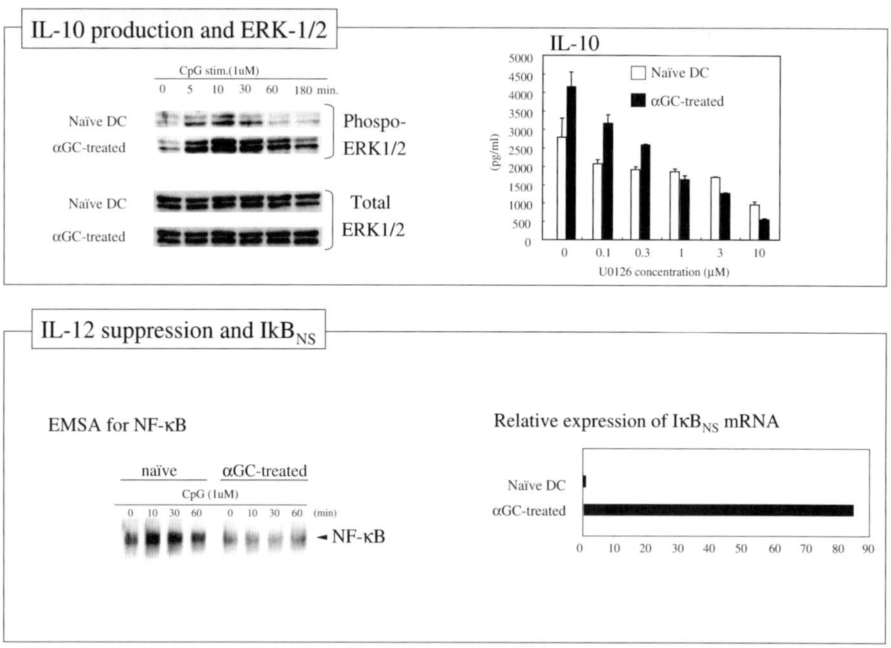

Fig. 3. Signal molecules responsible for changes in cytokine profiles in the regulatory DCs.

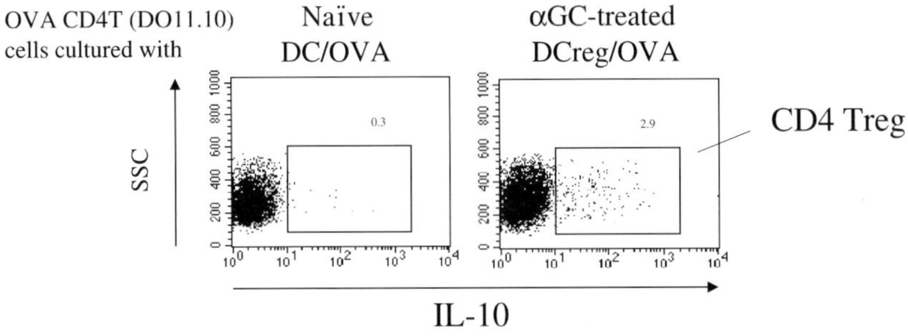

Fig. 4. Induction of IL-10 producing regulatory CD4 T cells by IL-10 producing regulatory DCs.

3.5. Induction of IL-10 producing regulatory CD4 T cells by IL-10 producing regulatory DCs

In order to investigate the final effector mechanisms of Vα14 NKT cell-mediated regulatory cascade, the regulatory DCs were pulsed with OVA and co-cultured with naïve CD4T cells from OVA transgenic mice. Significant numbers of IL-10 producing CD4T cells were generated by the culture. Moreover, the transfer of antigen-pulsed regulatory DCs induced suppression of immune responses in the WT mice, while no suppression was obtained in IL-10-KO recipients, indicating that IL-10 from Treg cells is an effector molecule (Fig. 4).

4. Discussion

In the present study, we demonstrated the cellular and molecular mechanisms of the induction of regulatory DCs by Vα14 NKT cell activation in vivo. Repeated stimulation of Vα14 NKT cells with α-GalCer led to changes in their cytokine profile, producing IL-10 but no IFN-γ despite of their potential ability to produce large amounts of both IL-10 and IFN-γ under naïve physiological conditions. Interestingly, these Vα14 NKT cells induced regulatory DCs characterized by immature phenotypes of cell surface molecules, high IL-10 and low IL-12 production, survived and maintained for a long time, more than 30 days. Therefore, Vα14 NKT cell mediated regulatory mechanisms is useful for further application for treatment of autoimmune diseases or allergic disorders. Further discussions are demonstrated in Ref. [5].

References

[1] M. Kronenberg, L. Gapin, The unconventional lifestyle of NKT cells, Nat. Rev., Immunol. 2 (2002) 557.

[2] M. Taniguchi, et al., The regulatory role of Vα14 NKT cells in innate and acquired immune response, Annu. Rev. Immunol. 21 (2003) 483.

[3] Y.N. Naumov, et al., Activation of CD1d-restricted T cells protects NOD mice from developing diabetes by regulating dendritic cell subsets, Proc. Natl. Acad. Sci. U. S. A. 98 (2001) 13838.

[4] Y.G. Chen, et al., Activated NKT cells inhibit autoimmune diabetes through tolerogenic recruitment of dendritic cells to pancreatic lymph nodes. J. Immunol. 174 (2005) 1196.

[5] S. Kojo, et al., Induction of regulatory properties in dendritic cells by Vα14 NKT cells. J. Immunol. (in press).

International Congress Series 1285 (2005) 184–188

www.ics-elsevier.com

NKT cells regulate the development of asthma

Dale T. Umetsu *, Toshinori Nakayama, Masaru Taniguchi, Mitchell Kronenberg, Rosemarie H. DeKruyff, Omid Akbari

Division of Immunology, Children's Hospital Boston, Harvard Medical School, Boston, MA, United States

Abstract. Using NKT cell-deficient CD1d knockout and Jα281 knockout mice, we demonstrated that allergen-induced airway hyperreactivity (AHR), a cardinal feature of asthma, failed to develop in the absence of NKT cells. The failure of NKT cell-deficient mice to develop AHR was not due to an inability of these mice to develop Th2 responses and was reversed by adoptive transfer of tetramer purified NKT cells. These studies are the first to show that pulmonary NKT cells critically regulate the development of asthma and Th2-biased respiratory immunity against nominal exogenous antigens. In addition, our studies suggest that therapies that target NKT cells may be clinically effective in limiting the development of AHR and asthma.

Keywords: NKT cells; Asthma; Allergy; Airway hyperreactivity

Asthma is a major public health problem that has increased dramatically in prevalence over the past two decades [1]. Asthma is an immunological disease that is caused by Th2-driven inflammation, and is characterized by increased mucus production in the bronchioles, and by an inflammatory process in the peribronchial space that consists of eosinophils, basophils, mast cells and Th2 lymphocytes [2]. Although activation of mast cells can precipitate acute asthma, most people believe that $CD4^+$ Th2 cells secreting IL-4, IL-5 and IL-13 play the major role in orchestrating the inflammation in asthma. Th2 cells cause asthma, because IL-4 enhances isotype switch to IgE, because IL-5 enhances the growth and differentiation of eosinophils, and because IL-13 directly enhances airway hyperreactivity (AHR), a cardinal feature of asthma, and increases mucus production in the airways.

* Corresponding author.
E-mail address: dale.umetsu@childrens.harvard.edu (D.T. Umetsu).

0531-5131/ © 2005 Published by Elsevier B.V.
doi:10.1016/j.ics.2005.07.093

However, although Th2-driven immune responses are critically important in the development of asthma [3,4], a Th2 response in and of itself is not sufficient for the induction of asthma. Th2-biased allergen sensitization can occur independently of asthma, explaining why only about one third of individuals with allergic rhinitis (caused by Th2 responses in the upper respiratory tract) develop asthma (caused by Th2 responses in the lower airways) [5]. Therefore, additional elements intrinsic to the lower respiratory track may be required for localizing the Th2 response in the lungs, distinct from allergen sensitization per se, and for the full development of asthma to occur. These specific local elements within the respiratory tract have not been identified but may involve structural responses of the lower respiratory tract to repeated injury (e.g., airway remodeling) [6,7], or may involve immune system components localized to the lower respiratory tract.

NKT cells constitute a lymphocyte subpopulation that are abundant in the thymus, spleen, liver and bone marrow, and are also present in the airways. NKT cells have been discussed extensively at this meeting, and therefore, only a limited background will be provided here. Most NKT cells express an invariant TCR, called Vα14 in mice and Vα24 in humans. The invariant TCR of NKT cells recognizes glycolipid antigens presented in the context of nonpolymorphic, MHC class I-like molecules called CD1d on APCs. Because NKT cells produce large amounts of IL-4, we asked what role NKT cells play in the development of asthma.

1. AHR fails to develop in CD1d KO mice

To determine if NKT cells regulate asthma, we examined CD1d knockout mice, which lack the restriction element of NKT cells and, therefore, lack NKT cells. We compared the development of allergen-induced AHR in CD1d knockout mice with that in wild-type BALB/c mice, by sensitizing and challenging these mice with ovalbumin (OVA) to induce AHR. Wild-type BALB/c mice, when sensitized and challenged with OVA, as expected, developed severe AHR, as demonstrated by challenge of the mice with increasing concentrations of methacholine, which increases airway resistance. To our surprise, the CD1d knockout mice failed to develop AHR when sensitized and challenged in the same way. These findings were really quite striking, and therefore, we tried several different methods for inducing AHR, and several different antigens, including bovine serum albumin and *Aspergillus* antigen. In all cases, while the wild-type BALB/c mice developed severe AHR, the CD1d knockout mice had normal airway reactivity [8]. These findings have been confirmed by other laboratories [9].

2. Do CD1d KO mice have functioning airways?

The failure of the CD1d knockout mice to develop AHR could have been due to a number of possibilities, for example, an intrinsic inability of these mice to develop AHR. To rule this out, we administered rIL13, which directly affects bronchial smooth muscle and airway epithelial cells to the CD1d knockout mice [10]. We found that administration of recombinant IL-13 to the CD1d knockout mice induced severe AHR, as it did in wild-type BALB/c mice. These results indicated that the CD1d knockout mice had functioning airways.

3. Failure of Jα281 KO mice to develop AHR

That NKT cells were required for the development of AHR was confirmed by examining another NKT cell-deficient strain, Jα281 knockout mice. These mice lack the α-chain of the invariant TCR of NKT cells and, therefore, lack NKT cells. The Jα281 knockout mice, like CD1d knockout mice, when sensitized and challenged with OVA failed to develop AHR. The Jα281 knockout mice also had reduced airway eosinophilia, whereas the wild-type BALB/c mice, as expected, developed severe AHR and severe airway eosinophilia.

4. Direct measurement of airway resistance

To confirm the absence of AHR in NKT cell-deficient mice, AHR was also assessed by directly measuring airway resistance and its reciprocal, dynamic compliance in anesthetized, tracheostomized, intubated and mechanically ventilated mice. In mice sensitized and challenged with OVA, airway resistance increased in the wild-type BALB/c mice on challenge with methacholine but did not increase in the CD1d KO mice nor in the Jα281 knockout mice. Dynamic compliance decreased in the wild-type BALB/c mice on challenge with methacholine but did not change in the CD1d or Jα281 knockout mice. This indicated that AHR failed to occur in either the CD1d or Jα281 knockout mice. Although several previous studies have shown that β2-microglobulin knockout mice, which lack all class I restricted cells, including CD8 cells and NKT cells, can develop Th2 responses and allergen-induced AHR [11], it is possible that in the absence of $CD8^+$, class I restricted T cells, alterations in airway responsiveness develop that obviate the need for NKT cells. However, the absence of AHR measured in several different ways, induced by several different protocols [8], in different laboratories [9], in both CD1d knockout mice as well as in Jα281 knockout mice, strongly suggests that NKT cells are specifically required for the development of AHR.

5. Adoptive transfer of NKT cells reconstitutes AHR

To more clearly show that the lack of NKT cells was the specific cause for the failure of the CD1d knockout and Jα281 knockout mice to develop AHR, we reconstituted the Jα281 knockout mice with NKT cells. NKT cells were purified with CD1d tetramers loaded with α-GalactocylCeramide (α-GalCer) from wild-type BALB/c mice and adoptively transferred into the Jα281 knockout mice, which were then assessed for allergen-induced AHR. We found that recipient Jα281 knockout mice reconstituted with NKT cells developed severe AHR, whereas the unreconstituted mice had normal airway reactivity. Furthermore, we determined whether the production of IL-4, IL-13 or IFN-γ by the NKT cells required to reconstitute AHR. We therefore adoptively transferred NKT cells purified from IL-4 knockout, IL-13 knockout, IL-4/IL-13 double knockout, or wild-type mice, and then assessed the recipients for AHR. We found that NKT cells from wild-type BALB/c mice and from INF-γ knockout mice fully reconstituted AHR in the Jα281 knockout mice, whereas NKT cells from IL-4 knockout and IL-13 knockout mice partially reconstituted AHR. However, NKT cells from IL-4-IL-13 double knockout mice failed to reconstitute AHR in the Jα281 knockout mice. These results

indicated that the induction of AHR required the production by NKT cells of both IL-4 and IL-13, but not IFN-γ.

6. Discussion

Our results indicate that the development of AHR in mice is complex, and that the specific role of $CD4^+$, αβ TCR^+ T cells is not fully understood. Thus, our results indicate that a response by conventional $CD4^+$ Th2 cells is not sufficient for the development of allergen-induced AHR, and that NKT cells, which are either $CD4^+$ or double negative, and which produce IL-4 and IL-13 but not IFN-γ, are absolutely required for the development of AHR. These results are consistent with the fact that a Th2 response in the upper airways (e.g., allergic rhinitis) is not always accompanied by asthma and a Th2 response in the lower airways [5,6]. Both Th2 biased immune responses and IgE production can occur in NKT cell-deficient mice, indicating that Th2 cell differentiation and IgE synthesis do not require the presence of Vα14*i* NKT cells. However, NKT cell must provide an element in the lower respiratory tract required for the development of AHR that is not provided by Th2 cells, though the specific relationship between conventional Th2 cells and NKT cells is not clear.

The precise mechanisms by which antigen administration into the lungs activates NKT cells to induce AHR are also not clear. Because immunization of NKT cell-deficient mice with more aggressive protocols and with different antigens did not induce AHR, we do not believe that NKT cells simply influence the magnitude of the pulmonary Th2 response, but rather license Th2 cells that enter the pulmonary compartment to become competent for the induction of AHR. While the specific signals provided by NKT cells to the allergen-sensitized CD4 αβ TCR T cells are unknown, our model is unique in that NKT cell function could be induced without administration of α-GalCer, in contrast to most other models of autoimmunity or infection, in which a role for NKT cells required activation using α-GalCer [12–16].

In our system, we hypothesize that antigen encountered in the lung alters the mucosal environment of the respiratory tract, exposing self-glycolipid antigens that are recognized by the self-agonist selected NKT cells [17,18]. However, the glycolipid antigen in our system that activates NKT cells in vivo when OVA, BSA or *Aspergillus* antigen is administered into the lungs has not been identified. Nevertheless, agonist selected T cells in the mucus membranes are thought to survey for cells that express enhanced levels of self as antigens in response to stress induced by environmental stimuli. Such agonist selected T cells, as part of the innate immune system, then respond rapidly by producing cytokines [17]. Our studies therefore suggest that antigens other than α-GalCer can indeed activate Vα14*i* NKT cells, and that innate immune mechanisms involving Vα14*i* NKT cells exist within the lung that respond rapidly to inhaled antigen.

Finally, while observations in mice generally predict immunological processes that occur in humans, the clinical implications of these studies of NKT cells in mice for human asthma will depend on replication of these findings in human patients with asthma. Because of the striking conservation between the amino acid sequences mouse and human CD1d, it is very likely that the observed requirement for NKT cells in mice will be also seen in humans. Indeed, we currently have preliminary observations that indicate significant numbers of NKT cells are present in the lungs of human patients with asthma, suggesting that NKT cells play a very important role in human asthma.

References

[1] Forecasted state-specific estimates of self-reported asthma prevalence—United States, MMWR. Morb. Mort. Wkly. Rep. 47 (1998) 1022–1025.

[2] D. Umetsu, et al., Asthma: an epidemic of dysregulated immunity, Nat. Immunol. 3 (2002) 715–720.

[3] F.D. Martinez, et al., Asthma and wheezing in the first six years of life, New Engl. J. Med. 332 (1995) 133–138.

[4] B. Burrows, et al., Association of asthma with serum IgE levels and skin-test reactivity to allergens, N. Engl. J. Med. 320 (1989) 271–277.

[5] S. Illi, et al., The pattern of atopic sensitization is associated with the development of asthma in childhood, J. Allergy Clin. Immunol. 108 (2001) 709–714.

[6] P. Van Eerdewegh, et al., Association of the ADAM33 gene with asthma and bronchial hyperresponsiveness, Nature 418 (2002) 426–430.

[7] S. Holgate, et al., Epithelial–mesenchymal interactions in the pathogenesis of asthma, J. Allergy Clin. Immunol. 105 (2000) 193–204.

[8] O. Akbari, et al., Essential role of NKT cells producing IL-4 and IL-13 in the development of allergen-induced airway hyperreactivity, Nat. Med. 9 (2003) 582–588.

[9] M. Lisbonne, et al., Cutting edge: invariant V alpha 14 NKT cells are required for allergen-induced airway inflammation and hyperreactivity in an experimental asthma model, J. Immunol. 171 (2003) 1637–1641.

[10] M. Wills-Karp, et al., Interleukin-13: central mediator of allergic asthma, Science 282 (1998) 2258–2261.

[11] D.R. Brown, et al., Beta 2-microglobulin-dependent NK 1.1+T cells are not essential for T helper cell 2 immune responses, J. Exp. Med. 184 (1996) 1295–1304.

[12] E.E. Nieuwenhuis, et al., CD1d-dependent macrophage-mediated clearance of *Pseudomonas aeruginosa* from lung, Nat. Med. 8 (2002) 588–593.

[13] B. Wang, Y. Geng, C. Wang, CD1-restricted NK T cells protect nonobese diabetic mice from developing diabetes, J. Exp. Med. 194 (2001) 313–320.

[14] S. Hong, et al., The natural killer T-cell ligand alpha-galactosylceramide prevents autoimmune diabetes in non-obese diabetic mice, Nat. Med. 7 (2001) 1052–1056.

[15] S. Sharif, et al., Activation of natural killer T cells by alpha-galactosylceramide treatment prevents the onset and recurrence of autoimmune type 1 diabetes, Nat. Med. 7 (2001) 1057–1062.

[16] J. Cui, et al., Requirement for Valpha14 NKT cells in IL-12-mediated rejection of tumors, Science 278 (1997) 1623–1626.

[17] A. Leishman, et al., Precursors of functional MHC class I- or class II-restricted CD8alphaalpha(+) T cells are positively selected in the thymus by agonist self-peptides, Immunity 16 (2002) 355–364.

[18] A. Bendelac, et al., Mouse CD1-specific NK1 T cells: development, specificity, and function, Annu. Rev. Immunol. 15 (1997) 535–562.

International Congress Series 1285 (2005) 189–191

www.ics-elsevier.com

Potential of targeting natural killer T cells for the treatment of autoimmune diseases

Sachiko Miyake *

National Institute of Neuroscience, NCNP, Department of Immunology, 4-1-1, Ogawahigashi, Kodaira, Tokyo 187-8502, Japan

Abstract. Natural killer T (NKT) cells are potent immune modulators after stimulation with glycolipid ligand such as alpha-galactosylceramide (alpha-GC) through a rapid and massive production of a variety of cytokines such as IFN-gamma and IL-4. OCH, a sphingosine-truncated analogue of alpha-GC, induces the selective production of Th2 cytokines from NKT cells and inhibits Th1-mediated autoimmune disease models such as experimental autoimmune encephalomyelitis, type I diabetes and arthritis. The selective induction of Th2 cytokines is due to its unstable binding to CD1d and a short-lived stimulation to NKT cells which result in insufficient induction of c-Rel protein and following low level of IFN-gamma production. OCH induces less IFN-gamma production not only by NKT cells but also by NK cells due to an insufficient IL-12 production from dendritic cells. Lack of efficient IFN-gamma production and CD40L expression by NKT cells stimulated with OCH exert marginal IL-12 production by dendritic cells. © 2005 Published by Elsevier B.V.

Keywords: NKT cell; Glycolipid ligand; OCH; Th1/Th2; Autoimmune disease

1. Introduction

Natural killer T (NKT) cells are a unique subset of CD1-restricted T lymphocytes that express T cell receptor (TCR) and some NK receptors [1]. NKT cells express an invariant TCRalpha chain composed of Va14–Ja18 segments in mice and Va24–Ja18 segments in humans associated with TCRbeta chains using a restricted set of Vbeta. NKT cells recognize glycolipid antigens such as alpha-galactosylceramide (alpha-GC) presented by CD1d and rapidly secrete large amounts of cytokines including IL-4 and

* Tel.: +81 423412711 (5244); fax: +81 423461753.
E-mail address: miyake@ncnp.go.jp.

0531-5131/ © 2005 Published by Elsevier B.V.
doi:10.1016/j.ics.2005.07.092

IFN-gamma upon activation. Due to its potent ability to produce a variety of cytokines, NKT cells are involved in various kinds of immunoregulation including autoimmunity. We have recently demonstrated that OCH, a sphingosine-truncated analogue of alpha-GC, preferentially induced Th2 cytokines from NKT cells and administration of OCH suppressed EAE [2]. Here, we demonstrate that OCH is effective for the suppression of other Th1-mediated autoimmune diseases such as CIA and type I diabetes in NOD mice. We also show the molecular mechanism accounting for the unique property of OCH to selectively induce IL-4 by NKT cells.

2. Materials and methods

Diabetes was assessed by monitoring glucose levels in the blood using GLU-W (Fujifilm, Kanagawa, Japan) every week. To induce collagen-induced arthritis, mice were immunized intradermally at the base of the tail with 200 μg of bovine type II collagen (CII) (for SJL mice) (Collagen Research Center, Tokyo, Japan) emulsified with an equal volume of CFA, containing 250 μg of H37RA *Mycobacterium tuberculosis* (Difco, Detroit, MI). Cytokines were detected using ELISA. Proliferative response was measured by incorporation of ^{3}H thymidine (1 μCi/well) for the final 16 h of the culture analyzed with a beta-1205 counter (Pharmacia, Uppsala, Sweden).

3. Results

Administration of OCH suppressed diabetes in non-obese diabetic (NOD) mice and collagen-induced arthritis (CIA) by inducing T helper (Th) 2 bias of autoimmune T cells [3,4]. These results suggest that OCH is useful for a wide variety of Th1-mediated autoimmune diseases.

The NKT cell production of IFN-gamma is more susceptible to the sphingosine length of glycolipid ligand than that of IL-4, and the length of sphingosine chain determines the duration of NKT cell stimulation by CD1d-associated glycolipids. Furthermore, IFN-gamma production by NKT cells requires longer T cell receptor stimulation than required for IL-4 production by NKT cells stimulated either with immobilized anti-CD3 mAb or immobilized alpha-GC-loaded CD1d molecule. Interestingly, transcription of IFN-gamma but not that of IL-4 was sensitive to cycloheximide treatment, indicating the intrinsic involvement of de novo protein synthesis for IFN-gamma production by NKT cells. We determined c-Rel is preferentially transcribed in alpha-GC-stimulated, but not in OCH-stimulated NKT cells and is essential for IFN-gamma production by activated NKT cells [5].

OCH induced less IFN-gamma production than alpha-GC not only by direct effect on NKT cells, but also by indirect effect on NK cells. OCH injection induced one-tenth amount of serum IL-12 level compared with alpha-GC. Co-administration of OCH and low dose of IL-12 induced significantly higher production of IFN-gamma compared with either treatment alone. OCH treatment induced approximately one third of CD40L transcription compared with the effect of alpha-GC. OCH-induced IL-12 production was partially augmented by co-administration of anti-CD40 mAb. Furthermore, concomitant administration of IFN-gamma and stimulatory anti-CD40 mAb with OCH induced IL-12 production. These results suggested that the signals through CD40 and IFN-gamma provided by OCH-stimulated NKT cells did not lead to efficient production of IL-12 from dendritic cells, resulting in lack of IFN-gamma production from NK cells.

4. Discussion

Considering that CD1d molecule is non-polymorphic and remarkably well-conserved among the species, modified glycolipid antigen such as OCH for preferential induction of IL-4 production through NKT activation and subsequent Th2 polarization could be an attractive therapeutic reagent against Th1-mediated autoimmune diseases. However, the molecular mechanism accounting for the unique property of OCH to selectively induce IL-4 by NKT cells has not been clarified yet and littlc is known about the effect of OCH on extrinsic regulatory immune cells network for IFN-gamma production.

In this paper, we demonstrate the molecular mechanisms for the differential production of IL-4 and IFN-gamma by NKT cells stimulated with various glycolipid ligands including OCH. Sustained TCR stimulation and concomitant c-Rel expression by alpha-GC leads to the production of IFN-gamma, whereas short-term activation and marginal c-Rel transcription by OCH results in a preferential production of IL-4 by NKT cells. Finally, we showed the effect of OCH on surrounding immune network in which OCH induces less effective production of IFN-gamma and IL-12 by bystander cells possibly due to inefficient production of IFN-gamma and lower expression of CD40L by NKT cells. These results assure the supplemental reliability of the altered glycolipid ligand OCH for Th2 polarization and immune regulation in vivo and suggest that proper assessment of innate immune condition is required to estimate host responses when modulating NKT cell responses by OCH administration in vivo.

References

[1] S. Miyake, A. Chiba, T. Yamamura, Potential of targeting natural killer T cells for the treatment of autoimmune diseases, Mod. Rheum. 14 (2004) 279–284.

[2] S.* Miyake, K.* Miyamoto, T.* Yamamura, A synthetic glycolipid prevents autoimmune encephalomyelitis by inducing Th2 of natural killer T cells, Nature 413 (6855) (2001) 531–534 (*Equal contribution).

[3] M. Mizuno, et al., Synthetic glycolipid OCH prevents insulitis and diabetes inNOC mice, J. Autoimmun 23 (2004) 293–300.

[4] A. Chiba, et al., Suppression of collagen-induced arthritis by natural killer T cell activation with OCH, a sphingosine-truncated analog of alpha-galactosylceramide, Arthritis Rheum. 50 (1) (2004) 305–313.

[5] S. Oki, et al., The clinical implication and molecular mechanism of preferential IL-4 production by modified glycolipid-stimulated NKT cells, J. Clin. Invest. 113 (11) (2004) 1631–1640.

International Congress Series 1285 (2005) 192–201

www.ics-elsevier.com

A novel model for pathogenesis of autoimmune heart failure: The role of dendritic cells

Manu Rangachari [a,b], Urs Eriksson [c,d], Elisabeth H. Vollmann [e], Josef M. Penninger [a,*]

[a] *Institute for Molecular Biotechnology of the Austrian Academy of Sciences (IMBA), Vienna, Austria*
[b] *Graduate Programme in Immunology, University of Toronto, Toronto, Ontario, Canada*
[c] *Medicine A, Department of Internal Medicine, University Hospital, Basel, Switzerland*
[d] *Division of Experimental Critical Care Medicine, University Hospital, Basel, Switzerland*
[e] *Research Institute for Molecular Pathology (IMP), Vienna, Austria*

Abstract. Autoimmune diseases present a significant health challenge. Animal models of autoimmunity have shed great insight into both disease pathogenesis as well as into the workings of the immune system in general. Myocarditis is an autoimmune disease with epidemiological links to cardiotropic pathogens; however, many cases of the disease are sudden and unexplained. It has been proposed that a dysregulated adaptive immune response against cardiotropic pathogens can turn itself upon healthy human tissue, due to similarities between pathogenic and cardiac antigens. We discuss the critical role of dendritic cells (DCs) in the induction of myocarditis, and propose a model by which coincidental infection or cardiac tissue damage may represent the initial step in myocardial inflammation and subsequent myocarditis.

Keywords: Autoimmunity; Myocarditis; Molecular mimicry; Dendritic cell; Toll-like receptor; Heat shock proteins; Myocardial infarction

1. The adaptive immune system and mechanisms for its control

The mammalian adaptive immune system allows for the effective and rapid elimination of pathogens. The guiding principle of adaptive immunity is one of antigen specificity. Naïve T- and B-lymphocytes circulate between the bloodstream and lymphatic system, each bearing receptor specificity for a single antigen; the antigen must be processed and

* Corresponding author. Tel.: +43 1 79730454; fax: +43 1 79730 459.
E-mail addresses: josef.penninger@imba.oeaw.ac.at (J.M. Penninger), manu.rangachari@utoronto.ca (M. Rangachari).

0531-5131/
doi:10.1016/j.ics.2005.09.008

presented by specialized antigen-presenting cells (APCs) in order for it to be recognized by the lymphocyte. APCs encounter pathogens at peripheral sites of infection and subsequently undergo a maturation program. They present antigen conjugated to major histocompatibility complex (MHC) class I or class II molecules on their surface, and home to peripheral lymphoid tissue such as the lymph node or spleen. Lymphocytes proliferate massively upon antigen priming in the peripheral lymphoid tissue. The local milieu of cytokines and APC-provided receptor signals then dictates the lymphocytes' differentiation into effector immune cells that can direct an antigen-specific immune response. One study has suggested that the number of $CD8^+$ T cells specific for a single antigen can increase to 70 million per mouse just 11 days after viral infection [1]. Clearly, activation of adaptive immunity can result in a speedy and overwhelming response to infection.

The potency of the adaptive immune response does not come without negative consequences. Since antigens are typically protein-derived, the immune system requires regulatory mechanisms that can prevent lymphocyte activation and expansion against self-tissue (*autoimmunity*). Indeed, several such mechanisms are centrally programmed during lymphocyte development. Thymocytes that strongly react to self-antigen in the thymus are deleted in a process known as *negative selection*. Recent attention has also been paid to the development and function of regulatory T cells (T_{reg}), which can impair the responses of self-antigen-reactive effector T cells (Fig. 1).

Central tolerance is not always completely effective in eliminating self-reactive lymphocytes. For instance, in a transgenic model of murine arthritis, numbers of self-reactive T cells recognizing the immunogenic self-peptide were low in young mice yet increased with age [2]. Therefore, peripheral mechanisms of preventing autoimmunity are critical. One critical peripheral control on the activation of T cells is the requirement for costimulation. Briefly, a T cell requires two signals from an APC in order for it to proliferate—recognition of cognate antigen in the context of MHC, as well as recognition of costimulatory receptors present only on defined APCs. Recognition of antigen alone is insufficient to prime a naïve T cell. The costimulatory requirement thus restricts the ability of autoreactive T cells to respond inappropriately to bystander cells bearing self-antigen (Fig. 1).

The costimulatory interaction most relevant to the early activation of T cells is that between CD28 on the T cell and B7.1/B7.2 (CD80/CD86) on the APC. Ligation of CD28 upregulates expression of the T cell growth factor IL-2, promotes cell cycle entry, and increases glycolytic activity. CD28 is required to overcome proliferative repression mediated by Cbl-b, an essential negative regulator of T cell signaling [3]. The requirement for CD28-B7 signaling in T cell activation in vivo was shown by analyzing the development of experimental autoimmune encephalomyelitis (EAE) in mice deficient in CD28, B7.1 and B7.2. None of the strains developed this T cell-mediated autoimmune disorder [4].

Regulation of costimulatory molecule expression on the surface of APCs presents an additional level of peripheral control over immune responses. In the early 1990s, Janeway proposed that in order to be competent to activate T cells APCs require signals that can only be provided by pathogens. This would ensure that T cells respond only to pathogenically derived antigen [5]. Indeed, it has subsequently been shown that bacterially derived lipopolysaccharide (LPS) induces B7 expression on the surface of dendritic cells

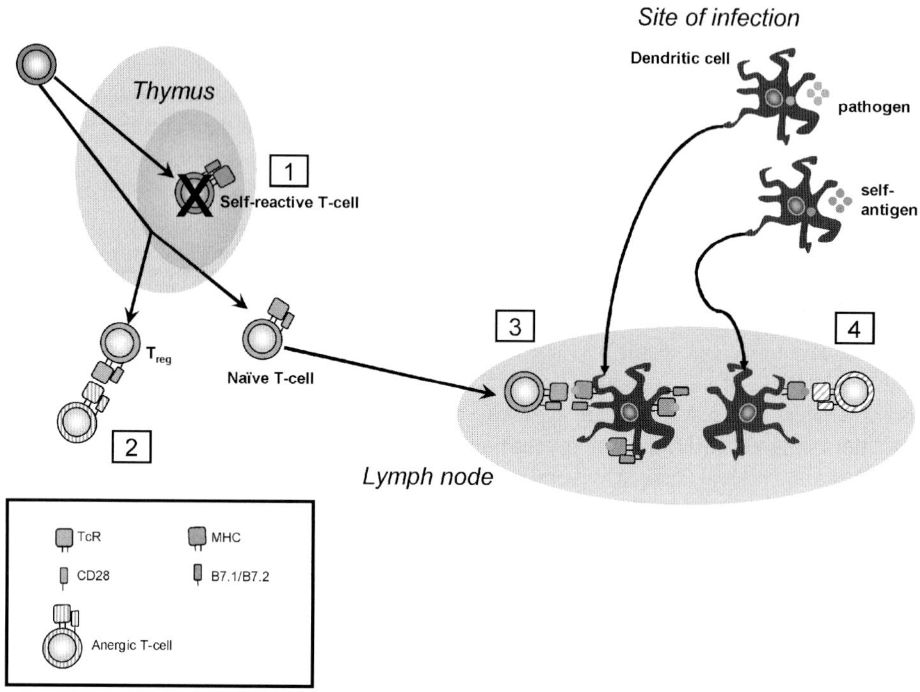

Fig. 1. Mechanisms of averting auto-immunity. Bone marrow precursors enter the thymus, where they undergo a T-cell development program that involves re-arrangement of their antigen-specific T-cell receptor (TcR). Cells whose TcR is strongly reactive to self-tissue are deleted in the thymus (1). The majority of naïve T-cells exiting the thymus are potential effector cells. A small population of selfreactive T-cells develop into regulatory T-cells (T_{reg}) that are characterized by the transcription factor FoxP3 and surface expression of CD25. T_{reg} cells can anergize effector T-cells through cell–cell contact as well as via soluble mediators (2). Peripheral tolerance can be controlled by the activation status of dendritic cells (DCs). DCs phagocytose sorrounding cells in the periphery; however, only those that receive pathogen-specific activation signals will be able to express costimulatory molecules and high levels of antigen/MHC, and thereby be able to stimulate T-cells (3). By contrast, Dcs that take up antigen without pathogenic stimulation will be able to present only low levels of antigen/MHC, and will not be able to express costimulatory molecules. These DCs will anergize T-cells rather than stimulate them (4).

(DCs), the type of APC chiefly responsible for T cell activation [6]. It is now known that pathogenic components such as LPS or dsRNA are recognized by Toll-like receptor (TLR) family members on the surface of APCs. TLR signals are crucial for the initiation of the APC maturation program—which involves an increase in surface antigen/MHC expression, the upregulation of costimulatory molecules such as B7.1 and B7.2, as well as the secretion of immunostimulatory cytokines such as IL-12 and TNFα. These events are necessary of the optimal induction of T cell responses. Ablation of TLR molecules or their related signaling components in murine DCs results in disruption of the maturation program [7].

It is therefore clear that the power of the adaptive immune system must be harnessed and used appropriately—namely against pathogens and not against self-tissue. A variety of regulatory mechanisms exist, ranging from centrally programmed clonal deletion of self-reactive thymocytes to the costimulatory requirement for peripheral activation of T cells

(Fig. 1). However, the existence of myriad autoimmune pathologies indicates that even these extensive mechanisms are not fool-proof. We examined one murine model of autoimmune disease, autoimmune myocarditis, and provide evidence that DCs can promote not only pathogen resistance but also autoimmunity.

2. Autoimmunity: the myocarditis model

Autoimmune diseases including, yet not limited to, type I diabetes, multiple sclerosis and lupus are a significant cause of morbidity and mortality worldwide. One such disease is myocarditis—the inflammation of the heart myocardium. Myocarditis is a leading cause of idiopathic dilated cardiomyopathy (DCM), in which destruction of the myocardium leads to clinical heart failure and frequently death. Myocarditis is a leading cause of unexpected death in people under the age of 40 [8].

Heart-specific pathogens are a major etiologic agent in myocarditis. These include cocksackievirus B3 (CB3), *Trypanosoma cruzi* and various strains of *Chlamydia* [9–11]. Enteroviral RNA can be detected in greater than one-third of patients with heart muscle failure, and the presence of enterovirus is a predictor of poor prognostic outcome [12]. Interestingly, however, patients with DCM frequently present autoantibodies against cardiac proteins, and peripheral blood lymphocytes from DCM patients could adoptively transfer disease to immunodeficient SCID mice [13,14]. Such findings have given rise to the hypothesis that while pathogenic attack may be responsible for an acute phase of myocarditis, post-infectious autoimmunity is responsible for chronic inflammation of the myocardium [15].

The high human cost of autoimmune disease, combined with the genetic tractability of the murine immune system, has made the study of mouse models of autoimmunity an area of intense interest. Several animal models of myocarditis exist. Some models, such as cocksackievirus-induced myocarditis, attempt to replicate human myocarditis by examining the consequences of the host–pathogen interaction on disease progression [16]. Indeed, the use of this model has uncovered an immunomodulatory role for the antiviral cytokine IFN-β in myocarditis [17]. Other models attempt to recreate the disease from the point of autoimmune induction. For several years, we have utilized a model of experimental autoimmune myocarditis (EAM) that involves immunizing mice from susceptible strains with a peptide derived from the murine cardiac myosin alpha heavy chain (myhcα) [18]. Mice develop severe myocarditis that reaches maximal severity at 21 days post-immunization. The immunological heart infiltrate consists predominantly of $CD11b^+$ macrophages, with lesser numbers of $CD4^+$ and $CD8^+$ T cells [11]. The induction of myocarditis has profound consequences on heart function: immunized mice display chronically impaired left-ventricular contractility and increased heart size [19].

While viral or bacterial infection can induce myocarditis, and while autoimmune mechanisms can promote chronic myocardial destruction, one is still left with the question of how the two are linked? One hypothesis postulates that heart-specific self-antigens may structurally mimic pathogenic ones, thereby leading the same T cells that cleared the initial infection to then attack the myocardium [11]. It is important to note that primed T cells do not require costimulation; antigen recognition alone is sufficient to induce effector responses. Further, heart-resident APCs from non-immunized mice present cardiac myosin-derived peptides in the context of MHC class II, and can induce the proliferation of myosin-specific T cell hybridomas in vitro [20]. It is therefore tempting to speculate that activated, pathogen-specific T cells, where home is the heart, are at the wrong place at the wrong time—that is, they are primed and able to respond to cardiac myosin. There is little homology between cardiac myosin-derived peptides and the sequences of known cardiotropic viruses [21]. However, significant homology exists between myosin and cardiotropic bacteria. We showed that several strains of *Chlamydia* contain peptides that are similar to the immunogenic myhcα peptide. Immunizing mice with these *Chlamydia*-derived peptides induced myocarditis. Further, mice infected with *C. trachomatis* develop autoantibodies directed against myhcα [22]. In a different model, Lewis rats immunized with the streptococcal M protein developed valvulitis and myocarditis. M protein-specific T cells could proliferate in response to cardiac myosin in vitro and could transfer myocarditis in vivo, indicating that this was a T cell-dependent autoimmune response [23].

3. An alternate view—the role of the DC

Much of the focus in the myocarditis field has been on the role of T cells in pathogenicity. This is not surprising given that transfer of myosin-specific $CD4^+$ T cells is sufficient for disease induction [15]. However, until recently the role of the innate immune system, and in particular DCs, had been largely ignored. DCs are not merely passive inducers of T cell activation; they actively modulate and shape T cell effector responses in vivo. DCs can exert this control through the differential expression of specialized costimulatory molecules—for example, B7RP-1/B7H-2 binds ICOS, a T cell receptor that promotes B cell germinal center formation and regulatory T cell induction [24–26]. DCs can also promote inflammatory T cell responses through production of IL-12, or can suppress T cell activation through production of IL-10 [27]. It has been shown some years ago that DCs harvested from immunized mice could induce autoimmune disease in naïve animals in models of thyroiditis and prostatitis [28,29]. Further, naïve DCs pulsed with the autoantigen thyroglobulin ex vivo could induce autoimmune thyroiditis in syngeneic recipients [30].

A potential role for DCs in the pathogenesis of myocarditis was first noted by Ludewig et al. while studying DC-mediated tumor immunotherapy [31]. They transplanted a β-gal-expressing tumor into mice that expressed the β-gal transgene in right ventricular cardiomyocytes. While treatment of these mice with β-gal-pulsed DCs resulted in rejection of the tumor, it also led to lymphocyte infiltration of the myocardium. While transgenic models are useful in delineating the minimal requirements for autoimmune pathology, it is clear that the high level of antigenic expression seen in such a system may not reflect a physiological situation. Nevertheless, further evidence for DC-mediated pathology came with analysis of IL-12p40$^{-/-}$ mice, which are resistant to myocarditis [32]. IL-12p40 is a subunit of IL-12 and IL-23, both of which are pro-inflammatory cytokines produced primarily by DCs [33]. These data, along with the finding that IL-12Rβ1$^{-/-}$ mice are also resistant, provided the first genetic evidence that signals emanating from DCs might be essential for the development of myocarditis [34].

We were able to show that IL-1R expression on DCs is critical for the development of myocarditis. Strikingly, while IL-1R$^{-/-}$ mice were resistant to disease, transfer of myhcα-pulsed IL-1R$^{+/+}$ bone marrow derived DCs (BMDCs) to IL-1R$^{-/-}$ host mice rescued disease susceptibility upon peptide immunization. While there was no apparent intrinsic defect in IL-1R$^{-/-}$ CD4^{+} T cells, adoptive transfer of CD4^{+} from immunized IL-1R$^{-/-}$ mice into SCID recipients did not cause disease. This indicates that improperly or incompletely activated DCs can program T cells to respond poorly in vivo [35].

We then asked whether myhcα-pulsed BMDCs could themselves induce disease in naive, non-transgenic mice. If successful, we wished to delineate the activation requirements of such pathogenic BMDCs. The Janeway hypothesis would predict that TLR stimulation of DCs, together with the presence of autoantigen, would be sufficient to induce autoimmunity. Indeed, ex vivo stimulation and myhcα-pulsing of BMDCs rendered them pathogenic [19]. Unstimulated, myhcα-pulsed, BMDCs could not induce disease, while stimulated BMDCs pulsed with an irrelevant peptide were also non-pathogenic. Notably, BMDCs stimulated with LPS alone could induce disease of only modest incidence and severity. However, the combination of LPS stimulation plus agonistic triggering of the CD40 receptor rendered BMDCs highly pathogenic. CD40$^{-/-}$ BMDCs were unable to induce disease. DCs typically receive CD40 signals from CD40L expressed on T cells, thus suggesting that DCs require two distinct signals in order to become autoaggressive—one mediated by pathogenic components, with the other provided by the adaptive immune system [19].

We also showed that while CD40 activation of BMDCs was indispensable, LPS could be replaced by other TLR ligands such as dsRNA, CpG or peptidoglycan [19]. This implies that myocarditis does not result from a specific type of pathogen but that it may be caused by a variety of bacterial or viral stimuli, with the common components being CD40 signaling and the presence of autoantigen. This finding also complements the known complex etiology of human myocarditis, with several known pathogenic culprits [9–11].

These data provided the first evidence linking pathogenic stimuli to autoimmunity in vivo. They also fit well with a theory of molecular mimicry as the driving force behind the autoimmune component of myocarditis. One could envision DCs being activated by cardiotropic viruses or bacteria while taking up self-antigen from cardiomyocytes damaged during the acute stage of the disease. These activated DCs could then present autoantigens to pathogen-specific T cells that had migrated to the heart to combat the causative infection. Indeed, LPS and CD40-activated BMDCs were able to induce disease when pulsed with apoptotic cardiomyocytes rather than with myhcα peptide [19].

However, the most provocative finding of our study was that TLR stimulation and antigen did not have to be concomitantly provided to BMDCs in order for autoimmunity to result. We found that injection of apoptotic cardiomyocytes directly into mice, followed by administration of either LPS or CpG, could cause the formation of inflammatory foci within the recipient hearts [19]. This uncoupling of pathogenic stimulus from the availability of antigen makes it tempting to speculate that the pathogenesis of autoimmune myocarditis does not absolutely require infection with a heart specific virus or bacteria; rather, disease could conceivably result if damage to cardiac tissue was accompanied by a coincidental infection at another site in the body.

4. A new model of pathogenesis

One could go further and propose that even infection is not required for the pathogenesis of autoimmune diseases such as myocarditis. Matzinger argues that the Janeway model, in which only pathogen-restricted signals can stimulate APCs to induce adaptive immunity, cannot explain non-infectious rejection of allogeneic transplants or tumor immunity. Rather, she proposes a broadened version of the Janeway model, in which the innate immune system can also be induced by endogenous "danger signals"—that is, either by normally intracellular components or by inducible stress signals such as heat shock proteins (Hsps) [36]. Indeed, Hsps can induce macrophages and DCs to produce inflammatory cytokines and upregulate activation markers. Tantalizingly, TLRs 2 and 4 have been suggested as receptors for Hsps—with TLR4 being chiefly known as the receptor for LPS [37]. One caveat to the study of Hsps as TLR ligands is that Hsp preparations in vitro may be contaminated with LPS or other pathogenic components [38]. Nonetheless, a recent study demonstrated that a verified low-endotoxin preparation of Hsp70 could be used as an adjuvant to peptide immunization in a transgenic model of diabetes [39]. Curiously, CD40 expression was required on host APCs in order for Hsp70-mediated autoimmunity to progress. However, CD40 expression was not required for LPS-mediated immunization. While LPS-mediated autoimmunity did require CD40 signaling in our study, this discrepancy might be explained by a lower APC activation threshold in transgenic models [19,39].

The induction of myocarditis as a result of cardiac tissue damage presents an attractive model. Ischaemic rat hearts release Hsp60 into the bloodstream [40]. Elevated Hsp70 levels have also been observed in the sera of patients who suffered acute myocardial infarction [41]. One could imagine a scenario in which myocardial infarction results in destruction of cardiomyocytes, and subsequent release of both Hsps and cardiac myosin. Resident DCs could phagocytose and present myosin-derived antigens, while Hsps could stimulate DC maturation and migration to the draining lymph node (Fig. 2).

Myocardial infarction may be induced in rodents through transient ligation of the coronary artery. This technique allows one to study the molecular players involved in infarction-related tissue damage and subsequent vascular remodeling. Transfer of splenocytes from post-infarct rats to normal ones can cause lymphocyte infiltration in the donors, suggesting that cardiac injury may be a causative factor in myocardial inflammation [42]. It would be interesting to see whether myocarditis-resistant mouse strains such as IL-1R$\alpha^{-/-}$ or CD40$^{-/-}$ would be protected from post-infarct myocardial inflammation. Alternately, in vivo blocking of these signals after infarction might represent a prophylactic therapy against cardiac damage-induced myocarditis.

It is important to note that our model of myocarditis induction via cardiac damage/coincidental infection is intended to complement, and not replace, the proposed role of immune molecular mimicry and cardiotropic pathogens. As noted previously, while homology between *Chlamydia*-derived peptides and the cardiac myosin antigen have been observed, no such relation has been noted for cocksackievirus [22,21]. However, cocksackievirus infection causes cardiomyocyte damage and death [43]. This could cause cardiac antigen release—in the presence of a potent immunostimulatory cocktail of Hsps and viral components (Fig. 2). The heart-specific tissue damage of cardiotropic

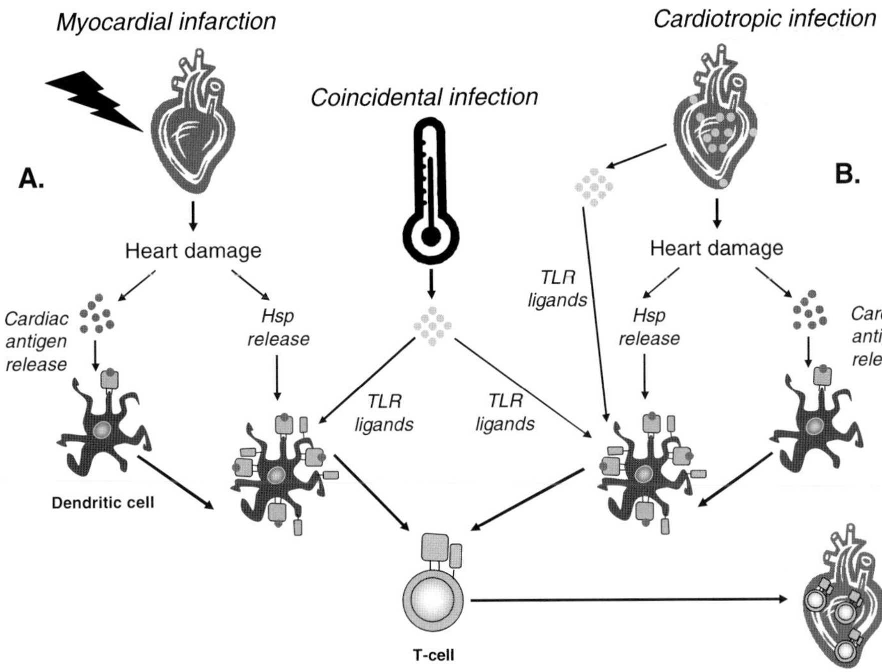

Fig. 2. DC-mediated models of myocarditis induction. Mice develop autoimmune myocarditis when injected with apoptotic cardiomyocytes followed by LPS [19]. This suggests that antigen uptake and DC stimulation via TLRs may be separable components of myocarditis induction. Moreover, this implies that the source of DC stimulation through TLR ligands need not necessarily be heart issue. (A) Myocardiotis could result from myocardial infarction or ischaemic heart disease, as damage to cardiomyocytes would result in release of heat shock proteins (Hsps) as well as cardiac antigen. Hsps can function as TLR ligands, suggesting that cardiomyocite damage would be sufficient for heart-resident DCs to take up antigen and present it along with costimulatory receptors. (B) Cardiotropic pathogens can effect cardiomyocyte damage. Cardiac antigens would be released, and release of TLR-stimulatory Hsps would be supplemented by pathogen-derived TLR ligands such as LPS and dsRNA. In both cases, coincidental infection at another site in the body could further induce DC maturation. Mature, cardiac antigen-pulsed DCs could then strongly stimulate cardiac antigen-specifec T-cells, leading to T-cell migration to the myocardium and subsequent effector functions and autoimmune heart damage.

pathogens could thus go a long way towards explaining their epidemiological link to myocarditis [9].

5. Conclusion

Autoimmune diseases are a major cause of morbidity and mortality that have only increased as worldwide standards of health care and sanitation have improved [44]. Animal models of autoimmunity allow for the pathogenesis of these diseases to be dissected systematically. Previous studies of myocarditis have demonstrated the essential role played by $CD4^+$ T cells, and have also established that bacterially derived peptides with homology to the cardiac antigen myhcα could induce disease in susceptible mice. We and others have demonstrated that DCs play a critical role in stimulating an autoimmune response against the heart. We have also shown that TLR stimulation plus CD40 triggering of DCs is essential for them to transfer autoimmunity to non-transgenic hosts. Surprisingly, we also revealed that autoimmunity could result merely from administering a pre-processed source of autoantigen (in the form of apoptotic cardiomyocytes) as well as a global TLR signal. This indicated that myocarditis might not necessarily result from the effects of a cardiotropic infection. Taken together with the existing model of molecular mimicry, our model may help to explain in part the complex etiology of myocarditis.

Finally, myocarditis and resultant DCM are notoriously refractory to diagnosis. While biopsies can now detect myocarditis in some living patients, the disease is frequently asymptomatic and only diagnosed post-mortem [8]. The asymptomatic nature of etiologic infections such as *Chlamydia* only makes the retrospective assignment of causation that much more difficult. While we offer a model for the induction of an autoimmune disease based on animal studies, it is clear that a complex web of factors may influence human disease induction and progression.

References

[1] D. Homann, L. Teyton, M.B. Oldstone, Differential regulation of antiviral T-cell immunity results in stable CD8+but declining $CD4^+$ T-cell memory, Nat. Med. 7 (2001) 913–919.

[2] V. Kouskoff, et al., Organ-specific disease provoked by systemic autoreactivity, Cell 87 (1996) 811–822.

[3] M. Rangachari, J.M. Penninger, Negative regulation of T cell receptor signals, Curr. Opin. Pharmacol. 4 (2004) 415–422.

[4] T.T. Chang, et al., Studies in B7-deficient mice reveal a critical role for B7 costimulation in both induction and effector phases of experimental autoimmune encephalomyelitis, JEM 190 (1999) 733–740.

[5] C.A. Janeway Jr., The immune system evolved to discriminate infectious nonself from noninfectious self, Immunol. Today 13 (1992) 11–16.

[6] T. De Smedt, et al., Regulation of dendritic cell numbers and maturation by lipopolysaccharide in vivo, JEM 184 (1996) 1413–1424.

[7] T. Kaisho, S. Akira, Dendritic-cell function in toll-like receptor- and MyD88-knockout mice, Trends Immunol. 22 (2001) 78–83.

[8] A.M. Feldman, D. McNamara, Myocarditis, N. Engl. J. Med. 343 (2000) 1388–1398.

[9] D. Fairweather, et al., From infection to autoimmunity, J. Autoimmun. 16 (2001) 175–186.

[10] G.A. DosReis, et al., The importance of aberrant T-cell responses in Chagas disease, Trends Parasitol. 21 (2005) 237–243.

[11] J.M. Penninger, K. Bachmaier, Review of microbial infections and the immune response to cardiac antigens, J. Infect. Dis. 181 (Suppl. 3) (2000) S498–S504.

[12] H.J.F. Why, et al., Clinical and prognostic significance of detection of enteroviral RNA in the myocardium of patients with myocarditis or dilated cardiomyopathy, Circulation 89 (1994) 2582–2889.

[13] A.L. Caforio, et al., Novel organ-specific circulating cardiac autoantibodies in dilated cardiomyopathy, J. Am. Coll. Cardiol. 15 (1990) 1527–1534.

[14] E. Omerovic, et al., Induction of cardiomyopathy in severe combined immunodeficiency mice by transfer of lymphocytes from patients with idiopathic dilated cardiomyopathy, Autoimmunity 32 (2000) 271–280.

[15] U. Eriksson, J.M. Penninger, Autoimmune heart failure: new understandings of pathogenesis, Int. J. Biochem. Cell Biol. 37 (2005) 27–32.

[16] S.L. Hill, N.R. Rose, The transition from viral to autoimmune myocarditis, Autoimmunity 34 (2001) 169–176.

[17] R. Deonarain, et al., Protective role for interferon-β in coxsackievirus B3 infection, Circulation 110 (2004) 3540–3543.

[18] C.L. Pummerer, et al., Identification of cardiac myosin peptides capable of inducing autoimmune myocarditis in BALB/c mice, J. Clin. Invest. 97 (1996) 2057–2062.

[19] U. Eriksson, et al., Dendritic cell-induced autoimmune heart failure requires co-operation between adaptive and innate immunity, Nat. Med. 9 (2003) 1484–1490.
[20] S.C. Smith, P.M. Allen, Expression of myosin-class II major histocompatibility complexes in the normal myocardium occurs before induction of autoimmune myocarditis, Proc. Natl. Acad. Sci. U. S. A. 89 (1992) 9131–9135.
[21] N.R. Rose, Viral damage or 'molecular mimicry'—placing the blame in myocarditis, Nat. Med. 6 (2000) 631–632.
[22] K. Bachmaier, et al., Chlamydia infections and heart disease linked through antigenic mimicry, Science 283 (1999) 1335–1339.
[23] M.W. Cunningham, T cell mimicry in inflammatory heart disease, Mol. Immunol. 40 (2004) 1121–1127.
[24] S.K. Yoshinaga, et al., Characterization of a new human B7-related protein: B7RP-1 is the ligand to the co-stimulatory protein ICOS, Int. Immunol. 10 (2000) 1439–1447.
[25] A. Tafuri, et al., ICOS is Essential for Effective T-helper-cell Responses, vol. 409, 2001, pp. 105–109.
[26] O. Akbari, et al., Antigen-specific regulatory T cells develop via the ICOS–ICOS-ligand pathway and inhibit allergen-induced airway hyperreactivity, Nat. Med. 8 (2002) 1024–1032.
[27] E.C. de Jong, H.H. Smits, M.L. Kapsenberg, Dendritic cell-mediated T cell polarization, Springer Semin. Immunopathol. 26 (2005) 289–307.
[28] S.C. Knight, et al., Induction of autoimmunity with dendritic cells: studies on thyroiditis in mice, Clin. Immunol. Immunopathol. 48 (1988) 277–289.
[29] S.G. Correa, C.M. Riera, P. Iribarren, Involvement of peritoneal dendritic cells in the induction of autoimmune prostatitis, J. Autoimmun. 10 (1997) 107–113.
[30] H. Watanabe, et al., Experimental autoimmune thyroiditis induced by thyroglobulin-pulsed dendritic cells, Autoimmunity 31 (1999) 273–282.
[31] B. Ludewig, et al., Immunotherapy with dendritic cells directed against tumor antigens shared with normal host cells results in severe autoimmune disease, J. Exp. Med. 191 (2000) 795–804.
[32] U. Eriksson, et al., Dual role of the IL-12/IFN-gamma axis in the development of autoimmune myocarditis: induction by IL-12 and protection by IFN-gamma, J. Immunol. 167 (2001) 5464–5469.
[33] P. Puccetti, M.L. Belladonna, U. Grohmann, Effects of IL-12 and IL-23 on antigen-presenting cells at the interface between innate and adaptive immunity, Crit. Rev. Immunol. 22 (2002) 373–390.
[34] M. Afanasyeva, et al., Interleukin-12 receptor/STAT4 signaling is required for the development of autoimmune myocarditis in mice by an interferon-gamma-independent pathway, Circulation 104 (2001) 3145–3151.
[35] U. Eriksson, et al., Activation of dendritic cells through the interleukin 1 receptor 1 is critical for the induction of autoimmune myocarditis, J. Exp. Med. 197 (2003) 323–331.
[36] C.C. Anderson, P. Matzinger, Danger: the view from the bottom of the cliff, Semin. Immunol. 12 (2000) 231–238.
[37] R.J. Binder, R. Vatner, P. Srivastava, The heat-shock protein receptors: some answers and more questions, Tissue Antigens 64 (2004) 442–451.
[38] M.F. Tsan, B. Gao, Endogenous ligands of toll-like receptors, J. Leukoc. Biol. 76 (2004) 514–519.
[39] D.G. Millar, et al., Hsp70 promotes antigen-presenting cell function and converts T-cell tolerance to autoimmunity in vivo, Nat. Med. 9 (2003) 1469–1476.
[40] G. Schett, et al., Myocardial injury leads to a release of heat shock protein (hsp) 60 and a suppression of the anti-hsp65 immune response, Cardiovasc. Res. 42 (1999) 685–695.
[41] B. Dybdahl, et al., Myocardial ischaemia and the inflammatory response: release of heat shock protein 70 after myocardial infarction, Heart 91 (2005) 299–304.
[42] A. Maisel, et al., Experimental autoimmune myocarditis produced by adoptive transfer of splenocytes after myocardial infarction, Circ. Res. 82 (1998) 458–463.
[43] M. Herzum, et al., Coxsackievirus B3 infection leads to cell death of cardiac myocytes, J. Mol. Cell. Cardiol. 26 (1994) 907–913.
[44] D.L. Sewell, et al., Immunoregulation of CNS autoimmunity by helminth and mycobacterial infections, Immunol. Lett. 82 (2002) 101–110.

ELSEVIER

International Congress Series 1285 (2005) 202–206

www.ics-elsevier.com

Semaphorins in the immune system

A. Kumanogoh, T. Shikina, K. Suzuki, M. Yamamoto, H. Takamatsu, N. Takegahara, S. Marukawa, I. Ishida, D.V.R. Prasad, T. Toyofuku, H. Kikutani *

Department of Molecular Immunology, Research Institute for Microbial Diseases, Osaka University, Osaka, Japan

Abstract. One of the Class IV semaphorins, Sema4A, is expressed constitutively on dendritic cells (DCs) and induced on Th1-polarized cells but not on Th2-polarized cells. Sema4A binds to Tim-2, a member of the T cell immunoglobulin domain and mucin domain (Tim) protein family, whose expression is induced on activated T cells, and enhances in vitro activation and differentiation of T cells. To determine functions of Sema4A in vivo, Sema4A$^{-/-}$ mice have been generated. Sema4A$^{-/-}$ DCs show a reduced ability to stimulate allogeneic T cells. T cells from Sema4A$^{-/-}$ also fail to differentiate into Th1 cells in vitro in Th1-inducing conditions, although they can differentiate into Th2 cells in Th2-inducing conditions. Indeed, Sema4A$^{-/-}$ mice display defects not only in T cell priming but also in Th1 differentiation. When wild type mice are injected with antigen-pulsed Sema4A$^{-/-}$ DCs, proliferation and IL-2 secretion of antigen-specific T cells are severely impaired. On the other hand, generation of Th1 cells but not Th2 cells is impaired in Sema4A$^{-/-}$ mice that have been injected with antigen-pulsed wild-type DCs. These findings indicate that both DC-derived Sema4A and T cell-derived Sema4A are necessary for T cell activation and differentiation; the former is required for T cell priming and the latter for Th1 differentiation.

Keywords: Semaphorin; Dendritic cell; T cell; Sema4A; Tim-2; Th1; Th2

1. Introduction

The semaphorin family comprises more than 30 soluble and membrane-bound proteins from viruses to human [1]. This family has been originally identified as axonal guidance cues that function during neuronal development [2]. However, emerging evidence indicates that members of this family play various roles not only in neuronal development

* Corresponding author. Tel.: +81 6 6879 8345; fax: +81 6 6875 4465.
E-mail address: kikutani@ragtime.biken.osaka-u.ac.jp (H. Kikutani).

0531-5131/
doi:10.1016/j.ics.2005.08.008

but also in angiogenesis, vascularization, oncogenesis, cardiogenesis and immune responses. In the immune system, several semaphorins are expressed. At least, two semaphorin molecules, Sema4A and Sema4D, have been shown so far to play critical roles in immune responses [3]. They exert their biological activities in quite unique ways different from those seen in the nervous system where semaphorins utilize member of the neuropilin or plexin families as receptors. For instance, Sema4D regulates activation of B cells and dendritic cells by turning off the negative signals of its receptor, CD72 [4], while Sema4A binds to Tim-2 and co-stimulates T cells [5]. Here, we show our recent findings on molecular and cellular mechanisms how Sema4A is involved in T cells priming and Th1 differentiation.

2. Expression and structure of Sema4A

Sema4A, a transmembrane-type semaphorin, originally identified as semB [6], contains an N-terminal signal sequence followed by a sema domain, an Ig-like domain, a lysine-rich stretch, a transmembrane region and cytoplasmic tail like other Class IV semaphorins. We have previously cloned Sema4A from a cDNA library prepared from mouse dendritic cells (DCs) [5]. Sema4A mRNA is detectable in the brain, spleen, lung, kidney, and testis of adult mice. The flow cytometry analysis using mAb against mouse Sema4A has revealed that Sema4A is constitutively expressed on the surface of bone marrow-derived and splenic DCs as well as of B cells. The expression of Sema4A is transiently induced on T cells that are activated in neutral or Th2 conditions, although it is hardly detectable on resting T cells. Interestingly, the strong Sema4A expression is maintained on the surface of both Th1-differentiating and Th1-differentiated T cells [7].

3. Sema4A receptor in the immune system

Another class IV semaphorin, Sema4D (CD100), utilizes Plexin-B1 as its receptor in the nervous system and CD72 in the immune system [4,8]. However, it is unknown whether Plexin molecules serve as a receptor for Sema4A. We have previously demonstrated that Sema4A binds Tim-2 in the immune system. Tim-2, a member of the Tim family is expressed on activated T cells [5]. Other members of the Tim family are also implicated in regulation of T cell responses [9]. For instance, the polymorphisms of Tim-1 have been reported to correlate well with susceptibility to mouse airway hypersensitivity and human asthma [10]. Tim-3 has been reported to be expressed preferentially on Th1 cells [11]. It is noteworthy that Sema4A can induce tyrosine-phosphorylation of the cytoplasmic region of Tim-2. This suggests that Tim-2 may transduce the signal of Sema4A.

4. Biological activities of Sema4A in the immune system

To determine the biological activity of Sema4A, we produced a soluble recombinant molecule as a fusion protein with the Fc portion of human IgG1 (Sema4A-Fc). Addition of Sema4A-Fc significantly enhanced in vitro proliferation as well as IL-2 production of T cells stimulated with anti-CD3. Administration of Sema4A also enhanced generation of IFN-γ or IL-4 secreting antigen-specific T cells in vivo. Anti-Sema4A could inhibit the ability of DCs to stimulate allogeneic T cells in mixed lymphocyte cultures and development of experimental autoimmune encephalomyelitis (EAE) in mice immunized with myelin-oligodendrocyte glycoprotrein (MOG) [5]. These observations suggest a critical role for Sema4A in T cell responses.

5. Generation of Sema4A$^{-/-}$ mice

To determine in vivo functions of Sema4A, Sema4A$^{-/-}$ mice were generated by gene targeting [7]. Sema4A$^{-/-}$ mice were born in a typical Mendelian pattern and appeared to develop normally. Apparent defects could not be observed in the nervous system of the mutant mice except for defective development of the retina. DCs from Sema4A$^{-/-}$ and wild-type mice could produce comparable amounts of IL-12 and express similar levels of co-stimulatory molecules and MHC class II molecules in response to CD40 or LPS stimulation. However, Sema4A$^{-/-}$ DCs poorly stimulated allogeneic T cells. Furthermore, in vivo priming of T cells was severely impaired in Sema4A$^{-/-}$ mice [7].

6. Defective Th1 differentiation in Sema4A$^{-/-}$ mice

Sema4A is abundantly expressed on Th1-differentiating cells but not Th2-differentiating cells, suggesting a possible role of Sema4A in Th1 differentiation. To determine a role of Sema4A in Th1 differentiation, naïve CD4$^+$ T cells prepared from Sema4A$^{-/-}$ and wild-type mice were stimulated with anti-CD3 and anti-CD28 in the Th1-inducing or Th2-inducing conditions for 5 days. Sema4A$^{-/-}$ T cells failed to differentiate into Th1 cells even when cultured in Th1-inducing conditions, which was accompanied by significantly reduced induction of T-bet, a transcription factor essential for Th1 differentiation. Furthermore, Th1 differentiation of Sema4A$^{-/-}$ T cells could be restored by addition of Sema4A-Fc or co-culture with wild-type T cells. These findings indicate that T cell-derived Sema4A acts as a ligand during Th1 differentiation.

To further analyze a role of Sema4A in Th1 differentiation in vivo, Sema4A$^{-/-}$ mice were intraperitoneally injected with *Propionibacterium acnes* (*P. acnes*), an agent known to induce Th1 responses. Seven days later, T cells were prepared form mice and restimulated with immobilized anti-CD3. T cells from wild-type mice produced a large amount of IFN-γ, whereas IFN-γ production was not observed in T cells from Sema4A$^{-/-}$ mice. Furthermore, development of delayed type hypersensitivity was also significantly impaired in Sema4A$^{-/-}$ mice immunized with protein antigens [7].

7. Enhanced Th2 responses in Sema4A$^{-/-}$ mice

When Sema4A$^{-/-}$ mice were infected with *Nippostrongylus brasiliensis* (*N. brasiliensis*), a strong Th2 inducer, they showed rather higher levels of serum IgE and IL-4 production [7]. To further analyze a role of Sema4A in Th2 responses, we produced Sema4A$^{-/-}$ BALB/c mice by backcrossing the mutant mice into BALB/c mice. To our surprise, a fraction of Sema4A$^{-/-}$ BALB/c mice developed typical atopic dermatitis, accompanied with high levels of serum IgE. Then, we painted the skin of Sema4A$^{-/-}$ BALB/c mice with picrylchloride. After picrylchloride treatment, Sema4A$^{-/-}$ BALB/c mice showed much severe dermatitis and higher levels of serum IgE compared with wild-

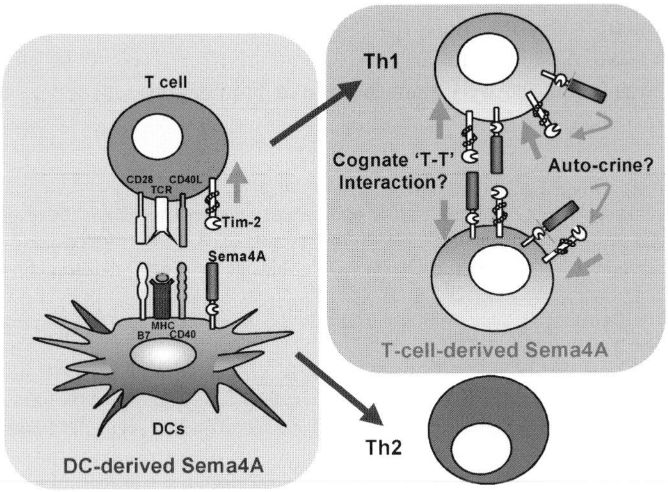

Fig. 1. Sema4A plays roles in T cell priming and Th1-differentiation.

type mice. These findings strongly suggested that enhanced Th2 responses are induced in the absence of Sema4A.

8. DC-derived Sema4A versus T cell-derived Sema4A

As described above, Sema4A is expressed not only on DCs but also on Th1-differentiating cells and required for T cell priming and Th1/Th2 regulation. This suggests a possibility that DC-derived Sema4A and T cell-derived Sema4A play distinct roles at different phases of T cell responses. To address this possibility, Sema4A$^{-/-}$ or wild-type DCs were pulsed with antigens and then transferred into Sema4A$^{-/-}$ or wild-type mice [7]. Antigen-specific Th1 and Th2 responses were markedly induced when wild-type mice were transferred with antigen-pulsed wild-type T cells, whereas generation of antigen-specific T cells were totally impaired in Sema4A$^{-/-}$ mice transferred with Sema4A$^{-/-}$ DCs. Transfer of Sema4A$^{-/-}$ DCs into either Sema4A$^{-/-}$ or wild-type mice resulted in impairment of proliferation and IL-2 production of T cells. On the other hand, transfer of wild-type DCs into Sema4A$^{-/-}$ mice, in which T cells lack Sema4A, resulted in reduced Th1 responses but rather enhanced Th2 responses. These results indicate that Sema4A on DCs is required for priming of antigen-specific T cells while Sema4A induced on activated or Th1-differentiating T cells may play a critical role in Th1/Th2 regulation (Fig. 1).

9. Conclusion

Here we have demonstrated that Sema4A play nonredundant roles in immune responses; particularly in T cell priming and Th1 differentiation. Particularly, our findings provide a novel mechanism for Th1/Th2 regulation. Therefore, Sema4A can be a potential target for potentiation or intervention in beneficial or pathological immune responses, respectively.

Acknowledgement

This work was supported by Uehara Memorial Foundation.

References

[1] Semaphorin Nomenclature Committee, Unified nomenclature for the semaphorins/collapsins, Cell 97 (1999) 551–552.
[2] M. Tessier-Lavigne, S.C. Goodman, The molecular biology of axon guidance, Science 274 (1996) 1123–1133.
[3] H. Kikutani, A. Kumanogoh, Semaphorins in interactions between T cells and antigen-presenting cells, Nat. Rev., Immunol. 3 (2003) 159–167.
[4] A. Kumanogoh, et al., Identification of CD72 as a lymphocyte receptor for the class IV semaphorin CD100: a novel mechanism for regulating B cell signaling, Immunity 13 (2000) 621–631.
[5] A. Kumanogoh, et al., Class IV semaphorin Sema4A enhances T-cell activation and interacts with Tim-2, Nature 419 (2002) 629–633.
[6] A.W. Puschel, R.H. Adams, H. Betz, Murine semaphorin D/collapsin is a member of a diverse gene family and creates domains inhibitory for axonal extension, Neuron 14 (1995) 941–948.
[7] A. Kumanogoh, et al., Nonredundant roles of Sema4A in the immune system: defective t cell priming and Thl/Th2 regulation in Sema4A-deficient mice, Immunity 22 (2005) 305–316.
[8] L. Tamagnone, et al., Plexins are a large family of receptors for transmembrane, secreted, and GPI-anchored semaphorins in vertebrates, Cell 99 (1999) 71–80.
[9] V.K. Kuchroo, et al., The TIM gene family: emerging roles in immunity and disease, Nat. Rev., Immunol. 3 (2003) 454–462.
[10] J.J. Mclntire, et al., Identification of Tapr (an airway hyperreactivity regulatory locus) and the linked Tim gene family, Nat. Immunol. 2 (2001) 1109–1116.
[11] L. Monney, et al., Thl-specific cell surface protein Tim-3 regulates macrophage activation and severity of an autoimmune disease, Nature 415 (2002) 536–541.

ELSEVIER

International Congress Series 1285 (2005) 207–211

www.ics-elsevier.com

Hyperactivation of gp130-mediated STAT3 signaling induces a rheumatoid arthritis-like disease that is dependent on MHC class II restricted CD4+ T cells

Masaaki Murakami [a,*,1], Shin-ichiro Sawa [a,1], Daisuke Kamimura [b], Hokuto Kamon [c], Hidemitsu Kitamura [b], Takaya Kawabe [a], Park Sung-Joo [a], Katsuhiko Ishihara [a], Toshio Hirano [a,b,c]

[a] *Depertment of Molecular Oncology Graduate School of Medicine, Osaka University, Japan*
[b] *Laboratory of Cytokine Signaling RIKEN RCAI, Japan*
[c] *Laboratory of Developmental Immunology Graduate School of Frontier Bioscience, Osaka University, Japan*

Abstract. Mice having a point mutation of IL-6 signal transducer, gp130, named gp130F759 induced a rheumatoid arthritis-like disease. The disease induction is totally dependent on mature lymphocytes, since no arthritis-like disease induced in a double mutant between gp130F759 and RAG2KO mice. We prepared several other double mutants including gp130F759/IgMKO, gp130F759/CD8KO, gp130F759/CIITAKO and gp130F759/CD4KO and analyzed the development of the arthritis. We found that development of the disease attenuated in gp130F759/CIITAKO and gp130F759/CD4KO, suggesting the MHC class II-restricted CD4+ T cells are important for the disease development. We showed memory/activated phenotype of CD4+ T cells increased in gp130F759 mice. Since activation of CD4+ T cells is mainly controlled by dendritic cells (DC) in vivo, we investigated this feature of DC in gp130F759 mice. We isolated DCs from superficial lymph nodes and observed that IL-6-mediated signaling suppresses maturation of DCs in vivo. However, total number of DCs in vivo significantly increased in gp130F759 mice compared with wild type controls. Thus, we hypothesize that the rheumatoid arthritis-like disease in gp130F759 mice is induced by an interaction between CD4+ T cells and DC under gp130F759 signal regulation.

Keywords: IL-6; gp130; Arthritis-like disease; CD4+ T cells; Dendritic cells

* Corresponding author.
E-mail address: murakami@molonc.med.osaka-u.ac.jp (M. Murakami).
[1] Equally contributed.

0531-5131/ © 2005 Published by Elsevier B.V.
doi:10.1016/j.ics.2005.07.096

1. Introduction

IL-6 is known as a proinflammatory cytokine produced by many kinds of cell populations in vivo [1]. We demonstrated that there are two signaling cascades from an IL-6 signal transducer gp130 [2]. One is STAT3-mediated signaling that is dependent on four YxxQ motifs in gp130's C-terminal portion and the other is Y759-mediated ERK/MAP kinase pathway. To investigate the roles for each of the two signaling pathways in vivo, we established knock-in mice named gp130FxxQ whose gp130 does not transduce STAT3-mediated signaling and gp130F759 whose gp130 transduces hyperactivation of STAT3 signaling [3]. Unexpectedly, gp130F759 mice spontaneously develop a rheumatoid arthritis-like disease within 1 year of age [4].

2. Results and discussion

2.1. MHC class II-restricted CD4+ T cells are critical for the development of the arthritis in gp130F759 mice

Because a background of gp130F759 mice was a mixture of 129 and C57BL6, we backcrossed them with C57BL6 8 times. We established several double mutant gp130F759 mice using RAGKO, CD8KO, IgMKO, CD4KO, and CIITAKO mice (all are C57BL6 background). No disease induced in gp130F759/RAGKO and gp130F759/CIITAKO (Fig. 1A). The disease development was significantly attenuated in gp130/CD4KO but a little bit enhanced in gp130/CD8KO (Fig. 1B). However, lack of B cells had no effect on the development of the disease (Fig. 1B). These results clearly demonstrated that MHC class II-restricted CD4+ T cells are critical for the development of the arthritis in gp130F759 mice.

2.2. Memory/activated phenotype of CD4+ T cells increased in gp130F759 mice

We investigated phenotype of CD4+ T cells in lymph nodes (LN) of gp130F759 mice. Memory/activated phenotype that was monitored by the expression levels of CD44 and CD62L increased in CD4+ T cells of gp130F759 mice compared with wild-type controls (Fig. 2A). The number of the memory/activated phenotype CD4+ T cells increased in age in gp130F759 mice (Fig. 2B).

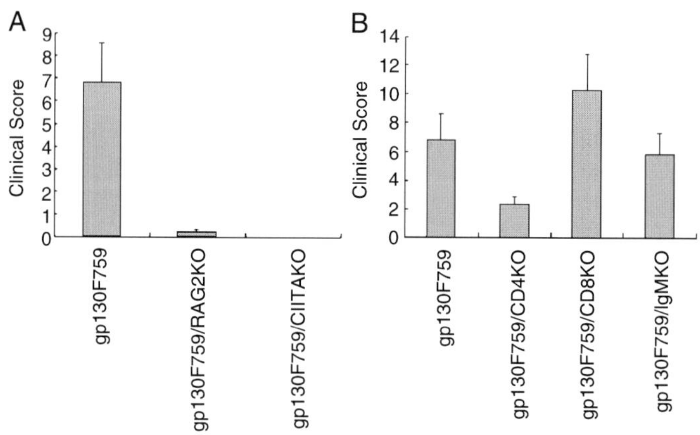

Fig. 1. MHC class II-restricted CD4+ T cells are critical for development of the arthritis in gp130F759 mice. Arthritis development of (A) gp130F759/RAGKO and gp130F759/CIITAKO and (B) gp130F759/CD4KO, gp130F759/CD8KO and gp130F759/IgMKO were investigated and compared with wild-type gp130F759 mice at 12 months after birth.

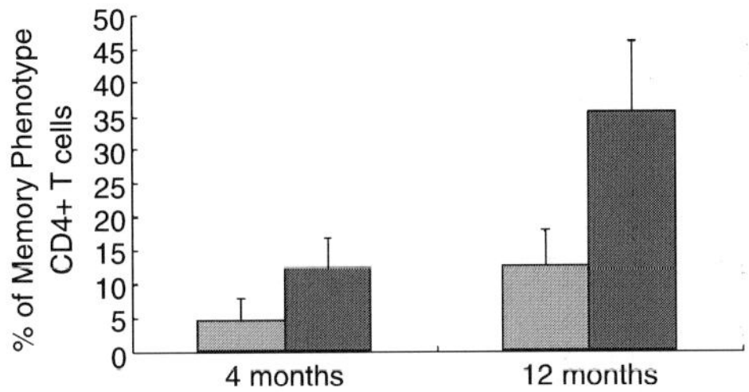

Fig. 2. Memory/activated CD4+ T cells increased in gp130F759 mice. Percentage of memory/activated CD44 high CD4+ T cells in spleen isolated from gp130F759, IL-6KO and wild-type control mice at 4 and 12 months after birth.

2.3. Phenotype of dendritic cells (DC) was changed in gp130F759 mice

Because one of the most important cell populations for CD4+ T cell homeostasis in vivo is DC, we investigated phenotype of DC in superficial LN of gp130F759 mice using expression levels of MHC class III and CD86 molecules. There are two types of DC in the LN; one is mature and the other is immature (Fig. 3, see control). Immature DC increased but mature ones decreased in gp130F759 mice (Fig. 3). On the other hand, immature DC decreased but mature ones increased in IL-6KO mice (Fig. 3).

2.4. Actual number of CD11c$^+$ DCs increased in gp130F759 mice

We next investigated whether actual number of DCs increased in gp130F759 mice. We harvested spleens from gp130F759, IL-6KO, and wild-type control and then counted CD11c$^+$ cells after collagenase treatment. As shown in Fig. 4, actual number of CD11c$^+$ DCs increased in gp130F759 mice compared with IL-6KO and control mice.

3. Materials and methods

3.1. Mice

C57BL/6 mice were obtained from (SLC) and mated with 129/B6-gp130$^{F759/F759}$ mice over 8 times (N8). C57BL/6 RAG2KO, IgMKO, CD4KO, CD8KO and C2TAKO mice were purchased from Jackson Laboratory and crossed with C57BL/6 background of

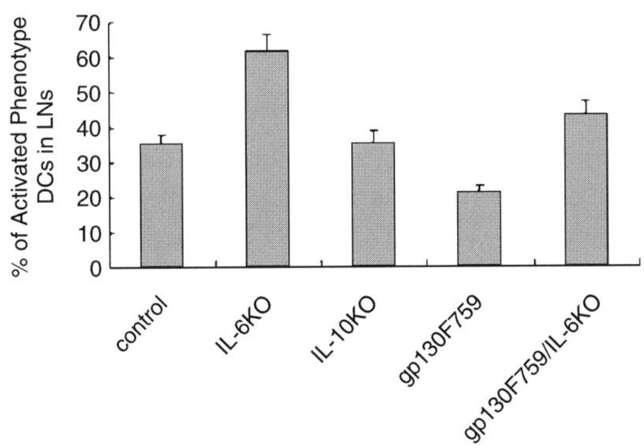

Fig. 3. IL-6 decreases the number of activated/mature DCs and increases the number of resting/immature DCs in the steady state. CD11c$^+$ DCs from about 10 weeks old gp130F759, IL-6KO and wild-type control mice were first purified from collagenase-treated superficial lymph nodes using anti-CD11c antibody-coated magnetic beads. The resulting population was analyzed for the expression of MHC class II and CD86 on the CD11c$^+$ cells.

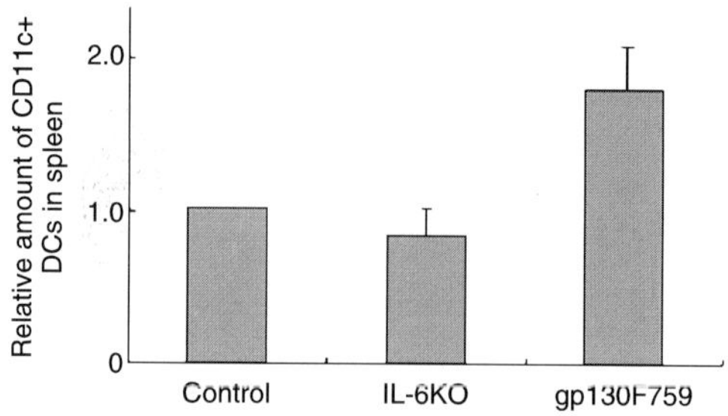

Fig. 4. Actual number of DCs increased in gp130F759 mice. CD11c$^+$ DCs from about 10 weeks old gp130F759, IL-6KO and wild-type control mice were first purified from collagenase-treated spleen using anti-CD11c antibody-coated magnetic beads. The resulting population was analyzed for the expression of CD11c molecules. Actual numbers of CD11c$^+$ are calculated.

gp130$^{F759/F759}$ mice (N8) to obtain double mutant mice. C57BL/6/Thy1.1 and C57BL/6 SJL, and from the Jackson Laboratory (ME, USA), and C57BL/6 IL-10 KO and C57BL6 D^{b}K^{b}KO mice from Taconic (Tokyo, Japan). gp130$^{F759/F759}$/IL-6 KO mice were generated by crossing gp130$^{F759/F759}$ mice with C57BL/6 IL-6 KO mice that were established previously [5]. All these mice were maintained at the Institute of Experimental Animal Sciences at Osaka University Medical School.

3.2. Antibodies, media, and reagents

Fluorescent- or biotin-conjugated antibodies and 2nd antibodies were purchased from BD PharMingen (San Diego, CA, USA) or e-bioscience (San Diego, CA, USA). RPMI 1640 (Sigma, USA) supplemented with 10% FBS (EQUITECH-BIO, USA), 2-mercaptoethanol (2-ME, 50 μM), L-glutamine (2 mM), penicillin (100 U/ml), streptomycin (100 U/ml), and sodium pyruvate (1 mM) was used as the complete culture medium. Recombinant mouse GM–CSF and IL-6 were purchased from Pepro Tech EC (London, UK). Recombinant human IL-6 was kindly provided by Ajinomoto Co. (Tokyo, Japan). LPS (*Escherichia coli* serotype:055:B5, 0111:B4) was purchased from Sigma.

3.3. Dendritic cell (DC) preparation from mice

For the analysis of surface molecules, the spleen or superficial lymph nodes were harvested from mice, treated with collagenase D (1 mg/ml) in complete culture medium for 30 min at 37 °C or room temperature, strained through 100-μm mesh (BD Falcon, Tokyo), and washed twice with cold plain RPMI medium. The washed cells were resuspended in cold MACS buffer (PBS containing 0.5% FBS and 2 mM EDTA) and treated with anti-CD11c antibody-coated microbeads (Miltenyi Biotec, Tokyo). CD11c$^+$ cell-enriched samples were prepared with an AutoMacs device (Miltenyi Biotec, Tokyo). Only anti-CD11c$^+$ and anti-CD3$^-$ cells were analyzed.

3.4. Assessment of arthritis

Clinical assessment of arthritis: Mice were inspected every week for up to 12 months and assessed for signs of arthritis as described before [4]. The arthritis score shown was the sum of the score as to 4 limbs graded 0 to 4. So the maximum arthritis score of the 4 limbs was 12.

3.5. Cell preparation, flow cytometry, and cell sorting

Lymphocyte suspensions were prepared from spleen and lymph nodes (inguinal, axillaries, cervical, and mesenteric) through 100 μm cell strainer (Falcon) into RPMI-1640 medium and washed. Erythrocytes were eliminated with 0.165 M NH_4Cl.

For cell surface staining, 10^6 cells were incubated with fluorescent mAbs for 30 min on ice, Cells were analyzed on the FACS Caliber (BD).

References

[1] T. Hirano, Interleukin 6 and its receptor: ten years later, Int. Rev. Immunol. 16 (1998) 249–284.

[2] T. Fukada, et al., Two signals are necessary for cell proliferation induced by a cytokine receptor gp130: involvement of STAT3 in antiapoptosis, Immunity 5 (1996) 449–460.

[3] T. Ohtani, et al., Dissection of signaling cascades through gp130 in vivo: reciprocal roles for STAT3- and SHP2-mediated signals in immune responses, Immunity 12 (2000) 95–105.

[4] T. Atsumi, et al., A point mutation of Tyr-759 in interleukin 6 family cytokine receptor subunit gp130 causes autoimmune arthritis, J. Exp. Med. 196 (2002) 979–990.

[5] S.J. Park, et al., IL-6 regulates in vivo dendritic cell differentiation through STAT3 activation, J. Immunol. 173 (2004) 3844–3854.

Author index

Keyword index